Edited by
Bruce J. Fried and
James A. Johnson

Human
Resources in
Healthcare

Managing
for Success

AUPHA Press, Washington, D.C.
Health Administration Press, Chicago, Illinois

Your board, staff, or clients may also benefit from this book's insight. For more information on quantity discounts, contact the Health Administration Press Marketing Manager at (312) 424-9470.

This publication is intended to provide accurate and authoritative information in regard to the subject matter covered. It is sold, or otherwise provided, with the understanding that the publisher is not engaged in rendering professional services. If professional advice or other expert assistance is required, the services of a competent professional should be sought.

The statements and opinions in this book are strictly those of the authors and do not represent the official positions of the American College of Healthcare Executives, of the Foundation of the American College of Healthcare Executives, or of the Association of University Programs in Health Administration.

06   05   04   03   5   4   3   2

Library of Congress Cataloging-in-Publication Data

Human resources in healthcare : managing for success / edited by Bruce J. Fried and James Johnson.
    p. cm.
    Includes bibliographical references and index.
    ISBN 1-56793-168-5 (alk. paper)
    1. Medical personnel.   2. Personnel management.   3. Public health personnel.   I. Fried, Bruce, 1952–   II. Johnson, James A., 1954–
    [DNLM: 1. Personnel Management—methods. WX 159 H91807 2001]
  RA410.6 .H85 2001
  362.1'068'3—dc21

2001039321

The paper used in this publication meets the minimum requirements of American National Standards for Information Sciences—Permanence of Paper for Printed Library Materials, ANSI Z39.48–1984. ♾ ™

Project Manager/Editor: Jane C. Williams; Acquisition Manager: Audrey Kaufman; Cover Designer: Anne Locascio

Health Administration Press
A division of the Foundation
  of the American College of
  Healthcare Executives
One North Franklin Street
Suite 1700
Chicago, IL 60606
(312) 424-2800

Association of University Programs
  in Health Administration
730 11th Street, NW
4th Floor
Washington, DC 20001
(202) 638-1448

CONTENTS

FOREWORD

Harry A. Nurkin, Ph.D., FACHE, president and CEO, Carolinas HealthCare System

Legendary business executive and former CEO of General Electric Company, Jack Welch, once said, "If you pick the right people and give them the opportunity to spread their wings—and put compensation as a carrier behind it—you almost don't have to manage them." One of the reasons for Welch's great success is that he believed that effectively managing a business depends on effectively recruiting, training, motivating, evaluating, and rewarding the workforce.

Healthcare, more than any other industry, depends on people to carry out its mission. Therefore, an organization's mission, strategic plans, and quality improvement initiatives are useless unless the organization has appropriate policies and procedures for managing people. Although healthcare organizations have become more sophisticated in technologies, financial management, quality improvement, and marketing, in most instances, they have not commensurately improved in the management of human resources. While employees are now viewed as "internal customers" and as "strategic assets," the practice of human resource management still lags behind that rhetoric.

Tomorrow's successful healthcare organization will be driven by a knowledge-based strategic workforce that clearly identifies and fully satisfies its customers. Tomorrow's successful healthcare managers, in turn, must understand this employee knowledge basis; that is, they should be aware of what employees know, how that knowledge is used, and how quickly new knowledge can be translated into customer-focused service. The collective knowledge, or intellectual capital, of a healthcare enterprise resides in the skills, experience, and creative potential of its employees. How to successfully manage these valuable assets is the focus of this book, *Human Resources in Healthcare: Managing for Success*, edited by Bruce Fried and James Johnson.

This book is a compilation of concepts and practical tools necessary for a manager to create a successful, customer-focused healthcare workforce. Fried and Johnson have assembled a diverse group of experienced authors who present both conceptual and pragmatic approaches to managing people.

Unlike previous literature that simply catalogs human resources management questions and problems, this book addresses the processes of identifying employees and enhancing their skills to become organizational assets that are more valuable than any technology.

Regardless of changes in regulations that affect revenue, healthcare businesses that will succeed in the future are those that win market share. Healthcare businesses that have gained and retained market share figured out long ago that the battleground for market share is neither technology nor quality, given that difference in technology or quality between competing healthcare entities rarely exists. This book does not de-emphasize the importance of the "science" of healthcare—that is, achieving and delivering high-quality healthcare products and services through use of scientific and innovative technology. However, it clearly reminds us of the great importance of the "art" of healthcare—that is, managing the human beings who provide the services and improve the products. The idea that managers should emphasize both the scientific and artistic components of the enterprise seems rather basic, but in reality, managers in general have demonstrated limited skill in dealing with human assets.

Although a plethora of human resources textbooks already exist, the human resources issues in the healthcare industry is unique enough to warrant a book that examines the idiosyncrasies of managing people in this environment. This book addresses the most difficult and challenging management responsibility—managing people successfully—with both conceptual and experiential clarity. It is stimulating, thought provoking, challenging, detailed, complex, and holds the attention of the reader. I highly recommend it to those who want to succeed as healthcare managers.

PREFACE

ealthcare has undergone remarkable changes in the past decades, including advances in technology, availability of information, and the advent of new forms of organizations and financing mechanisms. Despite these changes, healthcare remains, and will always remain, a people-oriented enterprise. Healthcare customers are people, and despite changes in the way care is provided, people always are central in the provision of care, whether that care is preventive, diagnostic, curative, chronic, or rehabilitative.

Despite what we as healthcare administrators and teachers know, or think we know, about managing people, the manner by which we manage and deal with people in our healthcare organizations remains rather primitive in many instances. One of the reasons that our management ways remain primitive is that many healthcare professionals become managers as a result of their success in clinical or technological areas. Physicians, nurses, and laboratory technicians who are highly effective in their particular discipline are frequently rewarded by promotion into the managerial ranks. The erroneous assumption behind those promotions is that the same skills required of the clinician or technician are applicable and relevant at the managerial level.

This book, *Human Resources in Healthcare: Managing for Success,* is written for healthcare management students and healthcare professionals who have, or in the future will have, responsibility for managing people in healthcare organizations. That audience includes virtually everyone from the supervisory to senior-management level in hospitals, health departments, physician practices, home care agencies, and other healthcare systems. Although the formal human resources department plays a key role in our organizations, the department does not "own" human resources management and is not capable of ensuring that the human resources practices implemented by managers are fair and equitable, effective and efficient, ethical, and legal. Human resources management is carried out at all levels in the organization and throughout the workday.

This book discusses the importance of systematic and strategic thinking about the organization's human resources function, focuses on ways to effectively implement human resources practices, and explores the traditions and beliefs that often stand in the way of implementation. Additionally, this book is linked with the casebook, *Human Resources and Organizational Behavior: Cases in Health Services Management* by Anne Kilpatrick and James Johnson (Health Administration Press 1999). The casebook provides numerous cases, culled from actual experience in healthcare settings, that illustrate many of the concepts in this book.

Chapter Overview

We attempt in this book to make readers aware of the wealth of information that healthcare managers must know to become effective managers of people. In putting this book together and working with the contributing authors, we quickly recognized that we had to make choices about which among the many human resources concepts to include and exclude. Our challenge was to produce a book that was conceptually sound, relevant to current and future healthcare managers, and written in a readable manner for a diverse audience.

One of our first tasks was to identify authors who have the expertise on certain human resources topics and who have the ability to write chapters that included essential and current information. Contributors to this book come from a diverse field, including academia, the health professions, law, business, and other healthcare-related areas. The result of our efforts is this foundation-setting book that covers a broad set of topics, which we hope will inspire and encourage readers to learn more from other resources such as books, journals, and the Internet.

We begin the book with a chapter by Myron Fottler on strategic human resources management. For many years, human resources was synonymous with "personnel" or managers who had a reputation for being passive and at times obstructionist in its relationship with internal customers or employees. The term "human resources" implies that the organization considers its work force as a strategic asset, although that term does not ensure such a proactive approach. Fottler presents a progressive perspective on human resources management: Human resources management has a key role in supporting the organization's mission and strategies.

Healthcare organizations employ a diverse set of professionals who presents unique management challenges. In Chapter 2, Kenneth White and Dolores Clement take us through the world of healthcare professionals, discussing their education, licensure, and changing role. In a similar vein, Chapter 3, by Eric Williams and Andrew Osucha, examines the emerging roles of physicians and argues that organizational change efforts can be more successful with physician participation.

Human resources management is embedded in a highly complex and changing web of legal and regulatory requirements, which affect virtually all aspects of managing and working with people. These legal issues are addressed in several chapters in this book. In Chapter 4, the primary focus is on equal employment opportunity issues and the most far-reaching and influential laws, including the Civil Rights Acts of 1964 and 1991 and the Americans with Dis-abilities Act. In Chapter 12, Beverly Rubin focuses on employee and employer rights, using employment law as a basis of discussion. This chapter addresses, among several other topics, the important and controversial areas of employ-ment contracts, employment-at-will, discipline, and privacy issues. Current legal requirements and court interpretations are impossible to provide in each of these chapters because changes happen constantly. We do, however, set out a framework for management practice based on those aspects of the law that we see as robust and unlikely to change dramatically in the foreseeable future.

Job analysis and job design are central aspects of human resources management; in fact, these processes affect everything we do in managing people. In Chapter 5, Myron Fottler discusses the importance of job analysis, job descriptions (see Appendix A for a sample job description), and job spec-ifications, and he provides some useful and useable approaches to conducting job analysis. He also presents the concept of job design and explains how the deliberate structuring of work can lead to improved individual, group, and organizational performance.

Our understanding of job requirements leads us to the next set of topics: recruitment and selection. In Chapter 6, we discuss the recruitment process and enumerate innovative methods of attracting people to the orga-nization. In the discussion of the selection process, we address issues of validity in selection tools as well as the relative reliability of measuring different human attributes.

Performance management is the process of assessing performance, pro-viding feedback to employees on their performance, designing strategies for improvement, and evaluating the effectiveness of those strategies. Chapter 7 provides a variety of approaches for evaluating performance, including 360-degree strategies. In this chapter, we argue that performance appraisal and management should be viewed as positive, rather than punitive, processes. In many instances, achieving this ideal perspective first requires an examination of the dominant organizational culture, which frequently views performance appraisal in a negative manner.

Training and employee development are important functions, not just to improve employee morale but to ensure that employees are knowledgeable and skilled for both current and future organizational needs. In the past, train-ing was often viewed as a "frill." The perspective in Chapter 8, on the other hand, is that training is a key part of an organization's competitive strategy. In this chapter, we discuss the importance of the learning organization and we present the training cycle necessary to improve individual and organizational performance.

Reward and compensation systems are key to employee motivation, retention, and performance; these topics are addressed in two chapters. Chap-ter 9, cowritten by John Crisafulli, provides an overview of the rewards and the purpose of an organization's compensation policy. Incentive plans, as well as the pros and cons of pay-for-performance schemes, are also discussed. In Chapter 10, Derek van Amerongen addresses the complex topic of physician compensation and the problems in redesigning physician compensation in different types of organizational settings. This topic is increasingly important because physicians are increasingly moving into employee and quasi-employee relationships with organizations.

Ensuring the health and safety of workers during work hours is a continuing concern in healthcare organizations, particularly given that the environment in which healthcare is provided teems with medical threats and given the litigiousness of U.S. society. In Chapter 11, Michael Ryan and Anne Kilpatrick provide a framework for implementing health and safety strategies in the workplace and stress how these strategies can be integrated into ongoing continuous quality improvement initiatives. They also provide a wide variety of additional resources related to health and safety issues (see Appendix B).

Organizational change is the norm in all organizations, and certainly continuous change is the rule in healthcare. In Chapter 13, Sharon Topping provides background information on the change process and impediments to successfully achieving organizational change. In addition, she also provides managers with specific strategies to help employees adapt to change, a task which is crucial in people management.

Unionization came relatively late to healthcare, but healthcare is now the biggest area of growth for the labor movement. Donna Malvey discusses unions, unionization process, and labor-management relations in Chapter 14. She gives particular attention to developments in the unionization of physicians and nurses and the implications of unionization for healthcare organizations.

Attention to customers is another concept that has come relatively late to healthcare, but certainly the concept is key to quality and competitiveness. In Chapter 15, Myron Fottler and Robert Ford discuss what is meant by customer focus and how human resources policies and practices need to change so that they become part of the healthcare organization's customer-focus strategies.

Acknowledgment

Bruce Fried would like to acknowledge many people for their tremendous support in putting this book together: Donna Cooper, from the Department of Health Policy and Administration, for working endlessly on editing drafts and corresponding with authors and our publisher. Audrey Kaufman, from Health Administration Press, for pushing to keep this project moving ahead. Jane Williams, also from Health Administration Press, for providing superb editorial support and keeping us on track. Laurie Gaydos and Diamanta Tornatore, students in the Department of Health Policy and Administration, for applying their excellent editing skills to many of the chapters in this book.

Thank you to Dean Harris for his invaluable guidance on many of the legal issues addressed in this book. Kerry Kilpatrick and Laurel Files, chair and associate chair of the Department of Health Policy and Administration, deserve my gratitude for always exhibiting faith in me and in this project. Of course, thanks to Arn Kaluzny for providing ongoing guidance throughout this project.

Thank you to my wife, Nancy, for her strong emotional and substantive support to my work. I am grateful to my children, Noah, Aaron, and Shoshana, for almost always letting me use the computer to work (perhaps because they were amazed that I was actually editing a book!). I owe major thanks to my parents, Pearl and George Fried, who have always encouraged and supported me.

Last but certainly not least, my thanks go out to all of the authors in this book who successfully produced excellent work and steadfastly responded to requests for clarification and rewrites.

James Johnson would like to thank his secretary, Mary Connolly, and his graduate assistant, Darryl Pauls, both from the Medical University of South Carolina.

Conclusion

We encourage you to think about how the concepts discussed in this book apply to the changing healthcare setting and to the healthcare organizations in which you work or have worked. Some of the material in this book is drawn from the general management literature and may require some modification to make it fit with the realities of your healthcare setting. We urge you to regularly consult the literature for changes and innovations in human resources management. To assist you in applying the concepts to the cases in the casebook, we have created a chart that will guide you in determining which chapters apply to which cases. Visit *http://www.ache.org/HAP.html* to see the chart.

We often think that the "hard" organizational problems are those issues that deal with finance, systems, and technology; on the other hand, we view human resources problems as "soft" and easily managed. We disagree with this designation. People management problems are the hard problems because if people's concerns and needs are not properly met, they are not motivated to perform and they are not supportive of the organization. Without this motivation and support, all of the organization's plans become compromised. We can find and develop solutions to people problems if we have an understanding of the unique features of a situation and if we use effective human resources management concepts and tools that are available to us. We hope this book provides some of those tools and opens your eyes to alternative ways of thinking about managing people in healthcare organizations.

Bruce J. Fried, Ph.D., and James A. Johnson, Ph.D.

This book is dedicated to Dr. Arnold D. Kaluzny who has guided me and countless others to live, work, teach, and conduct business with honesty and integrity. He has taught us to always strive to improve the quality of our organizations and hence the quality of life for the people who work in those organizations.

—*Bruce Fried*

I dedicate this book to the memory of my aunt, Dr. Marilyn Bearden Giles, who was very influential in my own education. She recently died of Alzheimer's.

—*James Johnson*

STRATEGIC HUMAN RESOURCES MANAGEMENT

Myron D. Fottler, Ph.D.

Learning Objectives

After completing this chapter, the reader should be able to:

- Define strategic human resources management
- Outline key human resources functions
- Discuss the significance of human resources management for present and future healthcare executives
- Describe the organizational and human resources systems that affect organizational outcomes

Introduction

Like most other service industries, the healthcare industry is very labor intensive. One reason for this reliance on an extensive workforce is that producing a "service," and storing it for subsequent consumption, is not possible. The production of the service that is purchased and the consumption of that service occur simultaneously. Thus, the interaction between consumers and healthcare professionals is an integral part of the provision of health services. Given the industry's dependence on healthcare professionals for service delivery, the possibility of heterogeneity of service quality must be recognized within an individual employee, given that skills and competencies change over time, and among employees, given that different individuals or representatives of various professions provide a service.

The intensive use of labor for service delivery and the possibility of variability in professional practice require the attention of industry leaders to be directed toward managing the performance of the persons involved in the delivery of health services. The effective management of people requires that healthcare executives understand the factors that influence the performance of individuals employed in their organizations. These factors include not only the traditional human resources management activities (i.e., recruitment and selection, training and development, appraisal, compensation, and employee relations) but also environmental and other organizational factors that impinge on human resources activities.

Strategic human resources management (SHRM) refers to the comprehensive set of managerial activities and tasks designed to develop and maintain a qualified workforce that contributes to organizational effectiveness

Strategic human resources management (SHRM) refers to the comprehensive set of managerial activities and tasks designed to develop and maintain a qualified workforce that contributes to organizational effectiveness as defined by the organization's strategic goals. SHRM occurs in a complex and dynamic milieu of forces within the organizational context. A significant trend in the past decade is for human resources (HR) managers to adopt a strategic perspective of their job and to recognize the critical linkages between organizational strategy and HR strategies (Fottler et al. 1990; Greer 2001).

This book explains and illustrates the methods and practices that can be used to increase the probability that competent personnel will be available to provide the services delivered by the organization and that the personnel will perform necessary tasks appropriately. Implementing these methods and practices means that requirements for positions must be determined, qualified persons must be recruited and selected, employees must be trained and developed to meet future organizational needs, and adequate rewards must be provided to attract and retain top performers. Of course these functions are performed within the context of the overall activities of the organization; they are influenced or constrained by the environment, the mission and strategies that are being pursued, and the systems indigenous to the organization.

Why study SHRM? How does this topic relate to the career interests or aspirations of present or future healthcare executives? Staffing the organization, designing jobs and teams, developing skillful employees, identifying approaches to improve performance and customer service, and rewarding employee success are as relevant to line managers as they are to HR managers. Successful healthcare executives need to understand human behavior, work with employees effectively, and be knowledgeable about numerous systems and practices available to build a skilled and motivated workforce. They also have to be aware of economic, technological, social, and legal issues that facilitate or constrain efforts to attain strategic objectives.

Healthcare executives do *not* want to hire the wrong person, to experience high turnover, to manage unmotivated employees, to be taken to court for discrimination actions, to be cited for unsafe practices, to have poorly trained staff undermine patient satisfaction, or to commit unfair labor practices. The material in this book can help the healthcare executive avoid mistakes and achieve results through others. Despite their best efforts, executives often fail because they hire the wrong people or they do not motivate or develop subordinates.

Healthcare organizations can gain a competitive advantage over competitors by effectively managing their human resources. Effective HR practices can enhance their competitive advantage by creating cost leadership (i.e., low-cost provider) and product differentiation (i.e., higher levels of service quality). A 1994 study examined the human resources management (HRM) practices and productivity levels of 968 organizations across 35 industries (Huselid 1994). The effectiveness of each organization's set of HRM practices was rated based on the presence of such things as incentive plans, employee grievance systems, formal performance appraisal systems, and employee participation in decision making. The study found that organizations with high HRM effectiveness ratings clearly outperformed those with low ones. A similar study of 293 publicly held companies reported that productivity was highly correlated with effective HRM practices (Huselid, Jackson, and Schuler 1997).

Based on "extensive reading of both popular and academic literature, talking with numerous executives in a variety of industries, and an application of common sense," Jeffrey Pfeffer (1994) identified 16 HRM practices that enhance an organization's competitive advantage:

1. Employment security
2. Selectivity in recruiting
3. High wages
4. Incentive pay
5. Employee ownership
6. Information sharing
7. Participation and empowerment
8. Teams and job design
9. Training and skill development
10. Cross-utilization and cross-training
11. Symbolic egalitarianism
12. Wage compression
13. Promotion from within
14. Long-term perspective
15. Measurement of practices
16. Overachieving philosophy

Most of the 16 HR practices will be described in more detail throughout the book. Although the list shows that effective HRM practices can strongly enhance an organization's competitive advantage, it fails to indicate *why* these practices have such an influence. In the following section we describe a model that attempts to explain this phenomenon.

Environmental Trends

Among the major environmental trends that affect healthcare organizations are the changing financing arrangements, emergence of new competitors, emergence of new technology, low or declining inpatient hospital occupancy rates, changes in physician-healthcare organization relationships, workforce demographic change and increased diversity, a capital shortage, increasing market penetration by managed care, increasing pressures for cost containment, and increasing expectations of patients. These trends resulted in increased competition, the need for higher levels of performance, and concern for organizational survival. Many healthcare organizations are closing facilities, undergoing corporate reorganization, instituting staffing freezes and/or reductions in workforces, providing greater flexibility in work scheduling, providing services with fewer resources, changing their organizational structures and/or job designs, outsourcing many functions, and developing leaner management structures with fewer levels and wider spans of control.

Healthcare organizations are pursuing a variety of major competitive strategies to respond to the current turbulent environment, including low-cost provision of traditional health services, provision of superior patient service through extra-high technical quality or customer service, specialization into a few key clinical areas (i.e., centers of excellence), or diversification with or outside healthcare (Coddington and Moore 1987; Blair and Fottler 1998). In addition, healthcare organizations are entering into strategic alliances (Kaluzny, Zuckerman, and Ricketts 1995) and developing or modifying their integrated delivery systems (Shortell et al. 1996; Fottler, Savage, and Blair 2000). Regardless of which strategies are pursued, all healthcare organizations are experiencing a decrease in staffing levels in many traditional service areas and an increase in staffing levels in new ventures, specialized clinical areas, and related support services (Wilson 1986; Hernandez, Fottler, and Joiner 1998). Hence, staffing profiles are increasingly characterized by a limited number of highly skilled and well-compensated professionals. Healthcare organizations are no longer "employers of last resort" for the unskilled, and at the same time, most are experiencing shortages of various nursing and allied health personnel.

The development of appropriate responses to this changing healthcare environment has received much attention during the past decade so that planning is now well accepted in healthcare organizations. However, *implementation* of plans has often been problematic: The process often ends with the development of goals and objectives but without strategies or methods of implementation or monitoring of results. Implementation appears to be the major difficulty in the overall management process (Porter 1980; Blair and Fottler 1998).

A major reason for this lack of implementation has been failure of healthcare executives to assess and manage the various external, interface, and internal stakeholders whose cooperation and support are necessary to implement any business strategy (i.e., corporate, business, or functional) successfully (Blair and Fottler 1990). A **stakeholder** is any individual or group with a "stake" in the organization. External stakeholders include patients and their families, public and private regulatory agencies, and third-party payers. Interface stakeholders are those who operate on the "interface" of the organization in both the internal and external environments, including members

*A **stakeholder** is any individual or group with a "stake" in the organization*

of the board of directors or the medical staff who have admitting privileges at several organizations. Internal stakeholders are those that operate within the organization, such as managers, professionals, and nonprofessional employees.

Involving supportive stakeholders, such as employees and human resources management, is crucial to the success of any plan. For example, if human resources managers are not actively involved, then the employee planning, recruitment, selection, development, appraisal, and compensation necessary for successful implementation are not likely to occur. As McManis (1987, 19) has noted: "While many hospitals have elegant and elaborate strategic plans, they often do not have supporting human resources strategies to ensure that the overall corporate plan can be implemented. But strategies don't fail, people do." Yet the healthcare industry spends less than one-half the amount that other industries spend on human resources administration (*Hospitals* 1989; Hernandez, Fottler, and Joiner 1998).

The SHRM Processes and Trends

According to Fottler and colleagues (1990), a strategic approach to human resources management includes:

- assessing the organization's environment and mission;
- formulating the organization's business strategy;
- assessing the human resources requirements based on the intended strategy;
- comparing the current inventory of human resources in terms of numbers, characteristics, or practices relative to the future strategic requirements;
- formulating a human resources strategy based on the differences between the assessed requirements and the current inventory; and
- implementing the appropriate human resources practices to reinforce the business strategy and attain competitive advantage.

Figure 1.1 provides some examples of possible linkages between strategic decisions and human resources management practices.

SHRM has not been given as high a priority in the healthcare industry as it has been given in many other industries. This neglect is particularly surprising in a labor-intensive industry that requires the right people in the right jobs at the right times and that undergoes shortages in some occupations (Cerne 1988). In addition, strong evidence suggests that organizations that utilize more progressive human resources approaches achieve significantly better financial results than comparable (but less progressive) organizations (Gomez-Mejia 1988; Huselid 1994; Huselid, Jackson, and Schuler 1997; Kravetz 1988).

Table 1.1 illustrates some strategic HR trends that affect job analysis, planning, staffing, training and development, performance appraisal, compensation, employee rights and discipline, and employee and labor relations.

FIGURE 1.1

Human
Resources
Implications of
Strategic
Decisions

Strategic Decisions	Human Resources Management Implications
Pursue low-cost competitive strategy	• Lower compensation • Givebacks in labor relations • Provide training to improve efficiency
Pursue service quality differentiation, and competitive strategy	• Recruit top-quality candidates • High compensation • Provide training in guest relations • Evaluate based on patient satisfaction
Pursue growth through acquisition strategy	• Select from acquired organization • Outplace redundant workers • Train new workers • Adjust compensation
Pursue growth through development of new markets	• Promote existing employees based on objective performance appraisal system
Purchase new technology	• Provide training
Offer new service and product line	• Recruit and select physicians and other personnel
Improve productivity/cost effectiveness through process improvement	• Encourage work teams to be innovative • Take risks • Assume a long-term perspective

These trends will be discussed in more detail in upcoming chapters. The "bottom line" for Table 1.1 is that we are moving to higher levels of flexibility, collaboration, decentralization, and team orientation, which are driven by the environmental changes and the organizational responses discussed earlier.

As illustrated by Figure 1.2, healthcare organizations are complex entities that require constant interaction with the environment. If they are to remain viable, these organizations must adapt their strategic planning and thinking to embrace changes in their external environments and missions. The internal components of the organization are then affected by these changes in that shifts in the organization's plans potentially necessitate modifications in the internal organizational systems and human resources process systems. Harmony, in turn, must be present among these systems. The characteristics, performance levels, and amount of coherence in operating practices among these systems influence the outcomes achieved in organizational and employee-level measures of performance.

Earlier Practice	Current Practice
Job Analysis/Planning	
Explicit job descriptions	Broad job classes
Detailed HR planning	Loose work planning
Detailed controls	Flexibility
Efficiency	Innovation
Staffing	
Supervisors make hiring decision	Team makes hiring decision
Emphasis on applicant's technical qualifications	Emphasis on "fit" of applicant and culture
Layoffs	Voluntary incentives to retire
Letting laid-off workers fend for themselves	Continuing support for terminated employees
Training and Development	
Individual training	Team-based training
Job-specific training	Generic training emphasizing flexibility
"Buy" skills by hiring experienced workers	"Make" skills by training less-skilled workers
Organization responsible for career development	Employee responsible for career development
Performance Appraisal	
Uniform appraisal procedures	Customized appraisals
Control-oriented appraisals	Developmental appraisals
Supervisor inputs only	Multiple inputs for appraisals
Compensation	
Seniority	Performance-based pay
Centralized pay decision	Decentralized pay decisions
Fixed fringe benefits	Flexible fringe benefits (i.e., cafeteria approach)
Employee Rights and Discipline	
Emphasis on employer protection	Emphasis on employee protection
Informal ethical standards	Explicit ethical codes and enforcement procedures
Emphasis on discipline to reduce mistakes	Emphasis on prevention to reduce mistakes
Employee and Labor Relations	
Top-down communication	Bottom-up communication and feedback
Adversarial approach	Collaboration approach
Preventive labor relations	Employee freedom of choice

TABLE 1.1
Strategic Human Resources Trends: From Earlier to Current Practices

FIGURE 1.2

Strategic
Human
Resources
Management
Model

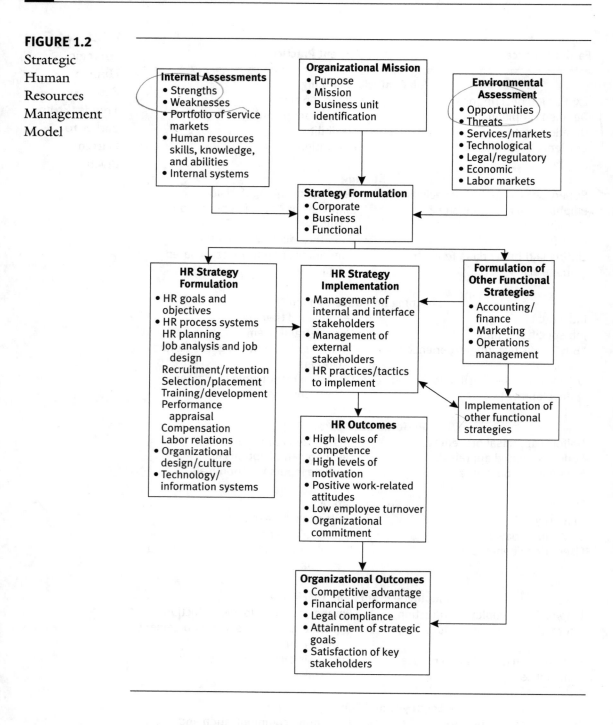

Internal Assessments
- Strengths
- Weaknesses
- Portfolio of service markets
- Human resources skills, knowledge, and abilities
- Internal systems

Organizational Mission
- Purpose
- Mission
- Business unit identification

Environmental Assessment
- Opportunities
- Threats
- Services/markets
- Technological
- Legal/regulatory
- Economic
- Labor markets

Strategy Formulation
- Corporate
- Business
- Functional

HR Strategy Formulation
- HR goals and objectives
- HR process systems
  HR planning
  Job analysis and job design
  Recruitment/retention
  Selection/placement
  Training/development
  Performance appraisal
  Compensation
  Labor relations
- Organizational design/culture
- Technology/ information systems

HR Strategy Implementation
- Management of internal and interface stakeholders
- Management of external stakeholders
- HR practices/tactics to implement

Formulation of Other Functional Strategies
- Accounting/ finance
- Marketing
- Operations management

Implementation of other functional strategies

HR Outcomes
- High levels of competence
- High levels of motivation
- Positive work-related attitudes
- Low employee turnover
- Organizational commitment

Organizational Outcomes
- Competitive advantage
- Financial performance
- Legal compliance
- Attainment of strategic goals
- Satisfaction of key stakeholders

Internal and External Environmental Assessment

Figure 1.2 identifies environmental assessment as a crucial element of SHRM. As a result of changes in the legal/regulatory climate, economic conditions, and labor market realities, healthcare organizations face constantly changing opportunities and threats. These opportunities and threats make particular services or markets more or less attractive from the organization's perspective. Among the environmental trends that currently affect the environment of healthcare organizations are increasing diversity of the workforce, aging of the workforce, labor shortages, changing worker values and attitudes, and technological change. Healthcare executives have responded to these external environmental pressures through various internal structural environmental changes, including the development of network structures, membership in healthcare systems, mergers and acquisitions, development of work teams, implementation of continuous quality improvement, telecommuting, employee leasing, and greater utilization of temporary or contingent workers.

Healthcare executives also need to make an internal assessment not only of their organizational strengths and weaknesses but also their internal systems, human resources skills, knowledge, abilities, and the portfolio of service markets. Management of human resources involves attention to the effect of environmental and internal components on the human resources process system. Because healthcare professionals play a critical role in delivering services in this labor-intensive industry, healthcare executives should be concerned with developing human resources policies and practices that are closely related to, influenced by, and supportive of the strategic goals and plans of their organization. Organizations, either explicitly or implicitly, pursue a strategy in their operations. Deciding on a strategy means determining the products or services that will be produced and the markets to which the chosen services will be offered. Once these selections have been made, the methods to be used to compete in the chosen market must be identified. The methods adopted are based on internal resources available, or potentially available, for use by executives.

As illustrated in Figure 1.2, strategies should be based on consideration of environmental conditions and organizational capabilities. To be in a position to take advantage of opportunities that are anticipated to occur, as well as to parry potential threats from changed conditions or competitor initiatives, managers must have detailed knowledge of the current and future operating environment. Cognizance of internal strengths and weaknesses allows managers to develop plans based on accurate assessment of the organization's ability to perform in the marketplace at the desired level.

SHRM does not occur in a vacuum; rather, it occurs in a complex and dynamic constellation of forces in the organization's context. A significant trend in recent years has been for HR managers to adopt a strategic perspective and recognize the critical linkages. As illustrated in Figure 1.2, the process starts with an understanding of the organization's purpose, mission, and business unit identification as defined by the board of directors and the top management team, and the process ends with the human resources function serving as a strategic partner to the operating departments. Under this new view of HRM, the HR manager's job is to help operating managers achieve their strategic goals by serving as a center of expertise for all employment-related activities and issues.

When HR is viewed as a strategic partner, talking about the single best way to do anything no longer makes sense. Instead, the organization must adopt HR practices that are consistent with its strategic mission, goals, and objectives. In addition, *all* healthcare executives are HR managers, so effective management of people depends on effective supervisors and line managers throughout the organization.

Mission and Corporate Strategy

An organization's *purpose* is its basic reason for existence. The purpose of a hospital may be to deliver high-quality clinical care to the population in a given service area. An organization's **mission** is how its board and top management have decided to fulfill its purpose. A mission specifies how the organization intends to manage itself to most effectively pursue the fulfillment of its purpose, and the mission statement often provides subtle clues about the importance the organization places on its human resources. In addition, the purpose and mission affect HR practices in obvious ways. A nursing home, for example, must employ nursing personnel, aides, and food service personnel to meet the needs of its patients.

*A **mission** specifies how the organization intends to manage itself to most effectively pursue the fulfillment of its purpose*

The first step in formulating a strategy is by performing *SWOT* (strengths, weaknesses, opportunities, and threats) *analysis*. Human resources play a fundamental role in SWOT analysis because the nature and type of people who work within an organization and the organization's ability to attract new talent represent significant strengths and weaknesses. With this information, the managers then attempt to use the organization's strengths to capitalize on environmental opportunities and to cope with environmental threats.

Most organizations formulate strategy at three basic levels: the corporate level, the business level, and various functional levels:

1. *Corporate strategy* is the set of strategic alternatives from which an organization chooses as it manages its operations simultaneously across several industries and markets.
2. *Business strategy* is a set of strategic alternatives from which an organization chooses to most effectively compete in a particular industry or market.
3. *Functional strategies* consider how the organization will manage each of its major functions (i.e., marketing, finance, and HR).

A key challenge for the HR managers when their organizations use a corporate strategy of growth is recruiting and training large members of qualified employees to provide needed services in growing operations as shown in Figure 1.1. New training programs may also be needed to orient and update the skills of new hires. The two-way arrows that lead from strategy formulation to human resources strategy formulation/implementation and vice versa indicate that their impact on the HR function should also be used in the initial formulation of strategy. When HR is a true strategic partner, all parties consult with and support one another.

The Human Resources Strategy

Once the organization's corporate and business strategies have been determined, managers can then develop a human resources strategy. This strategy commonly includes a staffing strategy (i.e., HR planning, recruitment, selection, and placement); a developmental strategy (i.e., performance management, training, development, and career planning); and a compensation strategy (i.e., salary structure and employee incentives).

A **staffing strategy** refers to a set of activities used by the organization to determine its future human resources needs, to recruit qualified applicants with an interest in the organization, and to select the best of those applicants as new employees. This strategy should be undertaken only after careful and systematic corporate and business strategies have been developed that mesh staffing activities with other strategies of the organization. For example, if retrenchment is part of the business strategy, staffing will focus on determining which employees to retain and what process to use in terminating the other employees.

*A **staffing strategy** refers to a set of activities used by the organization to determine its future human resources needs, to recruit qualified applicants with an interest in the organization, and to select the best of those applicants as new employees*

In addition, HR managers must also formulate an **employee development strategy** for helping the organization enhance the quality of its human resources; this strategy must also be consistent with the corporate and business strategies. For example, if the organization wishes to follow a strategy of differentiating itself from competitors through customer focus and service quality, then it will need to invest heavily in training its employees to provide the highest-quality service and its performance management must focus on measuring, recognizing, and rewarding performance leading to the high levels of service quality. Alternatively, if cost leadership is the selected strategy, the organization may invest less in training to keep overall costs low and focus whatever training is offered to reducing costs and enhancing productivity.

*An **employee development strategy** helps the organization enhance the quality of its human resources*

The **compensation strategy** must also complement the organization's other strategies. For example, if the organization is pursuing a strategy of related diversification, its compensation strategy must be geared toward rewarding employees whose skills allow them to move from the original business to related businesses (i.e., inpatient care to home health care). The organization may choose to pay a premium solely to a talented individual with skills that are relevant to one of the new businesses.

__Compensation strategy__ must be geared toward rewarding employees whose skills allow them to move from the original business to related businesses

Organizational Considerations

When attempting to formulate and implement HR strategy and the basic HR components discussed above, managers must also account for other key parts of the organization. The following four organizational components are important because they affect both how strategies are formulated and how they are implemented (Bamberger and Fiegelbaum 1996):

__Organizational design__ refers to the framework of jobs, positions, groups of positions, and reporting relationships among positions within an organization

1. **Organizational design** refers to the framework of jobs, positions, groups of positions, and reporting relationships among positions that is

used to construct an organization. Most healthcare organizations use a functional design whereby the organization groups its members into basic functional departments such as OB-GYN, surgery, emergency services, etc. Management roles are also divided into such functional areas as marketing, finance, human resources, etc; the top of the organizational chart is likely to reflect positions as CEO and vice presidents of marketing, finance, human resources, etc. To operate efficiently, and provide "seamless" service, this form of organization requires considerable coordination across the various departments.

In recent years, many healthcare organizations have been moving toward a *flat organizational structure* or the *horizontal corporation;* such a structure is created by eliminating levels of management, reducing bureaucracy, using wide spans of control, and relying heavily on teamwork and coordination to get work accomplished. These horizontal corporations are designed to be highly flexible, adaptable, streamlined, and empowered. The HR function in such organizations is typically diffused throughout the organization so that operating managers take on more of the responsibility for human resources activities and the HR staff plays a consultative role.

Corporate culture refers to the set of values that helps its members understand what the organization stands for, how it does things, and what it considers important

2. **Corporate culture** also affects how HR strategy is formulated and implemented. An organization's culture refers to the set of values that helps its members understand what the organization stands for, how it does things, and what it considers important. Because the corporate culture is the foundation of the organization's internal environment, it plays a major role in shaping the management of human resources, determining how well the organizational members will function together, and how well the organization will be able to achieve its goals.

Although no ideal culture exists for all organizations, a strong and well-articulated culture enables people to know what the organization stands for, what it values, and how to behave. A number of forces shape an organization's culture including the founder or founders, organizational affiliations, shared experiences, symbols, stories, slogans, heroes, and ceremonies. Managers must recognize the importance and origin of the organization's culture and take appropriate time to transmit that culture to others in the organization. Culture can be transmitted through orientation, training, consistent behavior (i.e., "walking the talk"), corporate history, and the telling and retelling of stories.

Culture may facilitate the work of either HR managers or line managers. If the organization has a strong, well-understood, and attractive culture, attracting and retaining qualified employees become easier to do. If the culture is perceived as weak or unattractive, attraction and retention become problematic. Likewise, the HR function can reinforce an existing culture by selecting new employees who have values consistent with that culture.

3. Technology also plays a role in the formulation and implementation of HR strategy. Healthcare organizations are quite different from manufacturing organizations in terms of how they perform each of the HR functions (i.e., criteria for hiring employees and methods of training employees); healthcare organizations typically emphasize educational credentials.

   Other aspects of technology are also important to HR in all settings. For example, automation of certain routine functions may reduce demand for certain human resources while increasing it for others, and computers and robotics are important technological elements that affect HRM. Rapid changes in technology affect employee selection, training, compensation, and other areas in the organization.

   Appropriately designed management information systems provide data to support planning and management decision making, and HR information is a crucial element of such a system. Such information can be used for both planning and operational purposes. For example, strategic planning efforts may require data on the future number of professionals in various categories who will be available to fill future positions. Internal planning may require such HR data to determine productivity trends, employee skills, work demands, and employee turnover rates. The use of an intranet (i.e., a miniature Internet operating within the boundaries of a particular organization) can improve service to all employees, help the HR department, and reduce many routine administrative costs (Gray 1997).

4. Workforce composition and trends are also an important part of the organizational environment of HRM. A number of workforce changes continue to emerge and affect HR strategy formulation and implementation. The American workforce has become increasingly diverse in numerous ways, including growth in older employees, women, Hispanics, Asians, African Americans, disabled, single parent, gays, lesbians, and people with special dietary preferences (Cox and Blake 1991). Previously, most employees followed a fairly predictable pattern of entering the workforce at a young age, maintaining a stable employment relationship for their workplaces, and then retiring at a fairly predictable age. Obviously, these patterns are no longer being maintained and continue to change and evolve as a result of demographic factors, improved health, and abolition of mandatory retirement.

Implementation

Successfully implementing a HR strategy generally requires the identification and management of key stakeholders (Blair and Fottler 1990, 1998). These stakeholders may be internal (i.e., employees); interface (i.e., physicians who are not employees); or external (i.e., third-party payers). The HR strategy (and all other strategies) can only be implemented through people, and such implementation requires motivational processes, communication processes, goal setting, and leadership.

Implementation also requires specific practices or tactics to implement the HR strategy that has been adopted. For example, if a healthcare organization has a business strategy to differentiate itself from competitors through a high level of focus on meeting customer (patient) needs, then it may formulate a HR strategy to provide all employees with training in "guest relations." However, that formulated strategy alone will not accomplish the objective; specific tactics for implementation need to be decided. For example, should this training be provided in-house or through external programs such as those available through the Disney Institute? How will each employee's success in applying the principles taught be measured and rewarded? The answers to such questions provide specific tactics to implement the strategic goal of differentiation on the basis of customer service.

Obviously, the organization will also formulate and implement other functional strategies in such areas as accounting/finance, marketing, and operations management. Organizational outcomes (positive or negative) are also a function of how well these functional strategies are formulated and implemented.

Outcomes

The outcomes achieved by a healthcare organization depend on the environment of the organization, the mission and strategies being pursued, the internal organizational systems, the human resources process systems, the consistency of operating practices across these internal systems, and how well all of the above are implemented. The appropriate methods for organizing and relating these elements are determined by the specific outcomes desired by the managers and major stakeholders of the healthcare organization. Although numerous methods exist for conceptualizing organizational performance and outcomes (Cameron and Whetten 1983; Goodman et al. 1977), the outcomes that may be useful for this discussion can be thought of as HR and organizational outcomes (see Figure 1.2).

Numerous HR outcomes should be associated with HR practices. An organization should provide its workforce with job security, meaningful work, safe working conditions, equitable financial compensation, and a satisfactory quality of work life. Healthcare organizations will not be able to attract and retain the numbers, types, and quality of professionals required to deliver health services if the internal work environments are unsuitable. In addition, employees are a valuable stakeholder group whose concerns are important because of the complexity of the way health services are delivered. The four measures of employee attitudes and psychological conditions are:

1. job satisfaction (Starkeweather and Steinbacher 1998);
2. commitment to the organization (Porter et al. 1974);

3. motivation (D'Aunno, Fottler, and O'Connor 2000);
4. level of job stress (DeFrank and Ivancevich 1998)

For long-term survival, a healthcare organization must have a balanced, exchange relationship with the environment. An equitable relationship must exist so that the exchange is mutually beneficial to the organization and to the elements of the environment with which it interacts. A number of outcome measures can be used to determine how well the organization is performing in the marketplace and how well the organization is producing a service that is valued by consumers, such as growth, profitability, return on investment, competitive advantage, legal compliance, attainment of strategic objectives, and satisfaction of key stakeholders. The latter may include such indices as patient satisfaction, cost per patient day, and community perceptions.

The mission and objectives of the organization will be reflected in the outcomes that are stressed by management and in the strategies, general tactics, and human resources practices that are chosen. Management makes decisions that, combined with the level of fit achieved among the internal organizational systems, determine the outcomes the organization can achieve. For example, almost all healthcare organizations need to earn some profit for continued viability. However, some organizations refrain from initiating new ventures that may be highly profitable if the ventures would not fit the overall mission of the organization for providing quality services needed by a defined population group.

Conversely, an organization may start some services that are acknowledged to be break-even propositions at best because the services are viewed as critical to the mission of the organization and the needs of the target market. The concerns of such an organization would be reflected not only in the choice of services offered but also in the human resources approaches used and the outcome measures viewed as important. This organization would likely place more emphasis on assessment criteria for employee performance and nursing unit operations that stress the provision of quality care and less emphasis on criteria concerned with efficient use of supplies and the maintenance of staffing ratios. This selection of priorities does not mean that efficiency of operations is ignored but that greater weight is placed on the former criteria.

The outcome measures used to judge the organization should reflect its priorities; one organization may emphasize patient satisfaction while another organization may place greater emphasis on economic return, profitability, and efficiency of operations. While quality of care also is important, the driving force for becoming a low-cost provider causes management to make decisions that reflect that resolve: maintenance or reduction of staffing levels is stressed, and prohibition of overtime is strictly enforced. Recruitment and selection criteria stress identification and selection of employees who will meet minimum criteria and expectations and, possibly, will accept lower pay levels.

In an organization that strives to be efficient, less energy may be spent on "social maintenance" activities designed for employee needs and to keep them from leaving or unionizing. Anticipate that the outcomes in this situation will reflect, at least in the short run, higher economic return and lower measures of quality of work life.

Conclusion

The intensive reliance on professionals for service delivery requires healthcare executives to focus attention on the strategic management of human resources in the delivery of services and to understand the factors that influence the performance of employees in their organization. To assist managers in understanding these relationships, this chapter presented a model of the association that exists among strategy, selected organizational design features, human resources management activities, employee outcomes, and organizational outcomes.

The outcomes achieved by the organization are influenced by numerous HR and non-HR factors. The mission determines the direction that is being taken by the organization and what it desires to achieve. The amount of integration of mission, strategy, HR functions, various behavioral components, and non-HR strategies defines the level of achievement that is possible. The remainder of the book addresses these challenges in more detail.

Discussion Questions

1. Differentiate corporate, business, and functional strategies. How does each relate to HR management? Why?
2. How may an organization's human resources be seen as either a strength or a weakness as part of SWOT analysis? What could be done to strengthen it in the event it was viewed as a weakness?
3. List factors under the control of healthcare managers that contribute to the reduction in number of applicants for training in health profession schools. Describe the steps that healthcare providers could take to improve this situation.
4. What are the organizational advantages of integrating strategic management and human resources management? What are the steps involved in such an integration?
5. Robert Levering and Milton Moskowitz published a best-selling book, titled *The Best 100 Companies to Work for in America*, based on review of HR practices in many organizations, among which was Beth Israel Hospital in Boston. Use a search engine to locate Beth Israel's web site address and see what information is contained at the site. What specific information interested you as a potential employee? How would you use this exercise to design a web site for a future employer? Why?

References

Bamberger, P., and A. Fiegelbaum. 1996. "The Role of Strategic Reference Points in Explaining the Nature and Consequences of Human Resource Strategy." *Academy of Management Review* 21 (4): 926–58.

Blair, J. D., and M. D. Fottler. 1990. *Challenges in Health Care Management: Strategic Perspectives for Managing Key Stakeholders.* San Francisco: Jossey-Bass.

———. 1998. *Strategic Leadership for Medical Groups.* San Francisco: Jossey-Bass.

Cameron, K. S., and D. A. Whetten. 1983. *Organizational Effectiveness: A Comparison of Multiple Models.* New York: Academic Press.

Cerne, F. 1988. "CEO Builds Employee Morale to Improve Finances." *Hospitals* 62 (11): 100.

Coddington, D. C., and K. D. Moore. 1987. *Market-Driven Strategies in Health Care.* San Francisco: Jossey-Bass.

Cox, T. H., and S. Blake. 1991. "Managing Cultural Diversity: Implications for Organizational Competitiveness." *Academy of Management Executive* 16 (1): 45–56.

D'Aunno, T., M. D. Fottler, and S. J. O'Connor. 2000. "Motivating People." In *Health Care Management, Fourth Edition,* edited by S. M. Shortell and A. D. Kaluzny. Albany, NY: Delmar.

DeFrank, R. S., and J. M. Ivancevich. 1998. "Stress on the Job." *Academy of Management Executive* 12 (3): 55–65.

Fottler, M. D., J. D. Phillips, J. D. Blair, and C. A. Duran. 1990. "Achieving Competitive Advantage Through Strategic Human Resource Management." *Hospital & Health Services Administration* 35 (3): 341–63.

Fottler, M. D., G. T. Savage, and J. D. Blair. 2000. "The Future of Integrated Delivery Systems: A Consumer Perspective." In *Advances in Health Care Management, Volume 1,* edited by J. D. Blair, M. D. Fottler, and G. T. Savage, pp. 5–32. Amsterdam: JAI/Elsevier Science.

Gomez-Mejia, L. R. 1988. "The Role of Human Resources Strategy in Export Performance." *Strategic Management Journal* 9: 493–505.

Goodman, P. S., J. M. Pennings, and associates. 1977. *New Perspectives on Organizational Effectiveness.* San Francisco: Jossey-Bass.

Gray, F. 1997. "How to Become Intranet Savvy." *HR Magazine* (4): 66–71.

Greer, C. R. 2001. *Strategic Human Resource Management.* Upper Saddle River, NJ: Prentice-Hall.

Hernandez, S. R., M. D. Fottler, and C. L. Joiner. 1998. "Integrating Management and Human Resources." In *Essentials of Human Resources Management in Health Services Organization,* edited by S. R. Hernandez, M. D. Fottler, and C. L. Joiner, pp. 1–20. Albany, NY: Delmar.

Hospitals. 1989. "Human Resources." *Hospitals* 63: 46–7.

Huselid, M. A. 1994. "Documenting HR's Effect on Company Performance." *HR Magazine* (1): 79–85.

Huselid, M. A., S. E. Jackson, and R. S. Schuler. 1997. "Technical and Strategic Human Resources Management Effectiveness as Determinants of Firm Performance." *Academy of Management Journal* 40 (1): 171–88.

Kaluzny, A., H. Zuckerman, and T. Ricketts. 1995. *Partners for the Dance: Forming Strategic Alliances in Health Care.* Chicago: Health Administration Press.

Kravetz, D. J. 1988. *The Human Resources Revolution: Implementing Progressive Management Practices for Bottom Line Success.* San Francisco: Jossey-Bass.

McManis, G. L. 1987. "Managing Competitively: The Human Factor." *Healthcare Executive* 2 (6): 18–23.

Pfeffer J. 1994. *Competitive Advantage Through People.* Boston: Harvard Business School Press.

Porter, L. W., R. M. Steers, R. T. Mowday, and P. V. Boulian. 1974. "Organizational Commitment, Job Satisfaction, and Turnover Among Psychiatric Technicians." *Journal of Applied Psychology* 59: 603–9.

Porter, M. E. 1980. *Comparative Strategy.* New York: The Free Press.

Shortell, S. M., R. R. Giles, D. A. Anderson, K. M. Erickson, and J. B. Mitchell. 1996. *Remaking Health Care in America: Building Organized Delivery Systems.* San Francisco: Jossey-Bass.

Starkeweather, R. A., and C. L. Steinbacher. 1998. "Job Satisfaction Affects the Bottom Line." *HR Magazine* 9: 110–12.

Wilson, T. B. 1986. *A Guide to Strategic Human Resource Planning for the Health Care Industry.* Chicago: American Society for Healthcare Human Resource Administration, American Hospital Association.

CHAPTER 2

HEALTHCARE PROFESSIONALS

Kenneth R. White, Ph.D., FACHE, and
Dolores G. Clement, Dr.P.H.

Learning Objectives

After completing this chapter, the reader should be able to:

- Understand the role of healthcare professionals in the human resources management function of healthcare organizations
- Define the elements of a profession, with an understanding of the theoretical underpinnings of the health professions in particular
- Describe the health professions, which include the majority of healthcare workers, and the required educational levels, scopes of practice, and licensure issues for each
- Relate knowledge of the health professions to selected human resources management issues and systems development
- Comprehend the changing nature of the existing and emerging health professions in the healthcare workforce, particularly the impact of managed care

Introduction

The training, education, and skills of healthcare professionals are essential in meeting the needs and demands of the population for safe, competent health services. These specialized techniques and skills healthcare professionals acquired through systematic programs of intellectual study are the basis for socialization into their profession. Additionally, the healthcare industry is labor intensive and distinguished from other service industries by the number of licensed and registered personnel that it employs and the variety of healthcare fields that it produces. These healthcare fields have emerged as a result of the specialization of medicine, development of public health, increased emphasis on health promotion and prevention, and technological development and growth. Because of this division of labor within medical and health services delivery, many tasks that were once the responsibility of medical providers have been delegated to other healthcare personnel. Such delegation of duties raises the following questions: Should healthcare providers other than those specifically trained to practice medicine be considered professionals in their own right? To what extent should their scope of practice be extended?

In this chapter, we define key terms, describe the roles of several healthcare professionals and their roles in the human resources management function, and discuss the issues that face healthcare professionals.

Professionalization

*A **profession** requires specialized knowledge and training that enable professionals to gain more authority and responsibility and to provide service that adheres to a code of ethics*

*An **occupation** also enables workers to provide services, but it does not require skill specialization*

Although the terms are often used interchangeably, a profession can be differentiated from an occupation. A **profession** requires specialized knowledge and training that enable professionals to gain more authority and responsibility and to provide service that adheres to a code of ethics. Similarly, an **occupation**, which is the principal activity that supports one's livelihood, also enables workers to provide services, but it does not require skill specialization. A professional usually has more autonomy in determining the content of the service he or she provides and in monitoring the workload needed to do so. In contrast, one in an occupation typically is supervised and adheres to a defined work schedule. A professional generally earns a salary, while an hourly wage rate is earned by one in an occupation. *Professionalization,* which often requires higher-education attainment, gives a person more work independence and mobility. On the other hand, an individual in an occupation may be merely functionally trained and, as a result, is less able to move from one organization to another.

The ever-evolving process of health services delivery necessitated the training of professionals who are empowered to make decisions in the absence of direct supervision. The proliferation of knowledge and the skills needed in the prevention, diagnosis, and treatment of disease have required the increase of educational levels necessary for practice. Undergraduate- and/or graduate-level degrees are now required for entry to a field, degrees which were considered "terminal" degrees as recently as a decade ago. Some professions, such as pharmacy and physical therapy, are moving toward professional doctorates (i.e., Pharm.D. and D.P.T., respectively) for practice.

A countervailing force against the increasing educational requirements of the health professions is ongoing change in the mechanisms for delivery and payment for services. With consolidation of the healthcare system and the rise of managed care, along with its demands for efficiency, fewer financial resources are available. As a result, healthcare organizations are pressured to replace more highly trained, and therefore more expensive, healthcare professionals with unlicensed support personnel. Fewer professionals are being asked to do more, and those with advanced degrees are required to supervise more assistants who are functionally trained for specified organizational roles.

Functional training produces personnel who can perform tasks but who do not know the theory behind the practice, and knowing theory is essential in becoming fully skilled and fully able to make complex decisions about patient care. Conversely, knowing the theory without having the experience also makes competent practice difficult. When educating potential healthcare professionals, on-the-job training or a period of apprenticeship is needed, particularly in addition to basic coursework. Dreyfus and Dreyfus (1996) contend that both theoretical knowledge and practiced response are needed in the acquisition of skill in a profession. They lay out five stages of abilities that an individual passes as he or she develops a skill:

1. *Novice.* At this stage, the *novice* learns tasks and skills that enable him or her to determine actions based on recognized situations. Rules and guidelines direct the novice's energy and action at this stage.
2. *Advanced beginner.* At this stage, the *advanced beginner* has gained enough experience and knowledge that certain behaviors become automatic, and he or she can begin to learn when tasks should be addressed.
3. *Competent.* At this stage, the *competent* individual has mastered the practiced response of definable tasks and processes and acquired the ability to deal with the unexpected events that might not conform to plans.
4. *Proficient.* At this stage, the *proficient* individual has developed the ability to discern a situation, intuitively assess it, plan what needs to be done, decide on an action, and perform the action more effortlessly than in the earlier stages.
5. *Expert.* At this stage, the *expert* can accomplish the goals without realizing that rules are being followed because the skill and knowledge required to reach the goal have become "second nature" to him or her.

Theoretical understanding is melded with practice in each progressive stage. Functional training can help an individual progress through the first three stages and provide him or her with *calculative rationality* or inferential reasoning ability to be able to apply and improve theories and rules learned. For skill development at the proficient and expert levels, *deliberative rationality* or ability to challenge and improve theories and rules learned is required. Healthcare professionals need to become experts in fields where self-direction, autonomy, and decision making for patient care may be required (Dreyfus and Dreyfus 1996).

Healthcare Professionals

The healthcare industry is the largest and most powerful industry in the United States. It constitutes over 6.5 percent of the total labor force and 13 percent of the gross domestic product. Healthcare professionals include physicians; nurses; dentists; pharmacists; optometrists; psychologists; non-physician practitioners, such as physician assistants and nurse practitioners; healthcare administrators; and allied health professionals. Allied health professionals is a huge group that consists of therapists, medical and radiologic technologists, social workers, health educators, and other ancillary personnel. These healthcare professionals are represented by their respective professional associations; Table 2.1 is a resource guide that lists professional associations.

Healthcare professionals work in a variety of settings, including hospitals; ambulatory care centers; managed care organizations (MCOs); long-term care organizations; mental health organizations; pharmaceutical companies; community health centers; physician offices; laboratories; research institutions; and schools of medicine, nursing, and allied health professions. According to the National Center for Health Statistics (Bureau of Labor Statistics 2000), healthcare professionals are employed by:

- hospitals (43.9 percent);
- nursing and personal care facilities (15.3 percent);
- physician offices and clinics (13.9 percent);
- dentist offices and clinics (5.9 percent);
- chiropractic offices and clinics (1.2 percent); and
- other health service sites (19 percent).

The Department of Labor recognizes about 400 different job titles in the healthcare sector; however, many of these job titles are not included in our definition of healthcare professionals. Almost one-third of all those employed in the healthcare sector probably belong in the support staff category (i.e., those employees who are part of the patient care team or involved in delivering health services). Although these approximately 1.5 million nurse aides/assistants, orderlies, and attendants are not discussed in this chapter, these occupations are important to mention because they represent important employment opportunities in the service-oriented economy that now characterizes the United States (Mick 1999). The primary reasons for the increased supply and wide variety of healthcare professionals include the following interrelated forces:

- technological growth;
- specialization;
- health insurance coverage;
- the aging of the population; and
- the proliferation of various healthcare delivery settings.

Healthcare professionals are discussed in greater detail in this chapter. We focus on nurses, pharmacists, selected allied health professionals, and healthcare administrators rather than on physicians, dentists, and other medically trained providers because the former group of professionals is at the center of the debate on increased delegation of duties.

Organization	Target Audience	Web Site
Health Professions		
Pew Health Professions Commission	Future health professions	www.futurehealth. ucsf.edu/press.html
Accrediting Organizations		
American Osteopathic Association (AOA)	Osteopathic hospitals and health systems	www.aoa-net.org
The Rehabilitation Accreditation Commission (formerly Commission on Accreditation of Rehabilitation Facilities [CARF])	Rehabilitation facilities	www.carf.org
Joint Commission on Accreditation of Healthcare Organizations (JCAHO)	Hospitals and health systems	www.jcaho.org
National Committee for Quality Assurance (NCQA)	Managed care plans	www.ncqa.org
American Association of Blood Banks (AABB)	Blood banks	www.aabb.org
American College of Surgeons: Commission on Cancer	Cancer programs	www.facs.org/dept/ cancer/coc/liaison.html
College of American Pathologists (CAP)	Clinical laboratories	www.cap.org

TABLE 2.1
Resource Guide for the Healthcare Professional

continued

TABLE 2.1
Continued

Organization	Target Audience	Web Site
Professional Associations		
American College of Healthcare Executives (ACHE)	Healthcare executives	www.ache.org
National Association of Health Services Executives (NAHSE)	African-American healthcare executives	www.nahse.org
Institute for Diversity in Health Management	Minority healthcare executives	www.institutefor diversity.org
Medical Group Management Association (MGMA)	Physician practice managers and executives	www.mgma.com
American College of Health Care Administrators (ACHCA)	Long-term care administrators	www.achca.org
American Association for Medical Transcription	Medical transcriptionists	www.aamt.org
American Association of Nurse Anesthetists (AANA)	Nurse anesthetists	www.aana.com
American Association for Respiratory Care (AARC)	Respiratory therapists	www.aarc.org
American Health Information Management Association (AHIMA)	Medical records and information management professionals	www.ahima.org
American Medical Technologists (AMT)	Medical technologists	www.amt1.com

continued

TABLE 2.1
Continued

Organization	Target Audience	Web Site
Professional Associations		
American Nurses Association (ANA)	Nurses	www.ana.org
American Occupational Therapy Association, Inc. (AOTA)	Occupational therapists	www.aota.org
American Organization of Nurse Executives (AONE)	Nurse executives	www.aone.org
American Physical Therapy Association (APTA)	Physical therapists	www.apta.org
American Society of Clinical Pathologists (ASCP)	Pathologists and medical technologists	www.ascp.org
American Society of Health-System Pharmacists (ASHP)	Pharmacists	www.ashp.org
American Society of Radiologic Technologists (ASRT)	Radiologic technologists	www.asrt.org
American Speech-Language-Hearing Association (ASHA)	Speech therapists, audiologists, and speech pathologists	www.asha.org
Healthcare Financial Management Association (HFMA)	Controllers, CFOs, and accountants	www.hfma.org
Health Information and Management Systems Society (HIMSS)	Health information managers	www.himss.org

continued

TABLE 2.1
Continued

Organization	Target Audience	Web Site
Professional Associations		
National Cancer Registrars Association (NCRA)	Cancer program registrars	www.ncra-usa.org
Trade Associations		
American Hospital Association (AHA)	Hospitals and health systems and personal membership groups	www.aha.org
Federation of American Hospitals (FAHS)	Investor-owned hospitals and health systems	www.fahs.com
Association of American Medical Colleges (AAMC): Council of Teaching Hospitals and Health Systems (COTH)	Academic medical centers	www.aamc.org/about/coth/start.htm
Catholic Health Association of the United States (CHA)	Catholic hospitals and health systems	www.chausa.org
American Association of Health Plans (AAHP)	Health plans	www.aahp.org

Nurses

Caregiving is the essence of nursing.[1] In today's nursing practice, caregiving means purposeful, intentional action that brings about change for the better (Berger and Williams 1999). Nurses also serve as patient advocates, multidisciplinary team members, managers, executives, researchers, and entrepreneurs.

Nurses comprise the largest group of licensed healthcare professionals in the United States. The National League for Nursing (2000) reports that the United States has 2.5 million *registered nurses (RNs)*, over 2.2 million (83 percent) of whom are employed in healthcare organizations. Approximately 60 percent of employed RNs, or 1.3 million, work in hospitals, while 17 percent, or 362,648, work in community or public health settings. Complementing this workforce are 370,000 *licensed practical nurses (LPNs),* or licensed vocational nurses (LVNs) as they are known in some states. According to the demographic profiles compiled by the National League for Nursing, most nurses are women; about 5.4 percent of RNs are men, although 13 percent of enrolled nursing students in 1997 were men; approximately 10 percent of RNs come from racial/ethnic minority backgrounds; and, in 1997, the average age of RNs was 44.5 years old.

RNs and LPNs

All U.S. states require nurses to be licensed to practice; the licensure requirements include graduation from an approved nursing program and successful completion of a national examination. Educational preparation distinguishes between two levels of nurses. RNs must complete an associate's degree in nursing (ADN), a diploma program, or a baccalaureate degree in nursing (BSN) to qualify for the licensure examination. ADN programs generally take two years to complete and are offered by community and junior colleges, and hospital-based diploma programs can be completed in about three years. The fastest growing avenue for nursing education is the baccalaureate preparation, which typically can be completed in four years and is offered by colleges and universities. LPNs, on the other hand, must complete a state-approved program in practical nursing and must achieve a passing score on a national examination. Each state maintains regulations and practice acts that delineate the scope of nursing practice for RNs and LPNs.

Among employed RNs, about 35 percent hold associate degrees, 35 percent have hospital-based program diplomas, and 30 percent possess BSN degrees. Additionally, 9 percent of these nurses hold master's-level degrees and less than one percent have doctorates. In addition to licensure and educational achievements, some nurses obtain certification in specialty areas such as critical care, infection control, emergency nursing, surgical nursing, obstetrical nursing, etc. The nursing field comprises many specialties and subspecialties; certification in these areas requires specialty education, practical experience, and successful completion of a national examination. Some nurses obtain certification in these specialty areas because certification helps them maintain their professional associations. To remain certified, continued employment, continuing education units (CEUs), or re-examination may be required.

APNs

An *advanced practice nurse (APN)* is a nurse with particular skills and credentials, which typically include basic nursing education; basic licensure; graduate degree in nursing; experience in a specialized area; professional certification from a national certifying body; and, if required in some states, APN licensure (National Council of State Boards of Nursing 2000). The APN specializes as a nurse practitioner (NP), certified nurse midwife (CNM), certified registered nurse anesthetist (CRNA), or clinical nurse specialist (CNS).

APNs generally have the ability to:

- perform comprehensive assessment;
- diagnose;
- manage health and illness problems;
- assess and intervene in complex systems;
- critically analyze research findings;
- lead in healthcare settings;
- cooperate and collaborate with other personnel; and
- be autonomous enough to make critical, independent judgments (Hickey, Ouimette, and Venegoni 1996).

Additional core competencies may be needed in each specialty area that an APN pursues. The largest number of APNs are NPs, who may further specialize in acute care or community settings or for particular client groups such as adults, children, women, or psychiatric/mental health populations.

Each state maintains its own laws and regulations regarding recognition of an APN, but the general requirements in all states include licensure as a registered nurse and successful completion of a national specialty examination. Some states permit certain categories of APNs to write prescriptions for certain classes of drugs. This *prescriptive authority* varies from one state to another and may be regulated by boards of medicine, nursing, pharmacy, or allied health. Some states require physician supervision of APN practices, although some managed care plans now include APNs on their lists of primary care providers.

APN specialization

Certified nurse midwives (CNMs) specialize in low-risk obstetrical care, including all aspects of the prenatal, labor and delivery, and postnatal processes. *Certified registered nurse anesthetists (CRNAs)* complete additional education to specialize in the administration of various types of anesthesia and analgesia to patients and clients. Often, nurse anesthetists work collaboratively with surgeons and anesthesiologists as part of the perioperative care team. *Clinical nurse specialists (CNSs)* hold master's degrees, have successfully completed a specialty certification examination, and are generally employed by hospitals as nursing "experts" in particular specialties. The scope of the CNS is not as broad as that of the NP; CNSs work with a specialty population under a somewhat circumscribed set of conditions, and the management authority of patients still rests with physicians. In contrast, NPs have developed an autonomous role in which their collaboration is encouraged, and they generally have the legal authority to implement management actions.

Pharmacists

In the foreseeable future, the pharmacy profession will continue to undergo extensive change. Until the latter part of the past decades, pharmacists performed the traditional role of preparing drug products and filling prescriptions; in the 1980s, however, pharmacists expanded that role. Pharmacists now act as an expert for clients and patients on the effects of specific drugs, drug interactions, and generic drug substitutions for brand-name drugs.

To be eligible for licensure, pharmacists must graduate from an accredited baccalaureate program in pharmacy, successfully complete a state board examination, and obtain practical experience or complete a supervised internship. After passing a national examination, a *registered pharmacist (R.Ph.)* is permitted to carry out the scope of practice outlined by state regulations. Recently, the trend in pharmacy has been to broaden education to include the terminal degree—*doctor of pharmacy (Pharm.D)*. Many pharmacy schools offer this program for those interested in research careers, teaching, higher administrative responsibility, or as members of the patient care team. This educational preparation also requires successful completion of a state board examination and other practical clinical experience, as outlined by state laws.

Allied Health Professionals

The term allied health professionals is generally not well understood because of its ambiguous definition (O'Neil and Hare 1990) and a lack of consensus about what such a role constitutes. In general, **allied health professionals** complement the work of physicians and other healthcare providers, although one may also be a provider. The U.S. Public Health Service defines an allied health professional as:

Allied health professionals complement the work of physicians and other healthcare providers, although one may also be a provider

> a health professional (other than a registered nurse or a physician assistant) who has received a certificate, an associate's degree, a bachelor's degree, a master's degree, a doctoral degree, or postbaccalaureate training in a science related to health care; who shares in the responsibility for the delivery of health care services or related services, including (1) services relating to the identification, evaluation and prevention of disease and disorders, (2) dietary and nutrition services, (3) health promotion services, (4) rehabilitation services, or (5) health systems management services; and who has not received a degree of doctor of medicine, a degree of doctor of osteopathy, a degree of doctor of veterinary medicine or equivalent degree, a degree of doctor of optometry or equivalent degree, a degree of doctor of podiatric medicine or equivalent degree, a degree of bachelor science in pharmacy or equivalent degree, a graduate degree in public health or equivalent degree, a degree of doctor of chiropractic

or equivalent degree, a graduate degree in health administration or equivalent degree, a degree of doctor of clinical psychology or equivalent degree, or a degree in social work or equivalent degree" (Health Professions Education Extension Amendments of 1992, Section 701 PHS Act).

A debate on the exclusiveness and inclusiveness of the U.S. Public Health's definition continues; some observers of healthcare consider nursing, public health, and social work to fall under the umbrella of allied health, but they are not included in this definition. Table 2.2 lists the major categories that comprise the allied health profession and the job titles that frequently fall under each category.

According to the 1999 National Occupational and Wage Estimates (Bureau of Labor Statistics 2001) for healthcare personnel, the allied health professions constitute 40.6 percent of the healthcare workforce in the United States. This number excludes physicians, nurses, dentists, pharmacists, veterinarians, chiropractors, and podiatrists. The allied health professions are the most heterogenous of the personnel groupings in healthcare. The National Commission on Allied Health (1995) broadly divided allied health professionals into two categories of personnel: (1) therapists/technologists and (2) technicians/assistants.

Some of the job titles presented in Table 2.2 may not fit into these two categories. In general, the therapist/technologist category represents those with higher-level professional training and who are often responsible for supervising those in the technician/assistant category. The therapist/technologists usually hold baccalaureate and higher degrees, and they are trained to evaluate patients, understand diagnoses, and develop treatment plans in their area of expertise. On the other hand, the technicians/assistants are most likely to have two years or less post-secondary education, and they are functionally trained with procedural skills for specified tasks.

Educational and training programs for the allied health profession are sponsored by a variety of organizations in different academic and clinical settings. They range from degree offerings at colleges and universities to clinical programs in hospitals and other health facilities. Prior to 1990, one-third of the allied health programs were housed in hospitals, although hospitals graduated only 15 percent of their students (O'Neil and Hare 1990). Junior or community colleges, vocational or technical schools, and academic health centers can all sponsor allied health programs. These programs can also be stand-alone when aligned with an academic health center, or they could be under the auspices of the school of medicine or nursing if a specific school of allied health professions does not exist. Dental and pharmacy technicians or assistants may or may not be trained in their respective schools or in a school of allied health professions.

TABLE 2.2
Major
Categories of
the Allied
Health
Profession and
Professional
Titles

Behavioral Health Services

Substance Abuse Counselor	Community Health Worker
Home Health Aide	Mental Health Assistant
Mental Health Aide	

Clinical Laboratory Sciences

Associate Laboratory Microbiologist	Laboratory Microbiologist
Chemist (Biochemist)	Laboratory Technician
Laboratory Associate	Microbiologist

Dental Services

Dental Assistant	Dental Hygienist
Dental Laboratory Technologist	

Dietetic Services

Assistant Director of Food Service	Dietitian
Associate Supervising Dietitian	Dietary Assistant

Emergency Medical Services

Ambulance Technician	Emergency Medical Services
Emergency Medical Technician	Specialist

Health Information Management Services

Director of Medical Records	Medical Record Specialist
Assistant Director, Medical Record Service	Senior Medical Record Systems
Health Information Manager	Analyst
Data Analyst	Coder

Medical and Surgical Services

Electroencephalograph Technician	Medical Equipment Specialist
Operating Room Technician	Biomedical Equipment Technician
Biomedical Engineer	Electrocardiograph Technician
Cardiovascular Technologist	Dialysis Technologist
Electrocardiograph Technician	Electroencephalograph Technologist
Surgical Assistant	Ambulatory Care Technician

Occupational Therapy

Occupational Therapist	Occupational Therapy Assistant
Occupational Therapy Aide	

continued

TABLE 2.2
Continued

Ophthalmic Services

Ophthalmic Dispenser	Optometric Technologist
Optometric Aide	

Physical Therapy

Physical Therapist	Physical Therapy Assistant

Radiological Services

Nuclear Medicine Technician	Radiation Technician
Ultrasound Technician	Medical Radiation Dosimetry
Nuclear Medicine Technologist	Diagnostic Medical Sonographer
Radiologic (Medical) Technologist	

Rehabilitation Services

Art Therapist	Dance Therapist
Exercise Physiologist	Music Therapist
Orthotics/Prosthetics	Orthopedic Assistant
Recreational Therapist	Recreation Therapy Assistant
Rehabilitation Counselor	Rehabilitation Technician
Addiction Counselor	Addiction Specialist
Psychiatric Social Health Technician	Sign Language Interpreter

Respiratory Therapy Services

Respiratory Therapist	Respiratory Therapy Technician
Respiratory Therapy Assistant	

Speech-Language Pathology/Audiology Services

Audiology Clinician	Staff Audiologist
Speech Clinician	Staff Speech Pathologist

Other Allied Health Services

Central Supply Technician	Medical Illustrator
Podiatric Assistant	Veterinary Assistant
Health Unit Coordinator	Chiropractic Assistant
Home Health Aide	

A vast number of the allied health programs are accredited by the Commission on Accreditation of Allied Health Educational Programs (CAAHEP) —a freestanding agency that replaced the American Medical Association's Committee on Allied Health Education and Accreditation (CAHEA) in 1994. The formation of CAAHEP was intended to simplify the accrediting process, to be more inclusive of allied health programs that provide entry-level education, and to serve as an initiator of more far-reaching change. Some key allied health professions, such as physical therapy and occupational therapy, still accredit programs through their own professional associations.

Healthcare Administrators

Healthcare administrators organize, coordinate, and manage the delivery of health services, provide leadership, and organize the strategic direction of healthcare organizations. The variety and numbers of healthcare professionals they employ; the complexity of health services delivery; and environmental pressures to provide access, quality, and efficient services make healthcare organizations among the most complex organizations to manage.

Healthcare administrators organize, coordinate, and manage the delivery of health services, provide leadership, and organize the strategic direction of healthcare organizations

Healthcare administration is taught at the undergraduate and graduate levels in a variety of settings, and these programs lead to a number of different degrees; the settings include schools of medicine, public health, healthcare business, and allied health professions. A bachelor's degree in health administration will allow individuals to pursue positions such as nursing home administrator, supervisor, or middle manager in healthcare organizations. Most students who aspire to have a career in healthcare administration will go on to receive a master's-level degree.

Graduate education programs in healthcare administration are accredited by the Accrediting Commission on Education for Health Services Administration (ACEHSA). Most common degrees include the Master of Health Administration (MHA); Master of Business Administration (MBA, with a healthcare emphasis); Master of Public Health (MPH); or Master of Public Administration (MPA). However, the MHA degree, or its equivalent, has been the accepted training model for entry-level managers in the various sectors of the healthcare industry (Shi and Singh 1998). The MHA program, when compared to a MPH program, offers core courses that focus on building business management (theory and applied management), quantitative, and analytical skills and that emphasize experiential training. In addition, some MHA programs require students to complete three-month internships or 12-month residencies as part of their two- or three-year curricula. Some graduates elect to complete post-graduate fellowships that are available in selected hospitals, health systems, MCOs, consulting firms, and other health-related organizations.

Nursing home administrator programs require students to pass a national examination administered by the National Association of Boards of Examiners for Nursing Home Administrators (NAB); this examination is a standard requirement in all states, but the educational preparation needed to qualify for this exam varies from state to state. Although more than one-third of the states still require less than a bachelor's degree as the minimum academic preparation, approximately 70 percent of the practicing nursing home administrators have, at a minimum, a bachelor's degree. As the population continues to live longer, the demand and educational requirements for long-term care administrators is estimated to increase, along with the growth of educational programs specific to this sector of the healthcare industry.

Considerations for Human Resources Department

The role of human resources management in healthcare organizations is to develop and implement systems, in accordance with regulatory guidelines and licensure laws, that ensure selection, evaluation, and retention of healthcare professionals. In light of this role, human resources personnel should be aware that each of the health professions, and often subspecialties within those professions, has specific requirements that allow an individual to qualify for an entry-level job in his or her chosen profession. The requirements of national accrediting organizations (e.g., JCAHO); regulatory bodies (e.g., CMS—formerly HCFA); and licensure authorities (e.g., state licensure boards) should be considered in all aspects of human resources management. We briefly discuss some of the issues that a healthcare organization's human resources department must consider when dealing with healthcare professionals.

Qualification

In developing a comprehensive employee compensation program, human resources personnel must include the specific skill and knowledge required for each job in the organization. Those qualifications must be determined and stated in writing for each job; the job description usually contains level of education, experience, judgment ability, accountability, physical skills, responsibilities, communication skills, and any special certification or licensure requirements. Human resources personnel needs to be aware of all specifications for all job titles within their organizations. This knowledge of healthcare professionals is necessary to ensure that essential qualifications of individuals coincide with job specifications, and it is also necessary for determining wage and salary ranges.

Licensure and Certification

A human resources department must have policies and procedures in place that describe the way in which licensure is verified on initial employment. Also, the department must have a system in place for tracking the expiration dates of licenses and ensuring licensure renewal. Therefore, the department must be conscientious about whether the information it receives is a *primary verification*, in which the information directly comes from the licensing authority, or a *secondary verification*, in which a potential employee personally submits a document copy that indicates licensure has been granted, including the expiration date. Certifications must be verified during the selection process, although certifications and licenses are generally not statutory requirements.

Many organizations accept a copy of a certification document as verification. If the certification is a job requirement, systems must be in place to track expiration dates and to access new certification documents.

Career Ladders

In selecting healthcare professionals, human resources personnel must consider past employment history, including the explanation of gaps in employment. To assess the amount of individual experience, evaluating the candidate's breadth and depth of responsibility in previous jobs is essential. Many organizations have *career ladders*, which are mechanisms that advance a healthcare professional within the organization. Career ladders are based on the Dreyfus and Dreyfus model of "novice to expert" (explained earlier in the chapter), and experience may be used as a criterion for assignment of an individual to a particular job category.

Educational Services

Healthcare professionals require continuous, life-long learning. Organizations must have in-house training and development plans for ensuring that their healthcare professionals achieve competency in new technologies and new programs and equipment and are aware of policy and procedure changes. Certain competencies must be renewed annually in areas such as cardiopulmonary resuscitation, safety and infection control, and disaster planning.

Coupled with organization-specific ongoing education, some professions and licensing jurisdictions may require continuing education that is profession specific. Healthcare organizations should be cognizant of fiscal resources necessary to support these educational requirements.

Practitioner Impairment

Healthcare professionals are accountable to the public for maintaining their high professional standards, and the governing body of healthcare organizations is by statute responsible for the quality of care rendered in the organization. This quality is easily jeopardized by an impaired practitioner. An **impaired practitioner** is a healthcare professional who is unable to carry out his or her professional duties with reasonable skill and safety because of a physical or mental illness, including deterioration through aging, loss of motor skill, or excessive use of drugs and alcohol.

*An **impaired practitioner** is a healthcare professional who is unable to carry out his or her professional duties with reasonable skill and safety because of a physical or mental illness*

The human resources department must periodically evaluate the performance of all healthcare professionals in the organization to ensure their *competence* (which is the basic education and training necessary for the job) and *proficiency* (which is the demonstrated ability to perform job tasks). Mechanisms must be in place to identify the impaired practitioner, such as policies and procedures that describe how the organization will handle investigations, subsequent recommendations for treatment, monitoring, and employment restrictions or separation. Each national or state licensing authority maintains legal requirements for reporting impaired practitioners.

In the coming decades, new challenges and opportunities, such as the issues described above, will face the human resources department of each organization as a result of ever-increasing changes in the health professions.

Changing Nature of the Health Professions

In the 1990s, we entered a new era of uncertainty in healthcare, one faced with a quickening pace of change (Begun and White 1999). Within this framework, new ways of thinking are rewarded as the meaning of "health" is redefined, the boundaries of healthcare professionals are reshaped, and the outcomes of healthcare professional interventions are measured in terms of quality of life. Changes in the organization and financing of healthcare services have shifted delivery from the hospital to the home and community, and technological advances have expanded job opportunities for healthcare practitioners. These shifts have changed the roles, functions, and expectations of the healthcare workforce and gave way to the emergence of the following issues.

Supply and Demand

Throughout the twentieth century, the nursing labor market cycled through periods of shortages and surpluses (Jones 2001). The beginning of the twenty-first century brought the nursing and allied health professions the challenge of keeping pace with the demand for their services. Indicators of demand include numbers of position vacancies and a rise in salaries. To fill positions, hospitals—the largest employers of nurses and allied health professionals— have raised salaries, provided scholarships, and given other incentives such as sign-on bonuses.

The supply of nurses and allied health professionals is reflected in the number of students in educational programs and those available for the health-care workforce. The aging of the nursing workforce (Buerhaus and Staiger 1999) and the decline in nursing school enrollees (AACN 2001) are threats to the future supply. Recruitment of nursing and allied health professions students has become a major focus of practitioners, professional associations, and academic institutions.

Alternative Therapies

Alternative therapies have gained more popularity, judging by the growing number of related titles on the topic in the lay press and academic literature. A turning point in the acceptance and increased respectability (Weber 1996) of alternative therapies was noted in a sentinel study of the prevalence in use of alternative or unconventional therapies (Eisenberg et al. 1993). In the study, Eisenberg and colleagues concluded that one in three adults relied on treatments and interventions that are *not* widely taught at medical schools in the United States; examples of these alternative interventions included acupuncture and chiropractic and massage therapies. This specialty area might be considered an emerging health profession.

Nonphysician Practitioners

With the advent of managed care, greater reliance has been placed on *nonphysician practitioners*. Collaborative practice models with nurse practitioners, physician assistants, pharmacists, and other therapists are appropriate to both acute and long-term health services delivery. Strides have been made in the direct reimbursement for some nonphysician healthcare provider services, which is an impetus for further collaboration in practice.

The consolidation and integration of the healthcare delivery system has not, however, eliminated slack and duplication of services. Although the changes attributed to managed care have led to the promotion and use of less-costly sites for care delivery, a larger impact on the division of labor among all healthcare professionals, and thus on health professions, may yet occur.

Licensure and Certification

The use of nonphysician practitioners at various sites might be viewed as an opportunity for the growth of nursing, pharmacy, allied health professions, and health administration. Alternatively, Hurley (1997) contends that it may lead to concerted efforts to repeal professional licensure and certification in healthcare. If policymakers jump on the bandwagon, this deregulation may lead to the demise of some health professions and may also lead to the proliferation of functionally trained, unlicensed personnel. The use of less highly educated personnel will have greater implications for the existence and growth of educational programs in the academic medical centers.

The use of unlicensed support personnel poses concerns about the intensity and quality of healthcare delivered. When fewer highly trained professionals are employed for oversight, the potential for adverse outcomes increases. Aiken, Sochalski, and Anderson (1996) found that, although the percentage of registered nurses has increased overall, fewer nurses per patient were available in the mid-1990s than a decade earlier to provide care for more acutely ill patients. The net effect was a relative increase in nonclinical personnel, which added stress for those who were expected to supervise unlicensed staff and care for sicker patients.

Entrepreneurship

Given the bureaucratic nature of organizations, the regulation of the healthcare industry, and additional constraints by payers and managed care, many healthcare professionals are choosing to pursue opportunities on their own. The service economy coupled with knowledge-based professions may encourage pursuit of new and different ventures for individuals who have the personality, skills, and tenacity to go into their own business. An entrepreneur must have a mix of management skills and the means to depart from a traditional career path to practice on one's own.

White and Begun (1998) characterize the entrepreneurial personality traits of a profession in terms of its willingness to take the risks associated with undertaking new ventures. Each profession might be categorized as defending the status quo, and therefore entails little risk (*defender professions*), or as looking for new and different opportunities with greater risk (*prospector professions*). White and Begun view the more entrepreneurial professions as more diversified in terms of processes and services delivered. The accrediting bodies of such entrepreneurial professions encourage educational innovation that might extend to nontraditional careers. Each of the health professions has, to greater or lesser extents, defender and prospector aspects.

Workforce Diversity

Each of the health professions must continue to monitor and encourage diversity in its membership because the demographic shifts that the United States is going through will have an impact on this nation's workforce composition in the coming decades. Although workforce diversity is a broad concept, it focuses on our differences in gender, age, and race; these aspects not only reflect the population that healthcare serves but also the people who provide the services. Some professions are dominated by one gender or the other, which is illustrated by the predominantly female field of nursing or the historically predominantly male field of health administration. The health administration profession, however, has made strides during the past decade as more females have entered the field. Labor shortages and employee turnovers are a common occurrence in the health professions, so the health professions must be cognizant of these trends so they can help balance those exiting with new entrants.

Changes in the ethnic and racial composition of the workforce are proportional to the changes in the size and age of the population (D'Aunno, Alexander, and Laughlin 1996). Because many healthcare professionals are racial/ethnic minorities, a concerted effort needs to be made to recruit and retain them because the diversity of the members of a profession should reflect the diversity of the members of the population.

Conclusion

Healthcare professionals are a large segment of the U.S. labor force. Historically, the development of healthcare professionals are related to the following trends:

- supply and demand;
- increasing use of technology;
- changes in disease and illness; and
- the impact of health services financing and delivery.

Nurses make up the largest sector of healthcare professionals, and the profession comprises various educational pathways and specialties. Pharmacists, allied health professionals, and healthcare administrators also make up diverse and specialized professional groups that play important roles in the U.S. healthcare system. The different levels of education, scopes of practice, and practice settings contribute to the complexity of this sector of the industry. The coming decades will be characterized by some reforms among the health professions because of increasing pressures to finance and deliver health services with higher-quality, lower-cost, and measurable outcomes.

Discussion Questions

1. Describe the process of professionalization. What is the difference between a profession and an occupation?
2. Describe the major types of healthcare professionals (excluding physicians and dentists) and their roles, training, licensure requirements, and practice settings.
3. Describe and apply the issues for human resources management and systems development to healthcare professionals.
4. How has managed care affected the health professions?
5. Who are nonphysician practitioners that provide primary care? What is their role in the delivery of health services?

Note

1. Begun and White (1999) characterize the nursing profession as a complex adaptive system of practitioners, professional associations, and educational institutions that interact with each other and are united by their common pursuit of the goals of the profession. The deeply held "dominant logic" or mindset of the nursing profession impairs the profession in times that it requires adaptation. Elements of the dominant logic of nursing include the ideology of professionalism, an emphasis on "caring," and a belief in oppressed status. With tenets of complex adaptive systems theory, Begun and White recommend application of nonlinear concepts for changing the dominant logic of nursing. Thus, new proficiencies, marketplace savvy, and attention to cost effectiveness of nursing services will emerge as nursing reshapes itself. This new way of looking at a health profession is helpful in conceptualizing new ways to adapt to and shape the environment of health services delivery.

References

Aiken, L. H., J. Sochalski, and G. F. Anderson. 1996. "Downsizing the Hospital Nursing Workforce." *Health Affairs* 15 (4): 88–92.

American Association of Colleges of Nursing (AACN). 2001. "Nursing School Enrollments Continue to Post Decline Though at Slower Rate." News Release. Washington, DC: AACN.

Begun, J. W., and K. R. White. 1999. "The Profession of Nursing as a Complex Adaptive System: Strategies for Change." In *Research in the Sociology of Health Care*. Greenwich, CT: JAI Press.

Berger, K. J., and M. B. Williams. 1999. "Nurses and Professional Nursing." *Fundamentals of Nursing, Second Edition*. Stamford, CT: Appleton and Lange.

Buerhaus, P. I., and D. O. Staiger. 1999. "Trouble in the Nurse Labor Market? Recent Trends and Future Outlook." *Health Affairs* 18 (1): 214–22.

Bureau of Labor Statistics. 2000. *Statistical Abstracts of the United States.* Washington, DC: U.S. Government Printing Office.

———. 2001. [Online information; retrieved 7/30/01]. http://stats.bls.gov/oes. 1999.

D'Aunno, T., J. A. Alexander, and C. Laughlin. 1996. "Business as Usual? Changes in Health Care's Workforce and Organization of Work." *Hospital & Health Services Administration* 41 (1): 3–18.

Dreyfus, H. L., and S. E. Dreyfus. 1996. "The Relationship of Theory and Practice in the Acquisition of Skill." In *Expertise in Nursing Practice: Caring, Clinical Judgment, and Ethics*, edited by P. Benner, C. A. Tanner, and C. A. Chesla. New York: Springer.

Eisenberg, D. M., R. D. Kessler, C. Foster, R. E. Norlock, D. R. Calkins, and T. L. Delbanco. 1993. "Unconventional Medicine in the United States." *New England Journal of Medicine 328* (24): 246–52.

Health Professions Education Extension Amendments of 1992, Section 701 PHS Act. Washington, DC: Government Printing Office.

Hickey, J. V., R. M. Ouimette, and S. L. Venegoni. 1996. *Advanced Practice Nursing: Changing Roles and Clinical Applications.* Philadelphia, PA: Lippincott.

Hurley, R. E. 1997. "Moving Beyond Incremental Thinking." *Health Services Research 32* (5): 679–90.

Jones, C. B. 2001. "The Future Registered Nurse Workforce in Healthcare Delivery." In *The Nursing Profession*, edited by N. L. Chaska, pp. 123–38. Thousand Oaks, CA: Sage.

Mick, S. S. 1999. "Health Care Professionals." In *Introduction to Health Services, Fifth Edition*, edited by S. J. Williams and P. R. Torrens. Albany, NY: Delmar.

National Commission on Allied Health. 1995. *Report of the National Commission on Allied Health.* Rockville, MD: Health Resources and Services Administration.

National Council of State Boards of Nursing. 2000. [Online information; retrieved 7/00]. www.ncsbn.org.

National League for Nursing. 2000. [Online information; retrieved 7/7/00]. www.nln.org.

O'Neil, E. H., and D. M. Hare (eds.). 1990. "Perspectives on the Health Professions." In *Pew Health Professions Programs*. Durham, NC: Duke University.

Shi, L., and D. A. Singh. 1998. *Delivering Health Care in America*. Gaithersburg, MD: Aspen.

Weber, D. O. 1996. "The Mainstreaming of Alternative Medicine." *Healthcare Forum Journal 39* (6): 16–27.

White, K. R., and J. W. Begun. 1998. "Nursing Entrepreneurship in an Era of Chaos and Complexity." *Nursing Administration Quarterly* 22 (2): 40–7.

CHAPTER 3

EMERGING ROLES FOR PHYSICIANS

Eric S. Williams, Ph.D., and Andrew Osucha, M.B.A.

Learning Objectives

After completing this chapter, the reader should be able to:

- Describe the variety of roles assumed by physicians and the forces associated with the emergence of these roles
- Discuss the human resources implications of new physician roles
- Appreciate the importance of physicians in aligning human resources strategy with organizational strategy
- Describe the importance of involving physicians in a variety of organizational change efforts

Introduction

At present, our healthcare system consists of a variety of actors and organizations embedded in a complex structure of tenuous, evolving relationships that sometimes defy understanding. Physicians are responding to these changes in a myriad of ways, including further management education through MHA or MBA degree programs and physician unionization. However, making sense of changes in the healthcare environment and the effects of such changes on healthcare professionals can be challenging. In this chapter, the adaptive process is examined through a framework of emerging physician roles. By expanding on the development of these roles within the context of an evolving healthcare system and Ulrich's (1997) four-part conceptualization of human resources management, we explore the implications of these adaptations and new roles.

In this chapter, we describe seven emerging roles of physicians and the human resources implications of these roles, discuss issues in managing physicians according to four key human resources management roles, and analyze the role of physicians in a variety of organizational change efforts.

Seven New Roles for Physicians

The role of the physician has clearly become more complex and has expanded to include a variety of new functions. As shown in Figure 3.1, seven physician roles have emerged in the wake of changes in the healthcare system. In this section, we summarize the key characteristics of these roles.

Coordinator of Services

The physician as coordinator of services across the continuum of care is rooted in what may be considered the traditional physician-patient relationship. A longstanding truism is that the most effective medical care is delivered in the context of a one-on-one relationship developed over time and sustained by mutual interest in the health of the patient. For primary care physicians (PCPs), this approach now involves more than just treating episodes of illness for individual patients; its focus now is on maintaining the health of a patient population. For younger patients, this approach may be limited to yearly physicals followed by appropriate preventive education and treatment. For older patients, particularly those with multiple chronic medical conditions, this approach may entail relatively frequent provider contact and more opportunity for intervention prior to costly medical crises. The fundamental change is that the individualized approach of the PCP has expanded to encompass patient populations.

Support for a population perspective may be facilitated through clinical pathways that extend beyond the clinical realm to encompass preventive care. Such pathways (e.g., guidelines, protocols, etc.) can be used as decision support devices and may eliminate expensive episodic care in favor of more cost-effective integrated care. Some elements of this approach are evidenced in various disease management programs.

Another aspect of the physician role as coordinator of care is the use of outcomes data rather than bureaucratic administrative controls to ensure physician accountability and performance. Outcomes such as patient satisfaction, immunization rates, Caesarian-section rates, and medical complication

FIGURE 3.1

Seven Emerging Roles for Physicians

1. Coordinator of services
2. Team player/manager
3. Businessperson
4. Community contributor
5. Technological sophisticate
6. Peer evaluator
7. Physician executive

rates might be used to measure performance. In addition, and perhaps more importantly, outcomes data may enable physicians and managers to improve the process of care.

The chief human resources implication of physicians as coordinators of care is the necessity that they work effectively with patients, other providers, and institutions to manage patient care within and across an integrated health system. Managing across the continuum requires physicians to have substantial interpersonal and organizational skills in addition to clinical acumen.

Team Player/Manager

The team player/manager role requires physicians to move from their traditional role as dominant players in healthcare to one in which they provide direction for the healthcare team. The rise of managed care, demands of other clinical professionals to have their perspectives included in clinical decision making, the increasing complexity of healthcare, and the need for increased coordination and integration across the system have all contributed to the decline of physician dominance (Starr 1982). In the current environment, the team player/manager role is more appropriate than a role in which the physician unilaterally makes clinical decisions. Physicians still retain great autonomy and authority, but viewing them as team players encourages them to draw on the expertise of other professionals.

As with the physician coordinator of services, team player physicians must work very closely with other members of the healthcare team. Such a role calls for a variety of skills beyond those found in the traditional clinical repertoire, including general management, conflict resolution, stress management, and political dexterity. Most importantly, physicians must develop the ability to help navigate the bureaucratic maze of healthcare.

Businessperson

Increasing enrollment of physicians in MHA and MBA programs provides evidence for the third emerging role of physicians: businessperson. This role does not necessarily require an advanced degree, but it does require physicians to become knowledgeable about the business of healthcare. At a minimum, physicians should understand:

- how strategy and policy are developed;
- how different types of healthcare financing options create incentives for providers;
- how to inspire, motivate, and gain commitment of associates;
- the impact of different organizational arrangements on the delivery of care; and
- the implications of organizing around clinical processes and the tools for process improvement.

Physicians thus trained are able to take a wider view of healthcare and to communicate effectively with managers. Further, this training may assist physicians in resolving the tension between clinical and business perspectives and help them to forge a new medical professionalism.

Community Contributor

The role of community contributor, as defined by Pathman and his colleagues (1998), involves the conceptualization of four aspects of community involvement for physicians:

1. Recognizing social and cultural issues in patient care
2. Coordinating community health resources in the care of patients
3. Identifying and intervening in community health problems
4. Participating as a leader in the community

The first aspect requires physicians to adapt their styles to better accommodate patient needs, paying particular attention to cultural, financial, and educational factors that affect health. The second and third aspects support the physician coordinator of services role because emphasis is placed on the value of preventive care and extension of care coordination across traditional clinical boundaries and into the community. The final aspect highlights the traditional role that many physicians have already assumed by serving on local health boards, participating in community activities, and working within their religious institutions. In total, the function of community collaborator stresses the importance of provider participation in community life.

Technological Sophisticate

Physicians are increasingly faced with the need to understand and process a vast amount of clinical and nonclinical information and to be familiar with a variety of new technological applications. This demand suggests a fifth role for physicians: technological sophisticate. Physicians must understand that innovations, such as computerized medical records, telemedicine, and digital medical imaging, are revolutionizing medical practice just as they are changing other aspects of life. The day is fast approaching when each physician may carry a personal data assistant that allows two-way teleconferencing, virtual viewing of medical images and electronic charts, Internet access to Medline and clinical databases, and e-mail. Additionally, all of these features will be available from virtually any place in the world.

Such advances can help physicians to work smarter, but only if they acquire basic technological skills. Like many members of the general population, many physicians have desktop systems that do not fulfill their potential utility because users lack technical knowledge. However, worklife may be fundamentally altered for those physicians willing to gain the necessary knowledge to become a part of the connected world and embrace the role of technological sophisticate.

Peer Evaluator

Traditionally physicians have self-governed through licensure, credentialing, board certification, and other means. More recently, government, managed care, and payers have taken an activist role in monitoring physician performance. Given the increasing availability of good outcomes-based measurement practices and information systems to support them, physicians may be able to reassert some of their traditional role in self-governance.

The role of peer evaluator suggests a partnership between physicians and others involved in measuring and improving physician performance. Admittedly, persistent low performance—poor patient satisfaction or bad clinical outcomes—should result in corrective action, but the real added value to physicians is the focus on improvement of both the physician through peer review and of the system through process improvement techniques (e.g., TQM, CQI, reengineering). Achieving these improvements requires physicians, through their businessperson role, to understand and apply process-improvement techniques for individual (peer) and system (clinical process) levels. In this way, physicians can reassert professional self-control and help improve system performance.

Physician Executive

The final role is a logical conglomeration of other roles, which results in the role of physician executive. The physician executive can be defined as a provider who has taken on major managerial responsibilities while maintaining a clinical identity; this can be quite challenging. Physician executives may be viewed as traitors by their colleagues and as "johnny-come-latelys" by nonphysician managers. However, the physician executive role may be of great value to an organization because such an individual can provide leadership that spans both arenas. The necessary skills are an amalgam of those embodied within the other physician roles, in addition to general management and executive leadership skill sets.

The first skill set, general management, comprises a broad range of business competencies. Essentially, the physician executive must have a sufficiently broad business sense to oversee operations, finance, accounting, marketing, and legal concerns. The second skill set involves executive leadership. As leaders of healthcare organizations, physician executives are responsible to a broad range of stakeholders. Effective leadership requires them to manage the often-conflicting requirements of diverse stakeholders, and it also involves developing and communicating a compelling vision for the organization and executing a strategy to move the organization toward its goals. This skill set is perhaps the most challenging of all the skills required in the seven emerging roles.

Developing these skill sets requires more than simple participation in continuing education courses. While physician executives must learn that they may need to seek advice and guidance from other professionals (e.g., attorneys, accountants), the physician executive of tomorrow will need to have some formal training in management.

Human Resources Implications of Emerging Roles for Physicians

In the book, *Human Resources Champions*, Ulrich (1997) proposes a four-part framework for conceptualizing the role of human resources management in organizations. His basic premise is that the human resources function extends far beyond the traditional operational HR role to include strategically managing human resources, overseeing the infrastructure of the organization, advocating for employees, and guiding change processes. In summary, these four roles are:

1. Strategic management of human resources
2. Management of the firm infrastructure
3. Management of employee contribution
4. Management of transformation and change

We apply this framework to the unique position of physicians in healthcare organizations and discuss how these four HR roles can be applied to the complex task of managing physicians as human resources.

Strategic Management of Human Resources

The strategic management of human resources reflects the notion that, like finance or manufacturing, human resources management must be part of the strategic thinking of any organization. Human resources strategies should support overall organizational strategy. This requires management to be knowledgeable about organizational strengths and weaknesses and the external environment and to develop a HR strategy that helps the organization achieve its goals. Ulrich suggests a thorough organizational diagnosis as the first step in this process.

For physicians, such a diagnosis begins with several basic observations. First, the competitive advantage of most healthcare organizations is rooted in the competency, commitment, and quality of its physicians. Second, cost control must begin with an examination of physician practice patterns because physicians are responsible for up to 80 percent of healthcare spending. Third, despite reduced autonomy, physicians remain the leader of the healthcare team; therefore, any organizational changes must involve physicians in planning and implementation.

The final observation is important to remember because any organizational assessment designed to promote the alignment of HR practices with business strategy must closely attend to the single most important source of human capital: the physician. Physicians must be assessed on four elements:

1. Attitudes and issues
2. Level of integration
3. Capabilities
4. Value added activities

Attitudinal assessments are typically confined to occasional employee surveys with standard questions on such topics as job satisfaction and communication. For strategic alignment purposes, assessing physician attitudes requires a more detailed treatment with specially designed survey instruments (Williams et al. 1999) that evaluate job satisfaction, job stress, organizational commitment, perceptions of physical health, and burnout. While this type of information is usually treated in a confidential manner, this information might also provide intervention opportunities for physicians who, for example, may be experiencing high levels of stress or burnout. Such an assessment instrument may be used in conjunction with a human resources information system that can track physician attitudes over time.

Physician Attitudes and Issues

The level of physician integration with the healthcare organization is to a large extent dependent on relationships of individual physicians and the organization (Shortell, Gillies, and Anderson 2000). The level of integration is highest if the physician is employed by the organization (e.g., a hospital-owned primary care practice) or is the owner (e.g., a partner in a multispecialty group practice). Contractual relationships are often associated with a lower level of integration. Contracts may be with groups of physicians in an independent practice association (IPA) or with individual physician practices.

Level of Physician-Organization Integration

Understanding the structure of the physician-organization relationship is merely one stage in a more detailed assessment of integration, which includes assessment of incentive alignment and physician participation in organizational life. The alignment of incentives begins with the identification of incentives facing the physician and the organization. The incentives of the organization can be determined by tax status (for-profit versus not-for-profit); mission, vision, and values of the organization; and the business orientation of the leadership. Such an assessment is broader than an assessment based on strictly financial grounds and affords a deeper understanding of the organizational incentive structure. This type of assessment may suggest additional policy options to better align incentives.

The assessment of physicians' incentives is much the same as it is for an organization. In assessing the organization's incentives, consideration should be given to values, business orientation, and motivations. Compensation arrangements—capitation, fee for service, and various hybrids—are a powerful way to align incentives because the payment methods may be used to modify physician practice patterns in ways that benefit both them and the organization. This is an absolutely essential element for incentive alignment, but motivation can also come from other sources such as training.

Physician-organization integration can also be assessed by the level of physician participation in organizational life. Physician participation in committees and task forces helps to create integration, but physicians, who are also culturally trained to be leaders, should be included in senior decisionmaking and policymaking bodies as well. Indeed, physicians and managers should be natural allies given that neither can effectively execute the core mission of healthcare organizations without participation of the other.

Physician Capability

Another area of assessment addresses the basic competency of an organization's physicians. The credentialing process is commonly used by healthcare organizations that contract with or employ physicians. In the credentialing process, the training and skills of the physician, along with any malpractice or licensure actions against him or her, are evaluated. However, the assessment of physician capability should also include an assessment of the ability of the organization to continually upgrade the capabilities and skills of its clinical staff through training and continuous medical education opportunities. This assessment is critical if the organization is to flexibly respond to the rapidly evolving medical marketplace.

Value-Added Activities

The final part of the organizational assessment focuses on examining value-added and non-value-added activities that physicians perform. Often, such an assessment is carried out as part of a continuous quality improvement (CQI) or reengineering effort. The knowledge of how physicians, nurses, administrators, and staff view non-value-added activities is sufficient for a simple assessment, and such information can be obtained through surveys and interviews with physicians. This assessment may determine the general level of value-added and non-value-added activities and may set the stage for quality-improvement efforts.

Management of Firm Infrastructure

Management of the firm infrastructure refers to the following traditional human resources roles:

- Recruitment and selection
- Performance appraisal
- Compensation
- Training/development
- Labor relations

Recruitment and Selection

Effective recruitment and selection of physicians is an increasingly important source of competitive advantage for healthcare organizations; however, recruitment is a costly endeavor. One study estimated that the cost of replacing a PCP ranged from $236,383 for a family practitioner to $264,345 for a general pediatrician (Buchbinder et al. 1999). Many intangible costs are associated with physician recruitment and selection, including increased staff workload, disrupted continuity of care, and greater stress. The costs of poor selection are even greater, so making the right hiring decision is critical.

The emergence of new and expanded selection criteria (see Figure 3.2) and improvements in recruitment and selection should also be considered. New criteria put a premium on recruiting and selecting physicians who are able to work with the organization. Accordingly, successful candidates must be well versed in both clinical and nonclinical matters and should:

- understand the business of healthcare while delivering quality care;
- be able to serve patients as knowledgeable navigators of the healthcare system;
- be able to improve the performance of themselves, their peers, and the healthcare system in general;
- be able to use the technical tools found in an increasingly networked world.

These new criteria can also be used to further improve the recruitment and selection process. In the years prior to the rise of managed care, the relative shortage of physicians made heavily recruiting physicians imperative for the healthcare organization. In those days, selection or credentialing was chiefly a bureaucratic exercise that involves record checking. Since the advent of managed care, however, this process has evolved to include quality and financial concerns. Our seven roles would add another dimension—one that includes the ability to successfully operate within the system. Interviews and background checks are insufficient in an increasingly competitive healthcare marketplace; organizational success depends on selecting physicians who will be able to deliver high-quality and cost-effective care.

Performance Appraisal

Performance appraisal is not typically carried out for physicians, except in activities associated with physician credentialing and recredentialing. Because these processes now include quality and economic concerns, the stakes are rising.

✓ Ability to coordinate across the total continuum of care

✓ Ability to work effectively with other members of the healthcare team

✓ Conversant in the business of healthcare

✓ Ability to create value for the community via own contributions

✓ Ability to use information technology in everyday work

✓ Ability to use performance information to improve the performance of self and the organization

✓ Ability to act as a physician leader

FIGURE 3.2
Selection, Recruitment, and Performance-Appraisal Criteria for Physicians (Developed from the Seven Emerging Physician Roles)

The selection criteria listed in Figure 3.2 can be applied to performance appraisal or credentialing, but other factors should also be considered when developing a performance appraisal system amid expanding physician roles. As healthcare systems become more intertwined, and performance occurs at multiple points within the healthcare system, performance information must be obtained from multiple sources, which will require a different style of recredentialing by healthcare systems and physician group practices. These sources of information may include physicians, their peers, and managers and would resemble a 360-degree performance appraisal system. Health plans may continue to perform recredentialing independently but may find partnering with their contracted healthcare organizations more efficient.

In addition to recredentialing by multiple stakeholders in the system, such activities might be performed within a CQI context. In his writings on quality improvement, Deming (1982) called for "fear to be driven out" of the organization. Similarly, the anxiety caused by review of physicians' performance might be replaced with an emphasis on performance improvement. In this context, appraisal would focus largely on current performance according to multiple indicators, addressing concerns and recognizing strengths.

This type of appraisal system could be developed from a currently operating recredentialing system. Modifications might include expanded evaluation criteria and broader stakeholder participation. Because this appraisal system would be based on the CQI approach, it might be administered under the auspices of the medical staff in conjunction with the CQI function. Regardless of the structure, an appropriate information system is essential. Information must be made available from multiple points within the healthcare system and enable the recredentialing body to make informed decisions.

Compensation

Compensation is one of the chief mechanisms used to align physician incentives with those of the organization. In a fee-for-service (FFS) system, the basic incentive is to provide more services. Under a capitated system, the incentive is to deliver the least amount of services to achieve a quality outcome. In practice, this incentive entails providing care in the most efficient manner. Most compensation systems, however, are ambiguous in the incentives created. Numerous subcategories (e.g., discounted FFS, global capitation), and combinations of these categories (e.g., capitated primary care physicians and FFS specialists), present challenges to individuals concerned with alignment of incentives.

The emerging physician roles presented in this chapter are most compatible with a fully capitated system. Incentive exists for independent action under a FFS system because individual services are paid for without regard to continuity and quality. In contrast, a system of capitation encourages cooperative action among providers in healthcare organizations because the entire organization is at risk and providers must work together to manage care and profit from their risk. Under capitation, the incentive is to minimize healthcare expenditures across the system, at acceptable levels of care quality, to maximize returns for the physician and healthcare organization. The physician as care coordinator and team manager can help to reduce inappropriate service use. Considerable incentive also exists for physicians in the role of peer evaluator to participate in CQI activities under a capitated system, while little incentive exists under FFS. Successful health services integration requires a capitated system and some sense of risk sharing on the part of physicians.

As health systems move toward greater integration across multiple units, more integration of training and professional development programs for physicians with those for other healthcare professionals is only logical. The restructuring of medical education, along with nursing, allied health, and health administration education, into an integrated health sciences school is an idea that requires further attention. The core of this integration effort could be a common curriculum shared by students from all healthcare disciplines, and it might feature multidisciplinary problem-based learning (Frankfort, Patterson, and Konrad 2000). This integration might facilitate the development of physicians as coordinators of care and team players. After completion of this shared curriculum, students could continue with more specialized education in medicine, nursing, allied health, and health administration. The value of this approach is that such training develops healthcare professionals whose education and skills mirror the needs of an integrated healthcare system.

Training and Development

Continuing medical education (CME) and internal training programs might also be used to support emerging physician roles. Much of the training for the seven new physician roles may be developed and offered for CME credit. However, this could only occur with the active participation of the American Medical Association (AMA) and other medical societies. Fortunately, an infrastructure is currently in place to help physicians develop skills in the seven emerging roles; many medical associations already offer programs in various management topics.

Until recently, the notion of physician unionization had only received peripheral attention. However, the idea entered mainstream consciousness on June 23, 1999 when, prompted by an increased sense of frustration and futility with managed care, the AMA House of Delegates rejected the advice of its leadership and voted to form a national labor organization to represent employed physicians and qualifying residents.

Labor Relations

Physicians who turn to unions for support typically feel they are not being treated fairly by the healthcare organizations for which they work. Managers must strive to create organizations that are supportive of physician autonomy and satisfaction to the highest degree possible under managed care. Such organizations might buffer physicians by using creative contracting or support personnel, or they might provide sufficient training and staff support so that physicians can better navigate the business of healthcare.

Management of Employee Contribution

According to Ulrich, management of employee contribution boils down to being an employee advocate, which requires at least three major activities:

1. understanding physicians as professionals;
2. building physician capacity for dealing with the changing demands of professional practice; and
3. building organizational structures and practices supportive of physicians.

Understanding physicians requires knowledge of the history of the medical profession, socialization, and professional values. The history of medicine is ancient, reaching far back into antiquity. The works of Starr (1982) and Freidson (1970) are helpful in understanding how medicine defines itself as a profession and how its members are socialized. More recent works might provide insight into how the profession is redefining itself in response to changes in healthcare markets (Irvine 1997; Relman 1997; Wynia et al. 1999).

The interaction between professional and business values among physicians is also important to understand; this interaction is often referred to as the concept of double agency (Angell 1993) and is manifested in the tension between cost and quality. Castellani and Wear (2000) further elaborate on double agency as "(a) the struggle to negotiate the cultural class between medicine and managed care, (b) the struggle to find a counterbalance to decentralization and its attack on medicine's power and ethics, and (c) the struggle to create new concepts of professionalism sufficient to overcome medicine's current narrative dysfunction." Reconciling professional and business values is extremely important because its practical manifestations envelop the day-to-day activities of physicians and managers. The manager as physician advocate can make a real difference through the development of physician and organizational resources to handle the changing healthcare environment.

Physician advocacy also involves building physician capacity for managing the demands of the healthcare marketplace. An advocate must be skilled in the management of stress, time pressure, and dissatisfaction, and an advocate must also help physicians to understand the business of medicine and must promote their development as businesspeople. Physicians should be familiar with the basics of leadership, contracting, health economics, conflict management, communication, strategy, and policy development. The organization must enable and motivate its physicians to acquire such skills.

The other important task of physician advocacy involves building an organization that supports physicians and other professionals. These tasks include articulation of how the interaction between professional values and business goals might be managed by appealing to values held by all healthcare professionals. These values should be manifested in the culture and practices of the organization. Policies that support continuing medical education, work-life balance, and collaboration reinforce the culture and values of the organization.

Perhaps the most important manifestation of this professional-supportive organization lies in the level of control that physicians have over clinical and administrative practices. Physicians should be relatively unencumbered when making the best decisions for the care of their patients. An organization should strive to negotiate contracts that permit this level of autonomy. Further, adequate resources, both human and material, should be available to assist physicians in coping with the administrative burdens of managed care; this level of support, however, does not come without caveats. Physicians must accept some level of oversight and understand demands for efficiency and quality. As Irvine (1997) suggests, one model of oversight includes personal oversight through use of clinical protocols and evidence-based medicine, peer oversight through local bodies, and external review through the use of stakeholder-based coalitions. An organization can support this oversight through the assumption of the utilization review process, as some physician groups have already done (Kerr et al. 2000).

Management of Transformation and Change

Among the HR functions identified by Ulrich, management of transformation and change is perhaps the most critical given the current state of healthcare. Managers are charged with helping the organization and its employees adapt to the changing environment—a task which calls for vision, decisiveness, good humor, and a steady hand. Ulrich identifies three types of change:

1. Initiative
2. Process
3. Cultural

Initiative change involves implementation of new programs, projects, or procedures. Process change refers to changes in the way work is done. Cultural change involves a reconceptualization of how business is done. Ulrich argues that managers as change agents must build organizational capacity to deal with these three types of change.

Initiative and Process Changes

Any initiative or process change in an organization affects physicians. However, for many reasons, physicians are not involved, or insufficiently involved, in planning process change. Consequently, change efforts are sometimes hampered, slowed, or implemented with inadequate attention to their impact on physicians. Ulrich identifies seven key success steps that may be applied to physician participation in initiative and process changes (see Figure 3.3).

The first step is leading change, and is typically assigned to the one who "owns" and heeds the call for initiative or process change. For projects that involve substantial clinical change, physician participation is essential and a

FIGURE 3.3

Seven Steps for
Managing
Initiative or
Process Change

1. Leading change
2. Creating a shared need
3. Shaping a vision
4. Motivating key stakeholders to embrace change
5. Changing system and structures to support change
6. Monitoring the change
7. Making change last

Source: Ulrich, D. 1997. *Human Resource Champions: The Next Agenda for Adding Value and Delivering Results.* Boston: Harvard Business School Press.

physician champion is essential. The physician champion must be able to influence colleagues, sell the change effort, and work with colleagues to lay the political groundwork for change.

The second step is creating a shared need for change. This factor is a particular challenge among physicians because of the diversity of interests among physicians. Issues might be uncovered in an organizational assessment and then evaluated with an eye toward identifying those issues that reflect the greatest level of shared need among physicians. Broad and intense needs will be those mostly likely to obtain a level of support necessary for effective change.

After identifying change leadership and shared needs, *the third step is shaping a vision.* The physician champion usually will be responsible for leading a discourse aimed at formulating this shared vision. However, the fourth success factor must be in place for this discussion to take place: *The physician champion must identify, involve, and motivate key stakeholders to commit to the initiative or process change.* This fourth step is largely synonymous with laying the political groundwork after a shared need is identified. The physician champion and others involved in initiative or process change must obtain the support of relevant stakeholder groups such as other physicians, nurses, patients, governmental bodies, and other healthcare organizations. After the groundwork has been laid, the vision can be articulated.

The fifth step is changing the system and structures. This step is where managers ensure that the initiative or process change becomes part of the organization's structure and systems, and this step may be the most challenging change factor because it demands change not only in the initiative or process but in the personnel and processes that support the change. If an organization has developed the flexibility to change, this transition will be smoother; if the organization lacks such flexibility, then this task may be particularly difficult.

The sixth step is monitoring the process. As the PDCA (Plan-Do-Check-Act) process suggests, monitoring how process change is occurring is important. The establishment of reliable and valid measures using industry or organizational benchmarks will ensure that the progress of the change can be monitored. The continuing attention of the physician champion and key stakeholders is also necessary for successful implementation of change. Maintenance of motivation can be ensured through the periodic reassessment of progress.

The seventh step is making change sustainable. When change is successful, declaring victory and moving on become a natural inclination. However, unless necessary systems are in place to support the change and the physician champion and key stakeholders continue to monitor it, slippage may occur.

The third type of change is cultural. Ulrich (1997) describes a five-step method of promoting cultural change (see Figure 3.4). Although physicians are an important part of healthcare organizations, true cultural change—a rearticulation of how business is done—involves every person in the organization. Thus, physicians should be involved and can provide leadership, but the concerned audience is far broader than the audience for a typical initiative or process change.

The first two steps involve defining and clarifying the concept of cultural change and articulating the necessity of cultural change; these two steps constitute the groundwork for cultural change. For physicians and most other employees in healthcare organizations, organizational culture is an amorphous phenomenon that is not well understood. The manager's job is to foster this understanding. Physicians must understand the interaction among professional values, practices, and culture on one hand and situational or practice characteristics on the other. When these forces complement each other, the organizational culture can be positive and supportive of physicians and nonphysicians alike; when these forces conflict, however, the organizational culture can be negative and corrosive. Understanding these forces and their interplay may better equip physicians to play important roles in this process.

Cultural Change

1. Define and clarify the concept of cultural change
2. Articulate why cultural change is important to organizational success
3. Assess the current organizational culture
4. Identify different approaches to creating cultural change
5. Develop an action plan for this change

FIGURE 3.4
Five Steps for Managing Cultural Change

Source: Ulrich, D. 1997. *Human Resource Champions: The Next Agenda for Adding Value and Delivering Results.* Boston: Harvard Business School Press.

Once the groundwork is laid, the third, fourth, and fifth steps of cultural change may be undertaken. *The third step is assessing the organizational culture, developing the vision of a future culture, and understanding the gap between the two.* Physicians can bring substantial clinical and operational insight to this assessment because (1) they bring a unique view of the broader practice of medicine as well as a perspective on how physicians respond to the current culture and (2) they understand the great value of best practices. Therefore, enlisting physicians in this assessment effort is important.

The fourth and fifth steps involve identifying different approaches to creating cultural change and developing an action plan. These steps are the most critical steps for physicians because if they do not understand, believe, or have input in this process, cultural change will be unsuccessful. Thus, their opinions and involvement must be actively solicited as they assume their newly emerging roles in the continually evolving world of healthcare.

Conclusion

In this chapter, we have presented seven roles that seem to be developing as physicians adapt to the changing healthcare environment. This list is not exhaustive and each role is obviously not mutually exclusive from the others; however, it does help to frame current developments among healthcare providers, along with the concomitant human resources implications.

Discussion Questions

1. An increasing proportion of physicians are becoming employees of organizations or are otherwise more tightly linked to the organization than in the past. How does this change the way in which a physician practices?
2. Much of the discussion about physician resistance to change is based on the training and socialization of physicians in previous generations. Given that younger physicians are being socialized in the managed care era, how likely will this traditional resistance pass?
3. Given the growing importance of outcomes in healthcare, do you see any problems associated with evaluating individual physicians' performance on the basis of their patients' health outcomes? How would you overcome these problems?
4. What are the strengths and weaknesses associated with having a physician executive as CEO versus a nonphysician trained in healthcare management?
5. Given the changing nature of physicians' work and the roles assumed by physicians, what advice would you give to a high school student who is considering medicine as a career?

References

Angell, M. 1993. "The Doctor as Double Agent." *Kennedy Institute for Ethics Journal* 3 (3): 279–86.

Buchbinder, S. B., M. Wilson, C. F. Melick, and N. R. Powe. 1999. "Estimates of Costs of Primary Care Physician Turnover." *The American Journal of Managed Care* 5 (11): 1431–8.

Castellani, B., and D. Wear. 2000. "Physician Views of Practicing: Professionalism in the Corporate Age." *Qualitative Health Research* 10 (4): 490–506.

Deming, W. E. 1982. *Out of the Crisis.* Cambridge, MA: The MIT Press.

Frankfort, D. M., M. A. Patterson, and T. R. Konrad. 2000. "Transforming Practice Organizations to Foster Lifelong Learning and Commitment to Medical Professionalism." *Academic Medicine* 75 (7): 708–17.

Freidson, E. 1970. *Professional Dominance: The Social Structure of Medical Care, First Edition.* New York: Atherton Press.

Irvine, D. 1997. "The Performance of Doctors, I: Professionalism and Self Regulation in a Changing World." *British Medical Journal* 314: 1540–2.

Kerr, E. A., B. S. Mittman, R. D. Hays, J. K. Zemencuk, J. Pitts, and R. Brook. 2000. "Associations Between Primary Care Physician Satisfaction and Self-Reported Aspects of Utilization Management." *Health Services Research* 35 (1): 333–49.

Pathman, D. E., B. D. Steiner, E. Williams, and T. Riggins. 1998. "The Four Community Dimensions of Primary Care Practice." *Journal of Family Practice* 46 (4): 293–303.

Relman, A. 1997. "Education to Defend Professional Values in the New Corporate Age." *Academic Medicine* 73 (12): 1229–33.

Shortell, S. M., R. R. Gillies, and D. A. Anderson. 2000. *Remaking Health Care in America: The Evolution of Organized Delivery Systems, Second Edition.* San Francisco: Jossey-Bass.

Starr, P. 1982. *The Social Transformation of American Medicine.* New York: Basic Books.

Ulrich, D. 1997. *Human Resource Champions: The Next Agenda for Adding Value and Delivering Results.* Boston: Harvard Business School Press.

Williams, E. S., T. R. Konrad, M. Linzer, J. McMurray, D. E. Pathman, M. Gerrity, M. D. Schwartz, W. Scheckler, J. Van Kirk, E. Rhodes, and J. Douglas. 1999. "Refining the Measurement of Physician Job Satisfaction: Results from the Physician Worklife Survey." *Medical Care* 37 (11): 1140–54.

Wynia, M. K., S. R. Latham, A. C. Kao, J. W. Berg, and L. L. Emanuel. 1999. "Medical Professionalism in Society." *New England Journal of Medicine* 341 (21): 1612–6.

THE LEGAL ENVIRONMENT

Bruce J. Fried, Ph.D.

Learning Objectives

After completing this chapter, the reader should be able to:

- Understand the impact of legal considerations on all human resources management activities and functions
- Discuss the concept of employment at will and the ways in which this concept has been eroded
- Understand the rationale for government intervention in the workplace to prevent discrimination
- Discuss the key features of major federal equal employment opportunity legislation
- Distinguish between the concepts of disparate impact and disparate treatment and the types of evidence required to demonstrate each form of discrimination
- Discuss key features of the Americans with Disabilities Act, including the concepts of undue hardship and reasonable accommodation
- Discuss sexual harassment as a form of employment discrimination, and describe the legal definitions of sexual harassment law
- Discuss strategies that organizations can use to prevent and identify discrimination in the workplace

Introduction

The healthcare workplace is a highly complex environment with a myriad of laws and regulations that further complicate it. While managers do not necessarily have to be lawyers, managers' awareness of key legal issues is essential because laws and regulations govern so much of the employee-employer relationship. Although managers have discretion in how they manage the workforce, adherence to legal requirements places significant constraints on their autonomy; therefore, managers and supervisors in large healthcare organizations must understand these legal requirements and constraints. While senior management in any organization may understand these legal issues, day-to-day human resources practice is the responsibility of lower-level managers who may not have the same degree of awareness. Attentiveness to legal requirements is important at all managerial levels, given that senior managers and board members are the ones charged liable if a violation occurs at any level of the organization. Compliance to legal requirements is good management practice, which is an even more compelling reason for managers to understand the workplace regulations. Most notably, this theory is true when it comes to equal employment opportunity. While "equal employment opportunity" is often viewed as a regulatory challenge or at worst a quota-based scheme, adherence to its mandated procedures is consistent with sound human resources practices. In the context of an overall skepticism about equal employment opportunity and affirmative action, whether or not companies are retreating from the progress made in recent years is not clear; that is, while much rhetoric persists about the possible obsolescence of affirmative action, companies in general do not appear to have fallen away from their legal and ethical obligations.

That said, noting the ambiguity in the definition and limits of protection of these laws and regulations is important. Virtually every employment-related law has been subject to extensive and far-reaching interpretation by the courts and quasi-judicial administrative agencies such as the National Labor Relations Board and the Equal Employment Opportunity Commission (EEOC). For this reason, employment law cannot be understood by simply reading the text of existing laws. Furthermore, as with all legislation, application of employment law may have unintended consequences, especially if implementation, interpretation, or use of a particular law, for example, is iinconsistent with the original intent of the lawmakers. An example of this inconsistency is evident in the Americans with Disabilities Act (ADA), which is discussed fully later in this chapter. Initially, the ADA was intended to increase the employment potential of individuals with disabilities; today, however, the majority of complaints filed under the ADA deal with on-the-job employee injuries.

This chapter provides an overview of equal employment opportunity requirements implied by current legislation; however, because of the constantly changing legal landscape, presenting the most current court rulings and agency regulations is difficult. This chapter is intended to sensitize the reader to the legal framework that governs the workplace, to communicate to the reader the importance of keeping up with current laws and regulations, and to make the reader understand that equal employment opportunity laws and good management practices are not at all incompatible.

Background and Historical Perspective

The legal environment affects virtually all aspects of human resources management; however, this was not always the case. Traditionally, the employee-employer relationship was guided by the **employment-at-will principle**, which assumes that both employee and employer have the right to sever the work relationship at any time without notice for any reason, no reason, or even a bad or immoral reason (Bouvier 1996; Levine 1994). Within this context, an employee may be terminated for trying to organize a union, for being a member of a particular race/ethnic group, or for refusing to participate in illegal activities. The employment-at-will principle was strengthened by the case *Adair v. United States* (2078 U.S. 161, 1908). While the federal courts today are not likely follow the precedent set in that case, the case does exemplify the concept of employment at will. In that case, Adair (a supervisor for a railroad) fired Coppage because Coppage was a member of a labor union. Adair was convicted of violating an 1898 federal statute that purported to prohibit carriers in interstate commerce from firing or otherwise discriminating against employees on the basis of their membership in a labor union. On appeal, Adair's conviction was overturned because the U.S. Supreme Court held that the federal statute was unconstitutional. Specifically, the court held that Congress violated the Fifth Amendment right to liberty and property by attempting to prohibit Adair from firing Coppage, and the court also held that the federal statute was beyond the authority of Congress under its power to regulate interstate commerce. In the language of the U.S. Supreme Court:

> "In the absence, however, of a valid contract between the parties controlling their conduct towards each other and fixing a period of service, it cannot be, we repeat, that an employer is under any legal obligation, against his will, to retain an employee in his personal service any more than an employee can be compelled, against his will, to remain in the personal service of another" (*Adair v. United States*, 2078 U.S. 161, 1908).

As documented in this chapter, employment at will has been dramatically eroded by a variety of laws and regulations during the twentieth century. Before we begin our review of specific equal employment opportunity legislation, let us address two key concepts—discrimination and workplace regulation.

Employment Discrimination: A Basis for Government Intervention

Much of the employment legislation enacted since 1900 seeks to limit illegal discrimination and promote fair practices in hiring, training, promotions, and other areas. Discrimination is not in and of itself illegal; for example, when an organization hires an individual, it probably discriminates in favor of

Employment at will assumes that both employee and employer have the right to sever the work relationship at any time without notice for any reason, no reason, or even a bad or immoral reason

those applicants who have the best qualifications and most experience for the position. By illegal discrimination, we mean discrimination against a particular individual or group of individuals based on non-job-related characteristics such as race, ethnicity, age, gender, sexual preference, or disability. As this chapter illustrates, a great deal of legislation is aimed at reducing non-job-related discrimination.

The passage of laws that address illegal discrimination is in effect a form of workplace regulation. Whenever any type of regulatory legislation is considered, the question arises whether or not such legislation is in fact required, or this question is asked: Can market forces perform these regulatory functions? According to some economists, illegal discrimination is ineffective and inefficient over the long haul. The organization that hires highly qualified individuals regardless of, for example, race, gender, or age wins over the organization that hires individuals based on its preferred race, gender, or age. What leads organizations to engage in illegal discriminatory practices? Some organizations and individuals have a "taste" for discrimination and may simply not want certain types of individuals in their workplaces. These organizations seem to be willing to pay for their preference with lower profits, diminished quality of service, and decreased market share that accompany the practice of hiring a preferred group (England 1994). Alternatively, employers may discriminate not because of their own tastes but as a result of their customers' or employees' tastes (Bergmann and Darity 1981).

Other employers, whether consciously or unconsciously, employ a more deliberate type of discrimination in their hiring or other employment decisions (England 1994); this practice is called **statistical discrimination.** For example, if an employer believes that newly married women in their early 20s are highly likely to leave work in the near future for family reasons, then the employer will apply this view to all female job applicants who fit this category. This view puts all members of a particular group at a disadvantage.

Statistical discrimination may be based on three distinct frameworks:

Statistical discrimination occurs when the employer makes a calculated decision about a particular individual based on the employer's perception about the larger group to which the individual belongs

1. *Perception about mean group productivity.* The employer may believe that individuals over age 50 tend to be less productive, so the employer may extend that belief to all job applicants over the age of fifty.
2. *Risk avoidance mechanism.* In its effort to avoid risk, the employer hires only individuals whose work performance is stable and predictable. An employer may believe that all young employees are disloyal and move from job to job or that older employees have a better work ethic. As a result, the employer may hire older individuals in lieu of younger job applicants.
3. *Imbalanced perception about the predictability of selection tools.* The employer may rely on selection tools, such as job qualifications, interview procedures, or various kinds of tests, that attempt to identify applicants who have the necessary knowledge, skills, and abilities to perform a

particular job. Unfortunately, some employers believe that these selection tools are more accurate or predictive for certain groups than for others.

As noted earlier, economic theories of discrimination suggest that discrimination sows the seeds of its own destruction and that employers who avoid illegal discrimination benefit. In the long run, nondiscriminatory employers gain a competitive advantage over employers who practice illegal discrimination because they have greater access to the most highly qualified job applicants. Unfortunately, these economic theories of discrimination have not been proven, and available evidence suggests that employers' "taste" for discrimination would continue were it not for government intervention in the labor market. Furthermore, societal beliefs and attitudes that form much of the basis for discriminatory practices do not readily change. Because the political environment has been impatient to wait out the glacial pace of social attitude change, the government entered the labor market arena in the 1960s to reduce discriminatory practices. Since that time, the government has continued its efforts and maintained a fairly consistent trajectory.

Workplace Regulation: The Evolution of Equal Employment Opportunity Legislation

"Equal employment" is defined broadly in the legislation and includes fairness in promotions, compensation and benefits, training opportunities, and other employment activities. To accomplish these aims in fairness, the federal government has utilized constitutional amendments, legislation, executive orders, and court and quasi-judicial bodies. Table 4.1 provides a summary of the major constitutional provisions, laws, and executive orders that support equal employment opportunity; however, this list does not include a number of other federal laws as well as countless state and local ordinances.

Equal employment opportunity refers to governmental attempts to ensure that all individuals have an equal chance at obtaining employment, regardless of their age, race, religion, disability status, or other non-job-related characteristics

The 1960s heralded the beginning of equal employment opportunity legislation; however, much of this legislation is based on constitutional amendments. The Thirteenth Amendment, which outlawed slavery, could be cited as the earliest form of workplace regulation. The Fourteenth Amendment forbade states from taking life, liberty, or property without due process of law and prevented states from denying unequal protection of the laws. This amendment, passed immediately after the Civil War, was originally intended to protect African Americans; it has, however, been used in cases of alleged reverse discrimination such as in the case of *Bakke v. California Board of Regents* (17 FEPC 1000, 1978), in which a Caucasian applicant to medical school alleged that he was not admitted because of a discriminatory quota system. The Supreme Court found in the applicant's favor, stating that the quota system had violated his right to equal protection under the law.

The 1960s was also a period of significant social activism in the United States. Federal legislation was passed that protected civil rights and ensured

TABLE 4.1
Sources of Equal Employment Opportunity Law

Source	Purpose	Covers	Administration
Fifth Amendment, U.S. Constitution	Protects against federal violation of "due process"	All individuals	Federal courts
Thirteenth Amendment, U.S. Constitution	Abolishes slavery	All individuals	Federal courts
Fourteenth Amendment, U.S. Constitution	Provides equal protection for all citizens and requires due process in state action	State actions (decisions or governmental organizations)	Federal courts
Civil Rights Acts of 1866 and 1871	Establishes the rights of all citizens to make and enforce contracts	All individuals	Federal courts
Equal Pay Act of 1963	Requires that men and women who perform equal jobs receive equal pay	Employers engaged in interstate commerce	EEOC and federal courts
Civil Rights Act of 1964 (+Title VII), amended in 1991	Prohibits discrimination on the basis of race, color, religion, sex, or national origin	Employers with 15 or more employees working 20 or more weeks per year, labor unions, and employment agencies	EEOC
Age Discrimination in Employment Act of 1967	Prohibits discrimination in employment against individuals 40 years of age and older	Employers with 15 or more employees working 20 or more weeks per year, labor unions, and employment agencies	EEOC

Law	Description	Coverage	Enforcement
Rehabilitation Act of 1973	Protects individuals with disabilities against discrimination in the public sector and requires affirmative action in the employment of individuals with disabilities	Government agencies and federal contractors and subcontractors with contracts greater than $2,500	Office of Federal Contract Compliance Programs (OFCCP)
Americans with Disabilities Act of 1990	Prohibits discrimination against individuals with disabilities	Employers with more than 15 employees	EEOC
Executive Orders 11246 and 11375	Prohibits discrimination by contractors and subcontractors of federal agencies and requires affirmative action in hiring women and minorities	Federal contractors and subcontractors with contracts greater than $10,000	OFCCP
Family and Medical Leave Act	Requires employers to provide 12 weeks of unpaid leave for family and medical emergencies	Employers with more than 50 employees	Department of Labor

equal opportunity in housing, voting, education, employment, and other areas; the following are the major federal equal employment opportunity laws:

- The Fair Labor Standards Act
- The Equal Pay Act of 1963
- Title VII of the Civil Rights Act of 1964 (which been amended several times, most recently in 1990)
- The Age Discrimination in Employment Act of 1967
- The Americans with Disabilities Act of 1990

Uniform Guidelines on Employee Selection Procedures is a federal document that provides basic guidance on compliance in virtually every human resources function

The basic premise of all equal employment opportunity laws is that employment decisions—including hiring, promotion, compensation and benefits, and training opportunities—should not be based on non-job-related characteristics such as age, gender, race, or disability. Because of the complexity of these laws, the federal government has produced a document, ***Uniform Guidelines on Employee Selection Procedures***, that summarizes and synthesizes the employment-related implications of these laws (*Federal Register* 1978).

The Fair Labor Standards Act and the Equal Pay Act of 1963

The Fair Labor Standards Act (FLSA) governs minimum wage, overtime payments, child labor, and equal pay

The Fair Labor Standards Act (FLSA) was originally passed in 1938 and has been amended many times. The major provisions of the FLSA are minimum wage, overtime payments, child labor, and equal pay; the two latter provisions are the most critical. The FLSA forbids the employment of children between 16 and 18 years of age in hazardous occupations such as mining, logging, woodworking, meatpacking, and certain types of manufacturing, and it severely restricts employment of minors under age 16. Minors aged 14 to 15 may work outside school hours under the following restrictions:

- Work may be allowed no more than 3 hours on a school day, 18 hours in a school week, 8 hours on a non-school-day, or 40 hours in a non-school-week.
- Work may not begin before 7 A.M. nor end after 7 P.M., except between June 1 and Labor Day when work must end at 9 P.M.

The Equal Pay Act of 1963 is an amendment to the FLSA. The act requires equal pay for all men and women who perform equal jobs

The amendment to the FLSA, the **Equal Pay Act of 1963**, requires equal pay for all men and women in the same organization who perform equal jobs. This act outlaws the once common practice of paying women less for doing the same job, which used to be commonly defended on the theory that a married man needed a higher salary to support his family. Sometimes determining what constitutes "equal work" is difficult. The Equal Pay Act specifies that two jobs are equal if they demand the same skill, effort, and responsibility and if they are performed under the same working conditions. If pay differences are the result of differences in seniority, merit, quantity or quality of work, or any other factor other than gender, then differences in compensation are allowable (Greenlaw and Kohl 1995).

Although the Equal Pay Act has been law for over a quarter century, substantial gaps in earnings between men and women still exist. In 1999, the median earning level for women was 72.2 percent of the median for men (median income was $36,476 for men and $26,324 for women). Substantial gains have been made since 1960, when women earned only 60.7 percent of men's earnings; in fact, in 1973, women earned only 56.6 percent of men's earnings. The improvement in women's wages relative to men's has been leveling off: Women's wages have decreased since 1997, when women's wages constituted 74.2 percent of men's wages (The National Committee on Pay Equity 2001).

Some other facts, according to the Business and Professional Women/ USA (2001) and The National Committee on Pay Equity (2001), worth noting about wage discrepancies between men and women include:

- At the current rate of change, the gender gap will not be eliminated until 2038.
- Women are less likely to receive additional compensation in forms other than salary, such as performance bonuses, stock options, and profit sharing.
- In 1999, women held 3.3 percent (77 out of 2,353) of the top-earning positions in *Fortune* 500 companies; while this is still miniscule, it represents a 175 percent increase since 1995.
- In 1998, for workers 20–24 years old, women's earnings were 82 percent of men's; whether this percentage represents a real change or if the wage gap does not set in until later is unclear.

Because of the difficulty in eradicating wage differences between men and women, some jurisdictions have adopted **comparable worth** legislation (Ledvinka and Scarpello 1991). Comparable worth is a concept that calls for equal or comparable pay for jobs that require comparable skills, effort, and responsibility and have comparable working conditions. In the healthcare environment, this concept is particularly salient because of the large concentration of female employees in certain occupations such as nursing. If the work of hospital nurses, for example, is only compared to work of other nurses within the same organization, remedying gender-based wage discrepancies would be difficult. If, however, the wages of nurses are compared to the wages of employees whose contribution or worth is comparable to that of nurses, gender-based wage disparities may be discovered.

Comparable worth calls for equal or comparable pay for jobs that require comparable skills, effort, and responsibility and have comparable working conditions

Title VII of the Civil Rights Act of 1964

Title VII of the Civil Rights Act of 1964 is clearly the most far-reaching and significant of all antidiscrimination statutes. The act prohibits discrimination in a variety of areas, including voting, public accommodations, public facilities, public education, and employment. In employment, the act bars discrimination in hiring, promotion, compensation, training, and benefits. Discrimination is specifically prohibited on the basis of race, color, religion, gender, or national origin.

Title VII of the Civil Rights Act of 1964 prohibits discrimination in a variety of areas, including voting, public accommodations, public facilities, public education, and employment

The Civil Rights Act was not passed without considerable opposition and debate. The major argument against the act was that it violated states' police power rights. An indication of the level of opposition to the act was an effort by some Southern lawmakers to insert into the act a provision that guarantees equal treatment for women (original drafts of the act did not deal with gender discrimination). This strategy was attempted under the assumption that while Northern congressmen and senators could support legislation that deals with discrimination based on race, the men who dominate Congress would never support a law that protects equal opportunity for women. Obviously, this strategy failed and the act was passed.

As amended by the *Equal Employment Opportunity Act of 1972* and the *Civil Rights Act of 1991,* the Civil Rights Act includes a wide range of organizations under its jurisdiction, including:

1. All private employers involved in interstate commerce that employ 15 or more people for 20 or more weeks per year
2. State and local governments
3. Private and public employment agencies
4. Joint labor-management committees that govern apprenticeship or training programs
5. Labor unions that have 15 or more members or employees
6. Public and private educational institutions
7. Foreign subsidiaries of U.S. organizations that employ U.S. citizens

Thus, with few exceptions (i.e., U. S. government-owned corporations, tax-exempt private clubs, religious organizations that employ persons of a specific religion, and organizations that hire Native Americans on or near a reservation), a large majority of employers in the United States are covered by the Civil Rights Act. Section 703a of the Civil Rights Act of 1964, Title VII, states that:

> (a) It shall be an unlawful employment practice for an employer to fail or refuse to hire or to discharge any individual, or otherwise to discriminate against any individual with respect to his compensation, terms, conditions, or privileges of employment, because of such individual's race, color, religion, sex, or national origin; or (2) to limit, segregate, or classify his employees or applicants for employment in any way which would deprive or tend to deprive any individual of employment opportunities or otherwise adversely affect his status as an employee, because of such individual's race, color, religion, sex, or national origin.

The Civil Rights Act is a far-reaching law with strong enforcement provisions, particularly after the 1991 amendments. Prior to 1991, Title VII limited damage claims to equitable relief such as back pay, lost benefits, front pay in some cases, and attorney's fees and costs. The 1991 amendments allow compensatory and punitive damages when intentional or reckless discrimination is proven. Compensatory damages may include future pecuniary loss, emotional pain, suffering, and loss of enjoyment of life. Punitive damages are intended to discourage discrimination by providing for payments to the plaintiff beyond actual damages suffered. Maximum damages are limited by the number of employees in the organization and range from $50,000 to $300,000 (*Employment Law Update* 1991a).

Uniform Guidelines on Employee Selection Procedures

Because of the complexity and changing interpretations of laws, employers are frequently uncertain about the legality of their employment practices. In response to these concerns, the federal government published guidelines to assist employers in the areas of hiring, retention, promotion, transfer, demotion, dismissal, and referral. The *Uniform Guidelines on Employee Selection Procedures* (*Federal Register* 1978) helps employers comply with federal antidiscrimination statutes. The basic guidelines are important to understand because they form the most readily accessible and useful interpretive rules for determining compliance.

The guidelines define the circumstances under which an employee selection procedure may be discriminatory:

> The use of any selection procedure which has an adverse impact on the hiring, promotion, or other employment or membership opportunities or members of any race, sex, or ethnic group will be considered to be discriminatory and inconsistent with these guidelines, unless the procedure has been validated in accordance with these guidelines (or, certain other provisions are satisfied) (*Federal Register* 1978).

This guideline implies that selection tools, such as job qualifications, tests, and interview procedures, must be job related and positively associated with job success. (The guidelines describe different methods of validating a test, and these methods are discussed more fully in Chapter 6.) A selection procedure may be found discriminatory if it measures factors that are unrelated to job success and in turn adversely affects a group or individual. The landmark case in this area was *Griggs v. Duke Power Company* (401 U.S. 424, 1971), in which an employee's request for a promotion was denied because he was not a high school graduate. Griggs, an African American, claimed that this job standard was discriminatory because it did not relate to job success and because the standard had an adverse impact on a protected class; a **protected class** refers to a group of individuals that falls under the protective umbrella of a particular law (e.g., women and minorities). The Supreme Court decided in favor of Griggs and established two important principles:

Protected class refers to a group of individuals (e.g., women and minorities) that is protected under a particular law

1. The court found that employer discrimination need not be overt or intentional to be present and illegal.

2. The court found that employment selection practices must be job related and that employers have the burden of demonstrating that employment requirements are job related or constitute a business necessity.

Disparate impact refers to the significant under-representation of members of the protected class as a result of the organization's employment policies and procedures

The *Griggs v. Duke Power Company* decision affirmed the concept of disparate impact. **Disparate impact** refers to a situation in which members of a protected class are significantly underrepresented because of the organization's employment policies and procedures. Again, the intent of the employer is irrelevant in disparate impact cases; the plaintiff merely has to demonstrate that the protected class is underrepresented because of the employer's policies. The most well-known method of demonstrating disparate impact is through the four-fifths (or 80 percent) rule; the **four-fifths rule** was developed in the *Uniform Guidelines* and has been accepted by the EEOC as a rule for assessing disparate impact cases.[1] The four-fifths rule states that discrimination is generally considered to have occurred if the selection rate for protected group members is less than 80 percent of the selection rate for the majority group. Consider the scenario in Figure 4.1, which illustrates the use of the four-fifths rule in determining disparate impact within an organization. The formula shows that the promotion rate for Hispanic nurses was 25 percent, while the promotion rate for Caucasian nurses was 40 percent. Because 25 percent (the promotion rate for Hispanics) is less than 80 percent of the 40 percent (the promotion rate for Caucasians), the formula concludes that the promotion rates have a disparate impact on Hispanic nurses. This figure, of course, is a simplistic illustration, and courts typically struggle with such disparate impact issues within the time frame required to obtain meaningful data and other factors (*Hazelwood School District v. United States* (433 U.S. 299, 15 FEP 1, 1977).

Four-fifths rule states that discrimination has occurred if the selection rate for protected group members is less than 80 percent of the selection rate for the majority group

FIGURE 4.1
Use of the Four-Fifths Rule in Determining Disparate Impact

Promotion Rate for Caucasian Nurses

Number of Caucasian nurses promoted	=	20
Number of Caucasian nurses applied	=	50
Promotion rate for Caucasian nurses	=	40%

Promotion Rate for Hispanic Nurses

Number of Hispanic nurses promoted	=	9
Number of Hispanic nurses applied	=	36
Promotion rate for Hispanic nurses	=	25%

Ratio of Promotion Rates

Promotion rate for Hispanic nurses	=	25%
Promotion rate for Caucasian nurses	=	40%

Formula: 25% / 40% = 62% (percentage is less than the 80% threshold)

A more common type of discrimination than disparate impact is disparate treatment. **Disparate treatment** exists when individuals in similar employment situations are treated differently because of their race, color, religion, sex, national origin, age, or disability. The most obvious case of disparate treatment is when an employer makes a hiring decision based on one of the above factors. Disparate treatment may also be more subtle, such as asking a female job applicant to demonstrate a particular skill when male applicants are not asked to do the same. The defining case in this area was *McDonnell Douglas Corp. v. Green* (411 U.S. 792, 80, 1973), in which a member of a protected class applied for a job and was rejected, but the company continued to advertise for this position. This case established the four-part guideline for determining disparate treatment:

Disparate treatment is when employees in the same organization are treated differently because of their race, color, religion, sex, national origin, age, or disability

1. The person is a member of a protected class.
2. The person applied for a job and was qualified.
3. The person was rejected for the job.
4. The position remained open to applicants with equal or fewer qualifications.

The most important difference between disparate impact and disparate treatment is that motive is irrelevant in disparate impact cases; in disparate treatment cases, on the other hand, the intent to discriminate must be proven. In a disparate impact case, the plaintiff must make the case that a particular employment practice disproportionately affects a particular group, and whether the employer intended to discriminate is irrelevant; in fact, disparate impact can be proven where employment practices appear quite innocuous. A minimum height requirement, for example, may appear quite neutral. However, height is not distributed equally among sexes and ethnic groups, and if this requirement is not linked to job performance, a disparate impact case can be made. With disparate treatment, discriminatory intent behind the employment procedure must be proven.

A number of legitimate defenses can be made against charges of disparate treatment. One defense is that while a qualified individual may have had the qualifications for a particular job, the employer hired someone with superior qualifications. Another defense is that a protected class characteristic (e.g., gender) is in fact a bona fide occupational qualification (BFOQ); a clear example of a BFOQ is requiring a woman to work as an attendant in a women's restroom. However, great debate continues about what constitutes a BFOQ, and court rulings are inconsistent in this area. The courts have rejected the argument that because most women cannot lift 50 pounds, all women should be eliminated for consideration for jobs that require heavy lifting. On the other hand, citing safety concerns in 1997, the U.S. Federal Court of Appeals defended the Federal Aviation Administration policy that requires pilots to retire at age 60 (Castaneda 1977). Thus, in certain instances, age can be a bona fide occupational qualification.

The Age Discrimination in Employment Act of 1967

The **Age Discrimination in Employment Act (ADEA) of 1967** forbids discrimination against men and women over 40 years of age by employers, unions, employment agencies, state and local governments, and the federal government. Like Title VII of the Civil Rights Act, enforcement of the ADEA is the responsibility of the EEOC. Most ADEA suits are brought on a disparate treatment theory of intentional discrimination because of age.

The Americans with Disabilities Act of 1990

Discrimination against individuals with disabilities was first prohibited in federally funded activities by the *Vocational Rehabilitation Act of 1973;* however, individuals with disabilities were not covered by Title VII of the Civil Rights Act of 1964. Thus, this group was not protected from employment discrimination until almost a decade later. Of the many federal equal employment opportunity laws, the ADA is unique in that it received unanimous support from both political parties.

The Americans with Disabilities Act (ADA) provides substantial protection to individuals with disabilities who are employed or potentially employable

The **Americans with Disabilities Act (ADA)** provides substantial protection to individuals with disabilities who are employed or potentially employable in work settings such as private sector organizations or a department or agency of state or local government that employs 15 or more employees.

The ADA prohibits discrimination against individuals with disabilities in all aspects of the employee-employer relationship, including job application procedures, hiring, termination, promotions, compensation, and training. The act is a far-reaching piece of legislation, which, on its passage, led most large organizations to examine, and in many cases modify, their procedures to ensure compliance.

The language of the ADA, like other legislation, is somewhat vague. It defines disability as "(a) a physical or mental impairment that substantially limits one or more of the major life activities, (b) a record of such impairment, or (c) being regarded as having such an impairment" (Americans with Disabilities Act 1990). Each of these definitions is obviously open to considerable debate and interpretation. Part (a) definition includes individuals who have serious disabilities, such as epilepsy, blindness, deafness, or paralysis, that affect their ability to carry out major life activities. Part (b) includes individuals with a history of a disability, such as history of cancer, heart disease, or mental disorder. Part (c) includes individuals who are regarded as having an impairment, including individuals who are burn victims and/or who have disfiguring conditions. For example, Part (c) protects a prospective employee from being denied employment because the employer feels that the prospective employee's physical appearance would elicit negative reactions from coworkers (*Employment Law Update* 1991b). While the ADA has broad definitions of a disability, it specifically *excludes* the following from its definition:

- Homosexuality and bisexuality (state and local legislation may provide protection against discrimination based on sexual orientation);
- Gender-identity disorders that do not result from physical impairment or other sexual behavior disorders (e.g., transvestitism, transsexualism);
- Compulsive gambling, kleptomania, or pyromania;
- Psychoactive substance abuse disorders; and
- Current illegal use of drugs.

One of the biggest areas of review by the EEOC has been the definition of a disability. In the area of obesity, for example, the EEOC has determined that the ADA only covers severely obese persons—individuals whose weight is in excess of 100 percent of the norm for their particular height or whose weight can be linked to a medical disorder. In addition, because almost 13 percent of all complaints filed with the EEOC between 1993 and 1997 were related to emotional and mental disorders, the EEOC released guidelines in 1997 that deal specifically with this type of issue.

The ADA does not require an organization to hire someone not qualified for a job; in fact, an employee or prospective employee must be qualified for the job to be protected under the ADA. According to the ADA, "the term 'qualified individual with a disability' means an individual with a disability who, with or without reasonable accommodation, can perform the essential functions of the employment position that such individual holds or desires" (Americans with Disabilities Act 1990). This definition requires the organization to have a good and defensible understanding of the essential functions of each of its jobs, and having this understanding requires the organization to have in place accurate and current descriptions of all its job functions.

The next dilemma that the ADA definition presents is how we define reasonable accommodation. The ADA specifically states that the employing organization is responsible for making reasonable accommodation to the physical or mental limitations of an individual with a disability who is otherwise qualified, unless this accommodation would impose an undue hardship on the organization. What is reasonable accommodation? **Reasonable accommodation** may be defined as attempts by employers to adjust, without undue hardship, the working conditions or schedules of employees with disabilities.[2] Reasonableness is determined on a case-by-case basis, and typically it includes relatively noncontroversial accommodations such as making existing facilities accessible to individuals with disabilities. However, it may also be reasonable to restructure jobs, alter work schedules, reassign individuals to different tasks, adjust training materials, and provide readers or interpreters.

Reasonable accommodation is an attempt by employers to adjust, without undue hardship to the organization, the existing working conditions to fit employees with disabilities

Determining what constitutes reasonable accommodation depends on determining what constitutes undue hardship for the organization. While no strict guidelines exist for determining the threshold of undue hardship, the law suggests comparing the cost of the accommodation with the employer's operating budget. In addition, the law stipulates that the overall size of the organization may be considered as well as the type of operation and the nature and cost of the accommodation. In actuality, the cost of most accommodations is not great. The U.S. General Accounting Office found that the actual cost of accommodation has been remarkably low: Over 50 percent of accommodations did not cost anything, while 30 percent cost employers less then $500 (McGill 1997). In addition, the EEOC has published a *Technical Assistance Manual* that suggests the following process for assessing reasonable accommodation:

- Look at the particular job involved and determine its purpose and essential job function.
- Consult with the individual with the disability to identify potential accommodations that may be needed; if several accommodations are available and possible, preference should be given to the individual's preferred accommodation.

Court rulings have sought to curtail what many consider abuses of the ADA; examples of these cases include *Schmidt v. Methodist Hospital of Indiana* (No. 9502772, Indiana 1996), *Zamudio v. Patla* (956 F.supp. 803, Illinois 1997), and *Howard v. North Mississippi Medical Center* (939 F.Supp. 505, Mississippi 1996) (Fiesta 1997). Policymakers and managers should understand the law so that they can anticipate and deal with both their intended and unintended consequences.

Sexual Harassment Law

Increased awareness of sexual harassment issues has come about as a result of feminism and the women's movement, greater societal attention to issues of diversity and accommodation in the workplace, and the increase in the number of women in the workplace at all levels. Certainly, several well-publicized cases that involved a Supreme Court justice nominee (i.e., Clarence Thomas), a U.S. senator (i.e., Bob Packwood), and former president (i.e., Bill Clinton) have increased the attention given to sexual harassment. Sexual harassment has long existed in the workplace; surprisingly, however, only in the recent past have employers and courts recognized its prevalence and its impact.

The major statute that governs sexual harassment is Title VII of the Civil Rights Act; under this statute, sexual harassment is considered a violation of an individual's civil rights. Although several Supreme Court cases have provided a richer explanation of sexual harassment (see Table 4.2 for a brief summary of the most important precedent-setting court cases in the last 25 years), many ambiguities still remain regarding what constitutes sexual harassment. Figure 4.2 enumerates the EEOC's definition of sexual harassment to help courts, employers, and employees understand the scope of the issue.

Two types of sexual harassment are recognized by the EEOC: (1) quid pro quo and (2) hostile environment. **Quid pro quo harassment** occurs

Quid pro quo harassment occurs when a job-related benefit is offered or made available to an employee in exchange for the employee's submission to sexual advances

Case	Key Finding and Precedent
Bundy v. Jackson, 641 F.2d 934, 24 FEP 1155, D.C. Cir. (1981)	A quid pro quo harassment case that extended the idea of discrimination to sexual harassment
Meritor Savings Bank v. Vinson, Supreme Court of the United States, 40 FEP 1822 (1986)	The Supreme Court ruled that sexual harassment can constitute unlawful sex discrimination under Title VII if the harassment is so severe that it alters the conditions of the victim's employment and creates an abusive working environment.
Ellison v. Brady, United States Court of Appeals, Ninth Circuit, 924 F.2d 872 (1991)	The Supreme Court ruled that sexual harassment must be viewed from the perspective of a "reasonable woman" and not people in general and that employers must take positive action to eliminate sexual harassment from the workplace.
Harris v. Forklift Systems, Inc. 114 S. Ct. 367 (1993)	An abusive work environment can be demonstrated even when the victim does not suffer serious psychological harm. This case adopted the idea that harassment occurs if a "reasonable person" would find that the behavior leads to a hostile or abusive working environment.

TABLE 4.2
Key Court Decisions on Sexual Harassment in the Workplace

FIGURE 4.2
Equal Employment Opportunity Definition of Sexual Harassment

Unwelcome sexual advances, requests for sexual favors, and other verbal or physical contact of a sexual nature constitute sexual harassment when:

1. submission to such contact is made either explicitly or implicitly a term of condition of an individual's employment;
2. submission to or rejection of such conduct by an individual is used as the basis for employment decisions that affect the individual; or
3. such conduct has the purpose or effect of unreasonably interfering with an individual's work performance or creating an intimidating, hostile, or offensive work environment.

Source: EEOC guideline based on the Civil Rights Act of 1964, Title VII.

when a job-related benefit is offered or made available to an employee in exchange for the employee's submission to sexual advances. A typical quid pro quo harassment is illustrated in a 1994 case that involves an employee at the University of Massachusetts Medical Center. The employee was awarded $1 million after she testified that her supervisor had forced her to engage in sex once or twice a week over a 20-month period as a condition of keeping her job

(Bureau of National Affairs 1994). The second, and more subtle type of sexual harassment, is hostile environment sexual harassment. **Hostile environment sexual harassment** occurs when sexual behavior of anyone in the work setting is perceived by an employee as offensive and undesirable. While the law is not explicit about what constitutes this type of harassment, some examples might include display of sexually suggestive pictures, exchange of sexually related jokes, and use of sexually explicit language in and around the work area.

While some cases of sexual harassment are relatively clear cut, other cases are harder to categorize or determine because the particular workplace and the individuals involved also have to be examined. For employers, an important concern that arises from sexual harassment charges is liability, given that courts have consistently found that employers are liable for the actions of their employees in civil rights cases. In sexual harassment cases, courts typically address three issues to determine whether harassment occurred, how severe were the consequences, and whether the employer is liable (Noe et al. 1996).

1. *The plaintiff cannot have invited or welcomed the sexual advances.* If the defendant can demonstrate that sexual interactions were mutually agreed to, then harassment cannot be confirmed. Defendants may attempt to prove that sexual behavior was invited (or at least not resisted) by making claims about the plaintiff's sexual history, wearing of provocative clothing, and so forth. However, courts typically do not focus on these issues but assume that sexual behavior simply does not belong in the workplace and is thus unwelcomed (Noe et al. 1996). In addition, courts look for repetitiveness in the harassment; a plaintiff is more likely to be successful if he or she can prove that the harassment was not just a one-time event but was in fact persistent and pernicious.

2. *The harassment needs to have been severe enough to have altered the terms, conditions, and privileges of employment or to have caused significant consequences for the employee.* Particularly in hostile environment cases, assessing objectively whether an environment is actually "hostile" or how harmful it may be is difficult, so courts have used two types of standards to help in this determination. A **reasonable woman** standard is used to assess and compare how a reasonable woman would react to similar circumstances faced by the plaintiff.. The second, and possibly less stringent, standard is the **reasonable person**, in which a reasonable man's or woman's reaction to similar circumstances is compared to that of the plaintiff's reaction. The use of a reasonable person standard versus a reasonable woman standard in determining the existence and severity of harassment is still under debate however. The Supreme Court has listed several questions to help courts maneuver through hostile environment sexual harassment cases:

Hostile environment sexual harassment occurs when sexual behavior of anyone in the work setting is perceived by an employee as offensive and undesirable

A reasonable woman standard is used to assess and compare how a reasonable woman would react to similar circumstances faced by the plaintiff

A reasonable person standard is used to assess and compare how a reasonable man or woman would react to similar circumstances

- How frequent is the discriminatory conduct?
- How severe is the discriminatory conduct?
- Is the conduct physically threatening or humiliating?
- Does the conduct interfere with the employee's work performance?

3. *Courts need to examine the extent of employer liability for the harassment.* Two questions are typically asked in determining liability: (1) Did the employer know about the harassment or should it have known? (2) Did the employer take steps to stop the behavior? In most instances, if the employer knew about the harassment and the behavior did not stop, courts will decide that the employer did not act appropriately to curtail the behavior. The issue of employer liability, like other aspects of sexual harassment law, is still very much in flux. For example, in a well-publicized case in Boca Raton, Florida, the Supreme Court ruled that employers are responsible for the misconduct of their supervisors even if the employer is unaware of supervisor behavior (*Faragher v. City of Boca Raton* [Florida 1998]).

For many years, sexual harassment was simply not recognized as an important workplace concern, which was the result of the general lack of sensitivity to the needs of women in the workplace. (While men are at times victims of sexual harassment, the vast majority of cases are related to men harassing women.) As we learn about the extent of sexual harassment and as we use the legal system to enforce existing laws, we also get a picture of the magnitude of this problem in the workplace, including the following:

- The EEOC reports that the number of sexual harassment charges filed with the EEOC has increased steadily between 1992 and 2000. In 1992, 10,532 charges were filed; in 2000, 15,836 were filed (Equal Employment Opportunity Commission 2001).
- The percentage of cases filed by males has increased from 9.1 percent of all charges in 1992 to 13.6 percent in 2000 (Equal Employment Opportunity Commission 2001).
- Monetary benefits from sexual harassment cases increased from $12.7 million in 1992 to $54.6 million in 2000 (Equal Employment Opportunity Commission 2001).
- In a study conducted as part of the Women Physicians' Health Study, 47.7 percent of women physicians reported experiencing gender-based harassment, and 36.9 percent reported sexual harassment (Frank, Brogan, and Schiffman 1998).
- Sexual harassment of women physician was more common in medical school (20 percent) or during internship, residency, or fellowship (19 percent) than in practice (11 percent) (Frank, Brogan, and Schiffman 1998).

- Sexual harassment is as prevalent or more so in healthcare than in other industries; one study indicates that nearly three-fourths of women in healthcare have been sexually harassed (Walsh and Borowski 1995; Sherer 1995).
- According to a 1990 study conducted by the American Medical Association, 81 percent of female medical students said they had been targets of sexual slurs and 50 percent said they were direct targets of sexual advances; the report also found that the worst harassment occurred in academic medical centers (Decker 1997).
- Over one-third of *Fortune* 500 companies have been sued for sexual harassment (Bernardin and Russell 1998).

While sexual harassment is unfortunately common in virtually all organizations, it is particularly problematic in healthcare organizations. As a response, the American Nurses Association's House of Delegates declared a resolution denouncing sexual harassment in the workplace and called on the industry to adopt and enforce sexual harassment policies (Mikulenak 1992). Why is sexual harassment so prevalent in healthcare organizations? Many factors contribute to this scenario. First, sexual harassment almost always feeds on the element of power and control. This element is present in healthcare organizations because of their hierarchical organizational structure and the traditional gender composition of their primary caregivers—doctors and nurses—where men fill most of the physician roles and women largely hold the nursing roles; therefore, men continue to maintain much professional and organizational authority over women. The majority of hospital employees are women, yet those in positions of authority (i.e., physicians, administrators, and board members) are, at least until relatively recently, predominantly men. This differential in authority is frequently the precursor to sexual harassment. Preventing sexual harassment in healthcare organizations is difficult because of the ambiguous, even disparate, degrees of supervision that employees are given. While every nurse and assisting staff member certainly has a formal supervisor in the organization, the supervision of physicians is not as clearly defined nor assigned. Thus, sexual harassment is particularly prevalent in one of the most organizationally complex healthcare organizations—academic medical centers. In addition, the fact that nurses levy the largest number of sexual harassment complaints is not surprising.

Second, the intimacy of relationships between employees may also account for the high prevalence of sexual harassment in healthcare organizations. Strong coworker relationships often form in the high-stress environment of healthcare, and this bond often creates a comfort level that provides a forum for sexual jokes and off-color humor. Discussion of the human body and sexuality is central to providing healthcare, and such discussion can evolve into an abusive, condescending, or suggestive manner of dialog.

The law and the courts are clear about management's responsibility for preventing and stopping sexual harassment. Various court rulings have reinforced the finding that employers can be held responsible for sexual harassment unless they take appropriate action in response to complaints. A review of sexual harassment court cases in 1992 (Terpstra and Baker) found that plaintiffs won virtually every case when the following situations held:

- when the harassment involved physical contact of a sexual nature;
- when sexual propositions were linked to threats or promises of a change in the conditions of employment;
- when the claimant notified management of the problem before filing charges;
- when the claims are corroborated; and
- when the organization had no formal sexual harassment policy that had been communicated to its employees.

The first line of defense against sexual harassment is the existence, or development, of a sexual harassment policy that is strongly supported by the organization's management. Typically this policy would include (Segal 1992):

- A written statement against sexual harassment, including a definition of sexual harassment and a strong statement indicating that it will not be tolerated.
- Instructions on how to report complaints, including procedures to bypass a supervisor if he or she is involved.
- Assurances of confidentiality and protection against retaliation.
- A guarantee of prompt investigation.
- A statement that disciplinary action will be taken against harassers up to and including termination.

Such a policy needs to also be reinforced with strong communications and training. Managers need to understand clearly the requirements for Title VII as well as their duty to provide an environment free of sexual harassment. In addition, managers also need to understand the investigative procedures to be used when charges occur. If charges are levied, management needs to respond immediately, and if these charges are proven to be true, the offender should be disciplined according to policy. As with any other human resources policy, discipline needs to be carried out consistently across similar cases and among managers and hourly employees alike (Sherman, Bohlander, and Snell 1998).

Implementing Equal Employment Opportunity Laws

The preceding section outlined the most important equal employment opportunity laws and other regulatory mechanisms. In this section, we examine the implications of implementing these laws for human resources management.

Human resources managers must consider two interrelated aspects of implementation (1) the legal requirements associated with meeting compliance, including, for example, establishing affirmative action plans and completing the annual AA-1 government reporting form; and (2) the compliance of the organization's human resources systems to existing laws, including job design, employee selection, and performance appraisal systems. The following are some factors to consider when implementing these laws while avoiding legal conflicts.

Employee Training on Proper Conduct

A certain amount of liability for employee conduct rests with the employer and, therefore, with the manager. This employee-employer relationship is governed by the legal concept of agency, in which the employer or the organization empowers its employee to perform duties, services, or work in the name of the employer. The employee's conduct while in this charge is a direct reflection of the employer's values and beliefs, so legally, the employee's actions are of potential equal liability to the employer. Specifically, the legal doctrine of **Respondeat Superior** holds the employer liable for the conduct of its employees because the employer enabled the employee and the employer is responsible for managing and supervising the employee (Furrow, Jost, and Johnson 1997). Therefore, training employees in appropriate conduct, and subsequently supervising that conduct, is of utmost importance. An employer cannot assume that employees are knowledgeable about equal opportunity, discrimination, and sexual harassment legalities. The employer should assume the burden of employee education to promote organizational compatibility and to avoid future litigation.

Respondeat Superior holds the employer liable for the conduct of its employees because the employer enabled the employee and the employer is responsible for managing and supervising the employee

Interview Questions

Sensitivity to legal doctrines and workplace regulations, as well as to cultural differences, when framing interview questions is a must for managers. If the appropriateness of an interview question is inconclusive, then not asking the question is a better option. Furthermore, all interview questions should be applicable to all interviewees. If a question can only be asked to a certain segment of interviewees, then the appropriateness of the question is dubious. Examples of these dubious questions include questions about possibilities for becoming pregnant and about retirement plans.

Defenses Against Discrimination

The best defense against lawsuits is creating and disseminating nondiscriminatory organizational policies; doing so serves multiple purposes:

• Specifying unacceptable behavior and its consequences at the onset of employment is likely to decrease future inappropriate behavior. It is an initial step in educating employees of what behavior is expected and accepted by the organization.

- Standard policies promote uniform conduct of employees, which thereby lends itself to fair and nondiscriminatory employee treatment. In other words, employees trained with uniform methods will inevitably conduct themselves in relatively similar manners.
- Publicizing desired employee conduct to employees and the public is a preemptive step against litigation for any organization. Legally, the organization must be able to distinguish between that which the employee does through autonomous choices and that which the employee does through organizational support or inattention. A set of policies permits the organization to delineate what behavior it endorses. However, simply having a set of policies in place is not a substantial defense. Organizational policies must be monitored and enforced for them to be effective, and this is a fact recognized by the courts. Tacit, unpoliced policies are ineffective defenses against discrimination.

Termination

Termination is rarely a happy event in an organization. Documentation of the circumstances surrounding the termination is as important as the reason for the termination itself. Barring extreme circumstances in which the well-being of the organization is jeopardized, an employee has the right to ample notice and explanation of employer dissatisfaction to be able remedy the problematic issues. Documentation of all incidents, requests for changes in conduct, employee evaluations, and employee responses to evaluations are the responsibility of the employer. Sufficient documentation of the choice to sever an employer-employee relationship is one of the best strategies to demonstrate the fair handling of a termination.

Many organizations implement a **termination-at-will** policy that, in theory, permits the employer or the employee to sever employment relations at any time and for any reasons. While these types of policies allow a heightened degree of employer discretion in termination matters, state and federal equal opportunity and discrimination standards supercede any private policies. A termination-at-will policy does not permit an employer to terminate an employee-employer relationship on non-work-performance grounds—that is, an employee has the right to contest a termination, even if a termination at will policy exists, if the employee believes that he or she was fired for discriminatory reasons. Furthermore, a prudent employer may regard termination at will policies lightly for any termination circumstance. Organizational termination-at-will policies have been likened to *termination-without-cause* clauses. Courts have pierced the veil of termination-without-cause policies even in cases when the termination was not of a discriminatory nature, which is the case with *Harper v. Healthsource New Hampshire, Inc.* (140 N.H. 770, 674 A.2d 962, 1996), in which a physician was terminated absent a stated reason. The termination of the physician without specifying a reasonable cause was found to be against public policy. Although this case stands alone in its

Termination at will, in theory, permits the employer or the employee to sever employment relations at any time and for any reasons

findings, the ruling was intended to discourage bad-faith decisions that might serve to endanger public welfare. In addition, terminating without stating a cause was said to hamper the employee from properly responding to the termination. With these findings in mind, an employer may not retain much protection in termination-at-will policies.

TABLE 4.3
Internet Resources for Federal Employment Law

Internet Address	Content
www.dol.gov	General site of the U.S. Department of Labor (DOL). The site contains labor statistics, online library, current news, a listing of programs and services, and contacts.
http://eeoc.gov	General site of the U.S. Equal Employment Opportunity Commission (EEOC). The site contains information regarding filing of charges, enforcement and litigation, enforcement statistics, small business information, and the Freedom of Information Act.
www.access.gpo.gov	General site of the U.S. Government Printing Office (GPO). The site allows access to any public document printed by the federal government.
www.nlrb.gov	General site of the U.S. National Labor Relations Board (NLRB), which is charged with administering the National Labor Relations Act. Its main duties include (1) the facilitation of fair relations between unions and employers and (2) the prevention and remedies of unfair labor practices by both parties.
www.business.gov	General site of the U.S. Business Advisor. This organization exists to provide guidance in all general business practices, which are overseen by the government in some capacity.
www.fmcs.gov	General site of the Federal Mediation and Conciliation Service (FMCS). The FMCS is an independent agency created by Congress to facilitate strong and stable labor-management relations. The site contains information regarding dispute mediation, preventative mediation, alternative dispute resolution (litigation alternatives), arbitration services, and labor management grants.

Conclusion

The complex legal environment surrounding human resources management is under constant federal scrutiny and reform. In addition, the legal requirements imposed on an organization shift according to industry and state specific regulations. To accommodate the complexity of the environment, managers must learn as much as they can about work environment regulations. While blanket policies and regulations are imposed on all employers, regulations that are specific to only a segment of employers may also exist; therefore, managers must strive to acquire knowledge specific to his or her situation. While this may appear a daunting task, the government has provided numerous resources from which managers may start (see Table 4.3).

In general, a wise manager is one who realizes the convoluted nature of his or her job and concedes to the necessity of ongoing education to help him or her execute thoughtful, deliberated choices. To make prudent, law-abiding decisions, the manager must be calculating, and doing so requires the manager to understand both the employer's and employees' rights.

Discussion Questions

1. Is affirmative action still necessary to ensure equal employment opportunity? Given the diversity in the United States, should we begin to think about class-based rather than race-based affirmative action?
2. Has concern about sexual harassment gotten out of hand, and has "political correctness" replaced common sense?
3. Why is mental disability so difficult to define in the context of the Americans with Disabilities Act?
4. Should there be a uniform definition of reasonable accommodation in the Americans with Disabilities Act?
5. Why is sexual harassment so prevalent in the healthcare environment? What can be done to break this historical pattern?
6. Have federal antidiscrimination laws gone too far? Should public policy in the United States seek a return to employment at will?

Notes

1. More refined versions of the four-fifths rule have been developed. In 1977, for example, the Supreme Court established a standard deviation analysis that numerous lower courts have followed. This method uses statistical analysis to determine whether the difference between the expected selection rates for protected groups and the actual selection rates could be attributed to chance (see *Hazelwood School District v. United States*, 433 U.S. 299, 15 FEP 1, 1977).
2. Note that the reasonable accommodation concept may also be applied to Civil Rights Act issues concerning accommodation of individuals with religious preferences.

References

Americans with Disabilities Act of 1990, Pub. L. No. 101–336. Codified at 42 U.S.C. section 12101 et seq.

Bergmann, B., and W. Darity. 1981. "Social Relations in the Workplace and Employee Discrimination." In *Proceedings of the Industrial Relations Association*, pp. 155–62. Association Meeting.

Bernardin, H. J., and J. A. Russell. 1998. *Human Resource Management: An Experiential Approach*. Boston: Irwin McGraw-Hill.

Bouvier, C. 1996. "Why At-Will Employment Is Dying." *Personnel Journal* 75 (5): 123–8.

Bureau of National Affairs. 1994. "Medical Center Employee Awarded $1 Million in Massachusetts Suit." *BNA's Employee Relations Weekly* 12: 111–2.

Business and Professional Women/USA. 2001. "BPW/USA's 101 Facts on the Status of Working Women." [Online article; retrieved 8/10/01]. http://www.bpwusa.org/content/FairPay/facts_and_figures/equalpayfacts.htm.

Castaneda, C. 1977. "Panel Backs FAA on Retire-at-60 Rule." *USA Today* (July 16): 11.

Decker, P. J. 1997. "Sexual Harassment in Health Care: A Major Productivity Problem." *The Health Care Supervisor* 16 (1): 1–14.

Employment Law Update. 1991a. "The New Civil Rights Act of 1991 and What It Means to Employers." *Employment Law Update* 6 (December): 1–12.

———. 1991b. "ADA: The Final Regulations (Title I): A Lawyer's Dream/An Employer's Nightmare." *Employment Law Update* 16 (9): 1.

England, P. 1994. "Neoclassical Economists' Theories of Discrimination." In *Equal Employment Opportunity: Labor Market Discrimination and Public Policy*, edited by P. Burstein. New York: Aldine de Gruyter.

Equal Employment Opportunity Commission. 2001. [Online article; retrieved 8/10/01]. http://www.eeoc.gov/stats/harass.html.

Federal Register. 1978. "Adoption by Four Agencies of Uniform Guidelines on Employee Selection Procedures." *Federal Register* (August 15): Part IV, 38295–309.

Fiesta J. 1997. "Labor Law Update—Part 3." *Nursing Management* 28 (8): 26–8.

Frank, E., D. Brogan, and M. Schiffman. 1998. "Prevalence and Correlates of Harassment Among U.S. Women Physicians." *Archives of Internal Medicine* 158: 352–8.

Furrow, B. R., T. S. Jost, and S. H. Johnson. 1997. *Health Law: Cases, Materials and Problems, Third Edition*, pp. 237–307. St. Paul, MN: Wadsworth.

Greenlaw, P. S., and J. P. Kohl. 1995. "The Equal Pay Act: Responsibilities and Rights." *Employee Rights and Responsibilities Journal* 8: 295–307.

Ledvinka, J., and V. G. Scarpello. 1991. *Federal Regulation of Personnel and Human Resource Management, Second Edition*. Boston: PWS-Kent.

Levine, M. J. 1994. "The Erosion of the Employment-at-Will Doctrine: Recent Developments." *Labor Law Journal* 45 (2): 79–89.

McGill, B. G. 1997. "ADA Accommodations Do Not Have to Break the Bank." *HR Magazine* (July): 85–91.

Mikulenak, M. 1992. "House Takes Stand Against Harassment, Discrimination." *The American Nurse* 1 (July-August): 13.

The National Committee on Pay Equity. 2001. "The Wage Gap Over Time: In Real Dollars, Women See a Widening Gap." [Online article; retrieved 8/10/01]. http://www.feminist.com/fairpay/f_change.htm.

Noe, R. A., J. R. Hollenbeck, B. Gerhart, and P. M. Wright. 1996. *Human Resource Management: Gaining a Competitive Advantage, Second Edition*, pp. 126–7. Boston: Irwin McGraw-Hill.

Segal, J. A. 1992. "Seven Ways to Reduce Harassment Claims." *HR Magazine* (January): 84–5.

Sherer, J. L. 1995. "Sexually Harassed." *Hospitals & Health Networks* 54.

Sherman, A., G. Bohlander, and S. Snell. 1998. *Managing Human Resources, Eleventh Edition*. Cincinnati, OH: Southwestern.

Terpstra, D. E., and D. D. Baker. 1992. "Outcomes of Federal Court Decisions on Sexual Harassment." *Academy of Management Journal* 35: 181–90.

Walsh, A., and S. C. Borowski. 1995. "Gender Differences in Factors Affecting Healthcare Administration Career Development." *Hospital & Health Services Administration* 40 (2): 263–77.

JOB ANALYSIS AND JOB DESIGN

Myron D. Fottler, Ph.D.

Learning Objectives

After completing this chapter, the reader should be able to:

- Define job analysis, job description, and job specification
- Discuss the relationship of job requirements (as developed through job analyses, job descriptions, and job specifications) to other human resources management functions
- Describe the steps involved in and the methods of collecting data for a typical job analysis
- Describe the relationship between job analysis and strategic human resources management
- Describe the changing nature of jobs and how jobs are being redesigned to enhance productivity

Introduction

In previous chapters, we have discussed the effects of the internal and external environments on the process of strategic human resources management; in particular, we have emphasized the importance of the legal environment. The interaction between an organization and its environment has important implications for the organization's internal organization and structure. For example, the environment affects how the organization organizes human resources to achieve specific objectives and perform different functions necessary in carrying out the organization's mission and goals. The organization will formally group the activities to be formed by its human resources into basic units referred to as jobs.

A **job** consists of a group of similar and related activities and duties. Jobs should be clear and distinct from each other to minimize misunderstandings and conflict among employees and to enable employees to recognize what is expected of them. Some jobs may require several employees, each of whom

*A **job** consists of a group of similar and related activities and duties*

87

*A **position** consists of different duties and responsibilities performed by only one employee*

will occupy a separate position. A **position** consists of different duties and responsibilities performed by only one employee; for example, a hospital may employ 40 registered nurses to fill 40 RN positions, but all of these positions govern only one job—that of the registered nurse. If different jobs have similar duties and responsibilities, they may be grouped into a *job family* for purposes of recruitment, training, compensation, or advancement opportunities; for example, the nursing job family may consist of registered nurses, nursing supervisor, and director of nursing services.

Healthcare organizations are continually restructuring and reengineering in an attempt to become more cost effective and customer focused; they put emphasis on smaller scale, less hierarchy, fewer layers, and more decentralized work units. As these changes occur, more managers want their employees to operate more independently and flexibly to meet customer demands. To do this, managers require decisions to be made by employees who are closest to the information and who are directly involved in the service delivery. The objective is to develop jobs and basic work units that are adaptable to thrive in a world of high-velocity change.

In this chapter, we enumerate the processes that may be used to conduct job analyses, emphasize that job analyses processes also provide the foundation for making objective and legally defensible decisions in managing human resources, discuss how healthcare jobs have been redesigned to contribute to organizational objectives and simultaneously to satisfy the needs of the employees, and review several innovative job design and job redesign techniques to enhance job satisfaction and organizational performance.

Definitions

*A **job analysis** is the process of obtaining information about jobs by determining the job's duties, tasks, and/or activities*

Job analysis is sometimes called the cornerstone of strategic human resources management because the information it provides serves so many human resources functions. **Job analysis** is the process of obtaining information about jobs by determining the job's duties, tasks, and/or activities. A **job description** is a written report about a job and the types of duties it includes. Because no standard format for job descriptions exists, the descriptions tend to vary in appearance and content from one organization to another; however, most job descriptions contain the job title, a job identification section, and a job duties section. In addition, the description may also include a job specification section, although a job specification may be prepared as a separate document. Appendix A is an example of a job description and performance development tool for the position of staff nurse in a hospital labor and delivery department.

*A **job description** is a written explanation of the duties of the job*

*A **job specification** describes the skills required to perform the job and the physical demands the job places on the employee*

A **job specification** describes the personal qualifications an individual must posses to perform the duties and responsibilities contained in a job description. Typically, the job specification describes the skills required to perform the job and the physical demands the job places on the employee.

Skills and qualification relevant to a job include education and experience, specialized knowledge or training, licenses, personal abilities and traits, and manual dexterities. The physical demands of a job refer to the condition of the physical work environment; work place hazards; and the amount of walking, standing, reaching, and lifting required to perform the job.

Job Analysis

Figure 5.1 indicates how job analysis is performed, including the functions for which it is used. The process involves undertaking a systematic investigation of jobs by following a number of predetermined steps specified in advance (Ash 1988). When completed, a written report is generated that summarizes information obtained from the analysis of 20 to 30 individual job tasks or activities. Human resources managers then use these data to develop job descriptions and job specifications. These documents, in turn, will be used to perform and enhance different human resource functions such as development of performance appraisal criteria or the content of training classes (Clifford 1994). The ultimate purpose of a job analysis is to improve organizational performance and productivity.

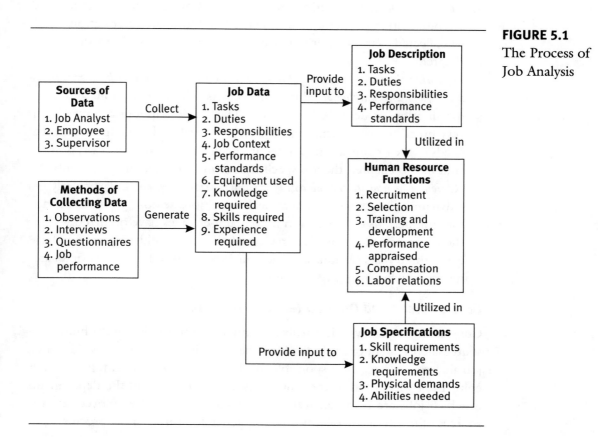

FIGURE 5.1

The Process of Job Analysis

Steps in Conducting the Process

The process of conducting a job analysis involves a number of steps. Although healthcare organizations may differ in the manner they conduct job analysis, the following steps provide a general guide (Anthony, Perrewe, and Kacmar 1993):

1. *Determine the purpose.* To increase the probability of a successful job analysis program, the purpose of conducting the job analysis should be explicit and tied to the organization's overall business strategy.
2. *Identify the jobs to be analyzed.* All jobs are analyzed if no previous formal job analysis has been performed. If the organization has undergone changes that have affected only certain jobs or if new jobs have been added, then only those jobs are analyzed.
3. *Explain the process to employees and determine their levels of involvement.* Employees should be informed of who will be conducting the analysis, why it is needed, whom to contact to answer questions and concerns, the schedule of events, and their roles in the process. In addition to good communication, a committee elected by employees may serve as a verification check and may reduce employee anxiety. Such committees can also help answer questions and concerns employees may have.
4. *Collect the job analysis information.* Managers must decide which method or combination of methods will be used and how the information will be collected. Various alternatives are discussed in the next section of this chapter.
5. *Organize the job analysis information into a form that will be useful to managers and employees.* This form consists of job descriptions and job specifications as described previously. The job descriptions can vary from very broad to very specific and precise; the level of detail depends on the needs of the organization as noted in the first step of the process. As noted later in this chapter, the job specifications must be relevant to the job.
6. *Review and update the job analysis information frequently.* Particularly in a dynamic environment such as healthcare, jobs seldom go unchanged for long periods of time. Even if no major changes have occurred within the organization, a complete review of all jobs should be performed every three years (Mathis and Jackson 1985). More frequent reviews are necessary when major organizational changes occur.

Data Sources and Data Collection Methods

Conducting job analyses is usually the primary responsibility of the human resources department or the individuals charged with these functions. Although job analysts are typically responsible for the job analysis program, they usually enlist the cooperation of the employees and supervisors in the departments in which jobs are being analyzed. These supervisors and employees are the sources of much of the job information generated through the process.

Job information is collected in several ways, depending on the purpose to be served by the organization. Typically, the organizational chart is reviewed to identify the jobs to be included in the analysis, and often, restructuring, downsizing, merger, or rapid growth initiates this review. A job may be selected because it has undergone undocumented changes in job content. As new job demands arise and the nature of the work changes, compensation for the job also may have to change, so the employee or the manager may request a job analysis to determine the appropriate compensation. The manager may also be interested in documenting change for recruitment selection, training, and performance appraisal purposes. Managers should consider a number of different methods to collect job analysis information because any one method is unlikely to provide all of the necessary information. Among the most popular methods of data collection are observation of tasks and behaviors of the jobholders, conducting interviews, use of structured questionnaires and checklists, and performance of a specific job.

Observations require job analysts to observe the employees performing their jobs. The observations may be continuous or intermittent, focusing only on a sampling of tasks performed; however, the usefulness of the observation may be limited in instances where the job does not consist of physically active tasks; for example, observing an accountant reviewing an income statement may not provide valuable information. Even with more active jobs, observation does not always reveal vital information such as the importance or difficulty of the task. Given the limited effectiveness of observation, incorporating additional methods for obtaining job analysis information is helpful.

Employees who are knowledgeable about a particular job (i.e., the employee performing the job, supervisors, or former jobholders) may be interviewed concerning the specific work activities that comprise the job. Usually a structured *interview* form is used to record information, and the questions asked correspond to the data needed to prepare a job description and job specification. Employees may be suspicious of the interviewer and his or her motives, especially if the interviewer asks ambiguous questions. Because interviewing can be a time-consuming and costly method of data collection, managers and job analysts may prefer to use the interview as a means to answer specific questions generated from observations and questionnaires.

The use of structured *questionnaires and checklists* is most efficient because it is a quick and inexpensive way to collect information about a job. If possible, having several knowledgeable employees complete the questionnaire for verification is desirable. Such survey data often can be quantified and processed by computer. Follow-up observations and interviews are not uncommon if a questionnaire or checklist is chosen as the primary means of collecting job analysis information. Although questionnaires and checklists provide the employer with a simplified method for obtaining job analysis information, the questionnaire must be extremely detailed and comprehensive so that valuable information is not missed. Compared to other methods, questionnaires are cheaper and easier to administer, but they are more time consuming and expensive to develop. Management must decide whether the benefits of a simplified method of data collection outweigh the costs of its construction.

Strategically, managers would favor methods of data collection that do not require a lot of work and upfront costs if the content of the job changes frequently. Another option may be to adopt an existing or widely used structured questionnaire, such as the Position Analysis Questionnaire (PAQ), the Management Position Description Questionnaire (MPDQ), and the Functional Job Analysis (FJA). Regardless of whether the questionnaire is developed in-house or purchased from a commercial source, rapport between analyst and respondent is not possible unless the analyst is available to explain items and clarify misunderstandings. Without such rapport, such an impersonal approach may have adverse effects on the respondents' cooperation and motivation.

Finally, the analyst can actually *perform the job* in question. This approach allows exposure to the actual job tasks as well as the job's physical, environmental, and social demands. This method is also appropriate for jobs that can be learned in a relatively short period of time; however, it is inappropriate for jobs that require extensive training and/or are hazardous to perform.

Relation to Other Human Resources Functions

Job analysis provides the basis for tying all the human resources functions together and for developing a sound human resources program. Not surprisingly, job requirements, as documented in job descriptions and job specifications, influence many of the human resources functions that are performed as part of managing employees. Therefore, when job requirements are modified, corresponding changes must be made in other human resources activities as well. Job analysis is the foundation for forecasting future needs for human resources and plans for such activities as training, transfer, or promotion. Frequently, job analysis information is incorporated into the human resources information systems (HRIS), which is discussed further in Chapter 6. The following are some functions affected by job analysis.

Recruitment and Selection Prior to recruiting capable employees, recruiters need to know the job specifications for the positions they need to fill; this information must include all of the knowledge, skills, and abilities required for successful job performance. The information in the job specifications is used in notices of job openings and provides a basis for attracting qualified applicants while discouraging unqualified applicants. Failure to update job specifications could produce a pool of applicants who are unqualified to perform one or more of the job functions. Until 1971, job specifications used as a basis for employee-selection decisions often bore little relation to the duties to be performed under the job description. Then in *Griggs v. Duke Power Company* (401 U.S. 424, 1971), the

Supreme Court ruled that employment practices must be job related. When discrimination charges arise, employers have the burden of proving that job requirements are job related or constitute a business necessity. Employers must now be able to show that the job specifications used in selecting employees for a particular job relate specifically to that job's duties.

Career Development/ Training

Any discrepancies between the knowledge, skills, and abilities demonstrated by the jobholders and the requirements contained in the job description and specification provide clues to training needs. *Career development* is concerned with preparing employees for advancement to jobs where their capabilities can be utilized to the fullest extent possible. The formal qualifications set forth in the job specifications for higher-level jobs serve to indicate how much more training and development are needed for employees to advance to these jobs.

Performance Appraisal

The requirements contained in the job description provide the criteria for evaluating the performance of the jobholder. Appraisal of employee performance, however, may reveal that certain performance criteria established for a particular job are not completely valid; these criteria must be specific and job related. If the criteria used to evaluate employee performance are overly broad, vague, and not job related, employers may find themselves accused of unfair discrimination.

Compensation

The relative worth of a job is one of the most important factors in determining the rate paid for performing a job. This worth is based on (1) the skill, effort, and responsibility demanded of the jobholder and (2) the conditions and hazards under which the work is performed.

Safety and Health

Information derived from job analysis is also valuable in identifying safety and health considerations. If a job is hazardous, the job description and specification should reflect this condition. Employers may need specific information about hazards (i.e., risk of contacting AIDS) to perform these jobs safely.

Labor Relations

Job analysis information is also important to the employee relations and labor relations functions. When employees are considered for promotion, transfer, or demotion, the job description provides a standard for comparison of talent. This standard prevents potential conflicts between employees and organizations and between each group's representatives. Regardless of whether the organization is unionized, information obtained through job analysis can often lead to more objective human resources decisions.

Legal Aspects

Although human resources managers consider job descriptions a valuable tool for performing human resources functions, several problems are frequently associated with these documents (Grant 1988). First, they are often poorly

written and provide little guidance for the jobholder. Second, they are generally not updated as job duties or specifications change. Third, they may violate
the law by containing specifications not related to job performance. Fourth,
the job duties they include are often written in vague, rather than specific,
terms. Fifth, they can limit the scope of activities of the jobholder in a rapidly
changing environment.

Today's legal environment has created a need for higher levels of speci-
ficity in job analysis and job descriptions. Federal guidelines now require that
the specific performance requirements of a job be based on valid job-related
criteria (Equal Employment Opportunity Commission 1978). Employment
decisions that involve either job applicants or employees and are based on
criteria that are vague or not job related are increasingly being challenged
successfully. Managers of small healthcare organizations, where employees
may perform many different job tasks, must be particularly concerned about
writing specific job descriptions.

When writing job descriptions, employers must use statements that
are terse, direct, and simply worded; unnecessary phrases and words should
be eliminated. Typically, the sentences that describe job duties begin with
verbs (see Appendix A for example). The term "occasionally" is used to describe those duties that are performed once, while the term "may" is used
for those duties performed only by some workers on the job. Excellent job
descriptions are of value to both employee and employer. They can be used to
help employees learn their job duties and to remind them of the results they
are expected to achieve. For the employer, the job description can serve as
a foundation for minimizing the misunderstandings about job requirements
that occur between supervisors and their subordinates. They also establish
management's right to take corrective action when the duties specified in the
job description are not performed at all or performed inappropriately.

The job analysis process is faced with several legal constraints largely
because it serves as a basis for selection decisions, compensation, performance appraisals, and training; these constraints are articulated in the *Uniform
Guidelines for Employee Selection Procedures* (Equal Employment Opportunity
Commission 1978) and several court decisions. The following are human
resources functions that are affected legally in the absence of a job analysis.

Selection   Section 14.c.2 of the *Uniform Guidelines* states that "there shall be a job analysis of the important work behaviors required for successful performance." To
determine "important work behavior," organizations should analyze job skills,
knowledge, and abilities that employees need to perform their jobs. After this
information is known, selection procedures can be developed (Thompson and
Thompson 1982).

When job analyses were not performed, the validity of selection decisions had been challenged successfully, which was the case in *Albermarle
Paper Company v. Moody* (422 U.S. 405, 1975). Numerous court decisions

regarding promotion and job analysis also exist. In *Rowe v. General Motors* (325 U.S. 305, 1972), the court ruled that a company should have written objective standards for promotion to prevent discriminatory practices. In *U. S. v. City of Chicago* (573 F.2nd 416, 7th Cir., 1978), the court ruled that the objective standards should describe the job for which the person is being considered for promotion. The objective standards in both cases can be determined through job analysis (Nobile 1991).

Career Development/ Training

Because training and career development can be quite costly, up-to-date job descriptions and specifications help to ensure that training programs and other assignments reflect actual job requirements of the higher-level positions. Good job analysis data also allow for more effective career planning because the relationships among jobs and job families are more clearly understood.

Performance Appraisal

Unless the job description and/or specifications are rewritten to be more specific and job related, the criteria for performance appraisal are too broad to yield a valid evaluation. The performance appraisal instrument then needs to be redone to reflect the updated and more valued information. More critical and less critical job requirements could then be specified with confidence.

Compensation

Before jobs can be ranked in terms of their overall worth to an organization or compared to jobs in other similar organizations through pay surveys, their requirements must be understood thoroughly. A job's worth is based on (1) the skills, knowledge, effort, responsibility, and ability that the job demands from its performers and on (2) the conditions and hazards under which the job is performed. Job descriptions and specifications provide such understanding to those who must make job evaluation and compensation decisions.

Labor Relations

Prior to the *Uniform Guidelines* and the associated court cases discussed previously, labor contracts required consistent and equitable treatment of unionized employees. The information provided by job analysis is helpful to both management and unions for contract negotiations and for avoiding or resolving grievances, jurisdictional disputes, and other conflicts. For these reasons, unionized employers have found preparing written job descriptions and job specifications advantageous.

The passage of the ADA has also had a significant impact on job analysis. When preparing job descriptions and job specifications, managers and supervisors must adhere to the legal mandates of the ADA (Mitchell, Alliger, and Morfopoalos 1997). The act requires that the essential physical and mental requirements (or *essential functions*) of the position should be stated within the job description. The purpose of essential functions is to match and accommodate human capabilities to job requirements.

Section 1630.2 (n) of the ADA states three guidelines for rendering a job function essential: (1) the position exists to perform this function; (2) a limited number of employees are available among whom the performance of

the function may be distributed; and (3) the function may be highly specialized, requiring needed expertise to complete the job. Managers who write job
descriptions in terms of essential functions reduce the risk of discriminating
on the basis of disability.

Job Analysis in A Changing Environment

The traditional approach to job analysis assumes that jobs remain relatively
stable and apart from incumbents who hold these jobs. It assumes jobs can
be meaningfully defined in terms of tasks, duties, processes, and behaviors
necessary for job success. Unfortunately, these assumptions discount technological advances that are often so accelerated that jobs that are defined today
may be obsolete tomorrow. In a dynamic environment where job demands
change rapidly, job analysis data can quickly become outdated and inaccurate;
obsolete job analysis information can hinder an organization's ability to adopt
to change.

Several approaches to job analysis may respond to the need for continuous change:

- Future-oriented approach. This strategic analysis requires managers to
  have a clear view of how job duties and tasks should be restructured to
  meet future organizational requirements. One study asked experts on a
  particular job to identify aspects of the job, the organization, and the
  environment that might change in the next few years and how these
  changes might affect the nature of the job (Schneider and Konz 1989).
  The data collected were then used to describe the tasks, skills, knowledge,
  and abilities needed for doing the job in the future.

  By including future-oriented information in job descriptions,
  healthcare organizations can focus employee attention on new strategic
  directions. For example, when one organization decided to change its
  strategic focus to increasing its "customer consciousness" orientation, job
  descriptions were amended to include tasks, skills, knowledge, and abilities
  related to customer contact and responsibilities. These new job
  descriptions focused more on "what we want to be doing in the future"
  (George 1990).

- Competency-based approach. This approach places emphasis on
  characteristics of successful performers rather than on standard job duties
  and tasks (Hunt 1996). These characteristics match the organization's
  culture and strategy and include interpersonal communication skills, ability
  to work as part of a team, decision-making abilities, conflict resolution
  skills, adaptability, and self-motivation (Carson and Stewart 1996). This
  approach serves to enhance a culture of continuous improvement because
  organizational improvement is its constant aim. Both future-oriented and
  competency-based approaches have potential challenges, including the

ability of managers to accurately predict future job needs, the necessity of job analysis to comply with EEOC guidelines, and the possibility of role ambiguity created by generic job descriptions.

- Generic job analysis. The traditional approach to job analysis serves to constrain desired change and flexibility by compartmentalizing and specifically defining presumably static job characteristics. It impedes shifting decision making downward in the organization, cross-training, employees, and getting employees involved in quality-improvement efforts (Blayney 1992). Reducing the number of job titles and developing fewer, more generic job descriptions can provide needed flexibility to manage unanticipated change. For example, Nissan Motor Company has only one job description for hourly production employees. The generic description gives the organization the opportunity to use employees as needed. Cross-training and multiple job assignments can occur in this environment. As noted above, however, employees may experience more conflict and ambiguity with generic job descriptions.

Most jobs are no doubt getting bigger and more complex. The last duty specified on a typical job description is "any other duty that may be assigned," and that is increasingly becoming *the* job description. This enlarged, flexible, and complex job description changes the way virtually every HR function is performed. For example, organizations can no longer recruit and select individuals who merely possess narrow technical skills required to perform the job; they must also seek competencies, intelligence, adaptability, and an ability/willingness to work in teams.

The rapid pace of change in healthcare makes the need for accurate job analysis even more important now and in the future. Historically, job analysis could be conducted and then set aside for a reasonable time. Today, however, job requirements are changing so rapidly that they must be constantly reviewed to keep them relevant. By one estimate, people may have to change their entire skill sets three or four times during their careers (Snyder 1996). If this projection is accurate, the need for accurate and timely job analysis is becoming even more important over time. Organizations that do not conduct job analysis to update their job requirements may recruit new employees who do not possess the needed skills or may not provide necessary training to update those skills.

Job Design

Job design is an outgrowth of job analysis and is concerned with structuring jobs to improve organizational efficiency and employee job satisfaction. It focuses on changing, eliminating, modifying, and enriching jobs to capture the talents of employees and to recognize their needs while improving organizational performance and achieving organizational objectives. Job

Job design is an outgrowth of job analysis and is concerned with structuring jobs to improve organizational efficiency and employee job satisfaction

design dictates the manner in which a given job is defined and how it will be conducted, which involves decisions such as whether the job will be handled by an individual or by a team of employees as well as the determination of where the job fits into the overall organization. It requires a conscious effort for the organizing of tasks, duties, and responsibilities into a unit of work to achieve a certain objective.

Each job design must also acknowledge the unique skills possessed by professionals and must incorporate appropriate professional guidelines or limitations required in a given profession. Most health professions have legal constraints concerning which functions and tasks that can be legally performed and under what type of supervision. For example, many technical caregiving functions require the expertise of either a physician or a medical professional under the direct supervision of a physician. Such constraints obviously reduce the flexibility of healthcare managers in designing jobs.

Specialization

As a result of technological change, increased specialization, and the emergence of the hospital as the central focus of the healthcare system, approximately 700 different job categories now exist in the healthcare industry. The most rapid growth areas in healthcare manpower are the recently developed categories—support services and allied health. More than two-thirds of all people employed in the industry are employed in nontraditional allied health or support service positions (U.S. Census Bureau 1998).

Researchers have concluded that specialization has inherent limitations and has been taken to extremes in healthcare (Fottler 1992). New approaches to organizing work and job design are needed because of the inherent disadvantages of specialization. The foremost criticism is that specialized workers may become bored and dissatisfied because their jobs may not offer enough challenge or stimulation. When boredom and monotony sets in, absenteeism rises, and the quality of work suffers. To counter the problems of specialization and to enhance productivity and employee job satisfaction, healthcare managers have implemented a number of job design and job redesign options to achieve a better balance between organizational demands for efficiency and productivity and individual needs for creativity autonomy. These alternative approaches include (1) job redesign (i.e., job enlargement and job enrichment); (2) employee empowerment; (3) work group redesign (i.e., employee involvement groups, employee teams); and (4) work schedule redesign.

Job enlargement expands the scope of a job horizontally, providing the same level of autonomy and responsibility, to provide greater variety of duties to the employee

Job enrichment expands a job vertically, adding and giving more autonomy and responsibility to the job and to the employee

Job Redesign

Job enlargement expands the scope of a job horizontally, providing the same level of autonomy and responsibility, to provide greater variety of duties to the employee. Alternatively, **job enrichment** expands a job vertically, adding and giving more autonomy and responsibility to the job and to the employee.

The position of the multiskilled health practitioner (MSHP) is a specific innovation in job redesign in that the position may either be enriched or enlarged. The **MSHP** is a "person cross-trained to provide more than one function, often in more than one discipline" (Vaughan et al. 1991). These combined functions can be found in a broad spectrum of healthcare-related jobs, ranging in complexity from the nonprofessional to the professional level and including both clinical and management functions. The additional functions (skills) added to the original worker's job may be of a higher, lower, or parallel level.

*The **MSHP** is a "person cross-trained to provide more than one function, often in more than one discipline"*

Most theories of job enrichment stress that unless a job is both horizontally and vertically enriched, the job makes little positive impact on motivation, productivity, and job satisfaction (Lawler 1986). Because the MSHP concept may involve horizontal, vertical, or both types of enrichment, whether or not it should be expected to enhance organizational outcomes is unclear, although research on the concept reveals that the outcomes have been positive in terms of enhanced productivity, job satisfaction, and patient satisfaction (Fottler 1996). However, those positive outcomes depend on many contingencies such as whether the "right" employees (i.e., those with higher-order needs for personal growth) are chosen for the program, implementation processes, available training opportunities, legal constraints, and continuing top-management commitment.

Employee Empowerment

Various job enlargement/job enrichment approaches such as the creation of the MSHP are programs by which managers and supervisors formally change the job of employees. A less-structured approach is to allow employees to initiate their own job changes through the concept of empowerment. Ann Howard of Development Dimensions International defines empowerment as "pushing down decision-making responsibility to those close to internal and external customers" (Simison 1999). To support empowerment, organizations must share information, knowledge, power to act, and rewards throughout the work force. Empowerment encourages employees to become innovators and managers of their own work and gives them more control and autonomous decision-making capabilities (Ettorre 1997).

Empowerment could involve employee control over the job content (i.e., functions and responsibilities), the job context (i.e., the environmental conditions under which the job is performed), or both (Ford and Fottler 1995). Most healthcare organizations are not ready for both and are advised to implement empowerment on an incremental basis. For empowerment to thrive and grow, organizations must encourage participation, innovation, access to information, accountability, and a culture that is open and receptive to change (Garcia 1997). Examples of organizations which have successfully implemented employee empowerment include Cigna Health Care, the State of Illinois, Mesa (Arizona) Community College, and the State of Kentucky.

Work Group Redesign

Teams *are groups of employees who assume a greater role in the service process; they provide a forum for employees to contribute to identifying and solving organizational problems*

Table 5.1 outlines the six forms of work groups or teams currently being used in healthcare. **Teams** are groups of employees who assume a greater role in the service process; they provide a forum for employees to contribute to identifying and solving organizational problems. With work teams, managers accept the notion that the group is the logical work unit to resolve organizational problems and concerns.

Regardless of which team structure is employed, several team processes have been identified with successful teams, including commitment to shared goals, consensus decision making, open and honest communication, shared leadership, a climate of trust and collaboration, a valuing of diversity, and

TABLE 5.1
Forms of
Employee
Teams in
Healthcare

Type of Teams	Description
Cross-Functional Teams	A group staffed by a mix of specialists (i.e., nurses, physicians, and managers) and formed to accomplish a specific objective. These usually are assigned rather than voluntary.
Project Teams	A group formed specifically to design a new service. Members are assigned by management on the basis of their ability to contribute to success. The group normally disperses after task completion.
Self-Directed Teams	Group of highly trained individuals who perform a set of interdependent job tasks within a natural work unit. Team members use consensus decision making to perform job duties, solve problems, or deal with internal or external customers.
Task Force Teams	A task force is formed by management to resolve a major problem. The group is responsible for developing a long-term plan for problem resolution that may include a change for implementing the proposed solution.
Process Improvement Teams	A group made up of experienced employees from different departments or functions and charged with improving quality, decreasing waste, or enhancing productivity in processes that affect all departments. Team members are normally appointed by management.
Virtual Teams	A group with any of the above purposes that uses advanced computer and telecommunication technology to link geographically dispersed team members.

acceptance of conflict and its positive resolution. A good team also requires (1) the employee selection process to partially consider the potential employee's interpersonal skills and (2) extensive training to be provided to team members (Bohlander and McCarthy 1996). In addition, a good team also sees it important for the manager to adapt the role of the leader (rather than supervisor) and not be threatened by the growing power of the team.

Work Schedule Redesign

The goal of work schedule redesign is to improve organizational productivity and morale by giving employees increased control over their work schedules. Various types of adjustments in work schedules alter the normal workweek of five eight-hour days in which everyone begins and ends the workday at the same time. Under the compressed workweek, the number of days in the workweek is shortened by lengthening the number of hours worked per day. The four day 40-hour week (4/40) is the most common form of compressed workweeks, and the 3/39 schedule is less common. The compressed schedule accommodates the employees' leisure-time activities and personal appointments. A potential disadvantage of the schedule redesign is that under the stringent rules of the Fair Labor Standards Act, nonsupervisory employees who work more than 40 hours a week must be paid overtime. In addition, long workdays may also increase the amount of manager and employee exhaustion and stress.

Flextime, or flexible working hours, allows employees to choose daily starting and quitting times, provided they work a certain number of hours per day or week and within the typical "core period" during the morning and afternoon in which all employees on a given shift are required to be on the job. In healthcare, flextime is most commonly taken by employees who perform clerical or management functions such as claims processing, health insurance, and human resources. However, flextime is less appropriate for patient care positions, which must be staffed at all times, and communication/coordination is a continuing challenge in such positions.

By allowing employees greater flexibility in work scheduling, employers can reduce some of the most common causes of tardiness and absenteeism (i.e., the normal time pressures of life). Employees can adjust their work schedules to accommodate their lifestyles, reduce pressure to meet a rigid schedule, and gain greater satisfaction. Employers can enhance their attractiveness for recruiting and retaining personnel while improving customer service as a result of higher levels of employee satisfaction; work productivity and quality might also be enhanced.

Job Sharing

Job sharing is an arrangement whereby two part-time employees share a job that otherwise would be held by a full-time employee; this arrangement is best suited for employees who wish to work part-time and older workers who wish to phase into retirement. Job sharers sometimes work three days a week to

Job sharing is an arrangement whereby two part-time employees share a job that otherwise would be held by a full-time employee

create an overlap day for face-to-face conferencing. It can also be scheduled to conform to peaks in the daily or weekly workload.

Job sharing can reduce absenteeism because employees have time to accommodate their personal needs that sometimes occur during work hours. However, in the beginning orientation, training, and development of two employees to perform the same job may require more time. The key to successful job sharing is good communication between partners through phone calls, e-mail, and voice mail. Kaiser Permanente (a HMO) has developed a job-sharing program for physicians in Northern California.

Telecommuting

Telecommuting is the use of personal computers, network connections, and fax machines to perform work at an employee's home that is traditionally done in the workplace

One of the most significant work schedule innovations is telecommuting (Conklin 1999). Telecommuting is the use of personal computers, network connections, and fax machines to perform work at an employee's home that is traditionally done in the workplace. An estimated 25 percent of the workplace were telecommuting either full-time or part-time in 2000. The most important reasons employers use telecommuting were to reduce costs (33 percent), improve productivity (16 percent), increase employee retention (16 percent), improve employee morale (15 percent), and improve customer service (11 percent) (Reilly 1997). In addition, it reduces overhead costs by eliminating or reducing office space.

Potential drawbacks of telecommuting include the potential loss of creativity as a result of lower levels of employee interaction, the difficulty of developing appropriate performance standards and evaluation systems, and the need to formulate an appropriate technology system for telecommuting (Capowski 1998). In addition, if some employees are denied the opportunity to work from home, they may pursue legal action and/or become dissatisfied employees. Telecommuting is obviously more appropriate for employers who are not engaged in direct patient care.

In sum, the healthcare industry can and does use all four work schedule design approaches discussed here for the positions that do not involve clinical care of patients. Positions that involve direct patient care must be staffed twenty-four hours a day, seven days a week. Compressed workweek or job sharing is the most appropriate work schedule adjustment for employees in such positions.

Conclusion

Job analysis is the collection of information relevant to the preparation of job description and job specifications. An overall written summary of the task requirements for a particular job is called a job description, and an overall written summary of the requirements an individual must possess to successfully perform the job is called a job specification. Job analysis information, developed in the form of job descriptions and job specifications, provides the basic foundation for all of the human resources management functions.

Some combinations of available job analysis methods (i.e., observation, interviews, questionnaires, and job performance) should be used because all have advantages and disadvantages. Key considerations regarding the choice of methods include the fit between the method and the purpose, cost, practicality, and an overall judgment concerning the appropriateness of the methods for the situation in question. The primary purpose of conducting job analysis should be described clearly to ensure that all relevant information is collected. In addition, time and cost constraints should be specified before choosing one or more of the available data collection methods.

Human resources managers should follow the following steps when conducting a job analysis: (1) determine purpose, (2) identify jobs to be analyzed, (3) explain the process to employees, (4) collect information, (5) organize the information into job descriptions and job specifications, and (6) review and update information frequently. Job descriptions and job specifications must be valid, accurate, and job related. Otherwise, the organization may face legal repercussions, particularly in the areas of employee selection, promotions, and compensation. The *Uniform Guidelines* and associated court cases provide guidelines for avoiding charges of discrimination in the development of job analysis data.

In today's rapidly changing healthcare environment, managers should consider the potential advantage of future-oriented job analysis approaches when change is more predictable and generic job analysis approaches when change is less predictable. Both are relatively new concepts that may have legal or practical limitations that must be considered before they are fully adopted. Various new approaches to job design are required as healthcare organizations strive to overcome the effects of excessive specialization. Among the most significant of these are job redesign approaches such as the multi-skilled health practitioners, employee empowerment, various team concepts, and work schedule redesign.

Discussion Questions

1. Why should healthcare managers conduct a job analysis? What purpose does it serve?
2. What are job descriptions and job specifications? What is their relationship to job analysis?
3. Which of the five methods of job analysis would you use to collect data for the position of a registered nurse in a large hospital. Why?
4. Describe the steps involved in the job analysis process.
5. How can the existence of a high-quality job analysis make a particular human resources function, such as employee selection, less legally vulnerable?

6. Are healthcare jobs static, or do they change over time? What might cause a job to change over time? What implications does this have for job analysis?

7. Describe and discuss future-oriented job analysis and generic job analysis approaches. How might each be used to help healthcare managers cope with a rapidly changing and competitive environment? What are some potential pitfalls of each approach?

8. What are the advantages and disadvantages of utilization of multiskilled health practitioners?

9. Access information on work teams at www.workteams.unt.edu. What types of work teams are most appropriate for achieving which objectives in the healthcare industry? Cite at least one successful team effort in healthcare.

10. Select one healthcare position with which you are familiar. What work schedule innovations make the most sense for this position? Why?

References

Anthony, W. P., P. L. Perrewe, and K. M. Kacmar. 1993. *Strategic Human Resource Management*. Fort Worth, TX: Dryden.

Ash, R. A. 1988. "Job Analysis in the World of Work." In *The Job Analysis Handbook for Business,* edited by S. Grael, pp. 3–23. New York: Wiley.

Blayney, K. D. (ed.). 1992. *Healing Hands: Customizing Your Health Team for Institutional Survival.* Battle Creek, MI: W. K. Kellogg Foundation.

Bohlander, G. W., and K. M. McCarthy. 1996. "How to Get the Most from Team Training." *National Productivity Review* 20 (3): 25–35.

Capowski, G. 1998. "Telecommuting: The New Frontier." *HR Focus* 75 (4): 2.

Carson, K. P., and G. L. Stewart. 1996. "Job Analysis and the Sociotechnical Approach to Quality: A Critical Explanation." *Journal of Quality Management* 1 (1): 49–56.

Clifford, J. P. 1994. "Job Analysis: Why Do It and How Should It Be Done?" *Public Personnel Management* 23 (3): 321–40.

Conklin, M. 1999. "9 to 5 Isn't Working Anymore." *Business Week* (September 20): 94–8.

Equal Employment Opportunity Commission, Civil Service Commission, Department of Labor, and Department of Justice. 1978. *Uniform Guidelines for Employee Selection Procedures. Federal Register* 43 (166): 38290–315.

Ettore, B. 1997. "The Empowerment Gap: Hope vs. Reality." *HR Focus* 74 (7): 1–6.

Ford, R. C., and M. D. Fottler. 1995. "Empowerment: A Matter of Degree." *Academy of Management Executive* 4 (31): 21–9.

Fottler, M. D. 1992. "The Evolution of Health Manpower Utilization Patterns in Health Services and American Industry: Implications for Implementing the Multiskilled Concept." In *Healing Hands: Customizing Your Health Team for Institutional Survival,* edited by K. D. Blayney, pp. 1–23. Battle Creek, MI: W. K. Kellogg Foundation.

———. 1996. "The Role and Impact of Multiskilled Health Practitioners in the Health Services Industry." *Hospital & Health Services Administration* 41 (1): 55–75.

Garcia, J. 1997. "How's Your Organizational Commitment?" *HR Focus* 74 (1): 22–34.

George, W. 1990. "Internal Marketing and Organizational Behavior: A Partnership in Developing Customer-Conscious Employees at Every Level." *Journal of Business Research* 20 (1): 63–70.

Grant, P. C. 1988. "Why Job Descriptions Don't Work." *Personnel Journal* 67 (1): 53–9.

Hunt, S. T. 1996. "Generic Work Behavior: An Investigation into the Dimensions of Entry-Level Hourly Job Performance." *Personnel Psychology* 49 (1): 51–83.

Lawler, E. E. 1986. *High Involvement Management*. San Francisco: Jossey-Bass.

Mathis, R. L., and J. H. Jackson. 1985. *Personnel/Human Resources Management*. St. Paul, MN: West Publishing.

Mitchell, K. E., G. M. Alliger, and R. Morfopoalos. 1997. "Toward an ADA-Appropriate Job Analysis." *Human Resource Management Review* 7 (1): 5–26.

Nobile, R. J. 1991. "The Law of Performance Appraisals." *Personnel* 35 (1): 1.

Reilly, E. M. 1997. "Telecommuting: Putting Policy into Practice." *HR Focus* 74 (9): 5–6.

Schneider, B., and A. M. Konz. 1989. "Strategic Job Analysis." *Human Resource Management* 28 (1): 51–63.

Simison, R. L. 1999. "Ford Rolls Out New Model of Corporate Culture." *Wall Street Journal* (January 13): A-1.

Snyder, D. 1996. "The Revolution in the Workplace: What's Happening to Our Jobs?" *Futurist* 30: 8.

Thompson, D. E., and T. A. Thompson. 1982. "Court Standards for Job Analysis in Test Validation." *Personnel Psychology* 35: 865–74.

U.S. Census Bureau. 1998. *Statistical Abstract of the United States*. Washington, DC: U. S. Government Printing Office

Vaughan, D. G., M. D. Fottler, R. W. Bamberg, and K. D. Blayney. 1991. "Utilization of Multiskilled Health Practitioners in U.S. Hospitals." *Hospital & Health Services Administration* 36 (3): 397–419.

Appendix A: Example of a Job Description and Performance Development Tool

Reprinted with permission from St. Vincent's Hospital, Birmingham, Alabama. 2001.

Job Title: STAFF NURSE   Department: 6 WEST

Cost Center Number: **6081**

Position Number: 2339/2381/2378   FLSA Status: Non-Exempt   Date Created: 07/01/00

Date Evaluation due:_____

Type of Evaluation: ____ 6 Month ____ Annual ____ Re-Evaluation ____ Pro-Rated Annual Due to Promotion

---

Associate's Name:_____   Employee Number: _____

SECTION I
JOB REQUIREMENTS

JOB SUMMARY

Assumes responsibility and accountability for a group of adult and geriatric/frail elderly medical/surgical patients for a designated time frame and assesses, prescribes, delegates, coordinates and evaluates the nursing care provided. Ensures provision of quality care for selected groups of patients through utilization of the nursing process, established standards of care, policies and procedures and interdisciplinary collaboration. Coordinates the plan of care to be provided by a multidisciplinary team throughout the continuum of care.

SUPERVISION

A. **SUPERVISED BY**:   Charge Nurse, 6 West
B. **SUPERVISES**:   No One
C. **LEADS/GUIDES**:   Unit associates / ancillary associates involved in the delivery of direct patient care or unit operations

JOB SPECIFICATIONS

A. **EDUCATION**
    -Required: Graduate of an accredited school of professional nursing
    -Desired: BSN

B. **EXPERIENCE**
    -Required: None
    -Desired: Previous clinical experience

C. **LICENSES, CERTIFICATIONS AND/OR REGISTRATIONS**: Current R.N. license in the State of Alabama; BLS-HCP prior to the completion of Hospital Education nursing orientation if not already current.

D. **EQUIPMENT/TOOLS/WORK-AIDS**: Medical equipment; computer terminal / printer; facsimile machine; copier; patient charts; personal computer; Pyxis⌐; HBOC Care Manager⌐ computerized documentation system; Dinamap⌐ monitor; Van Slyck⌐ patient classification system; Hill Rom COMposer⌐ system; ARJO⌐ patient lifting devices.

E. **SPECIALIZED KNOWLEDGE & SKILLS**: Must have knowledge of developmental tasks of adult and geriatric/frail elderly medical/surgical patients in all specialty and subspecialty categories, urgent and non-urgent in nature and be able to apply

6 West   Staff Nurse

knowledge in assessment and planning of patient care. Must possess excellent analytical and critical thinking skills in order to analyze data and behavior to develop and implement an appropriate plan of care. Desired operational knowledge of Windows] software and HBOC Pathways Care Manager] software.

F.   **PERSONAL TRAITS, QUALITIES, & APTITUDES:** Demonstrates personal traits / behavior consistent with the Core Values of St. Vincent's Hospital. Must be self-directed / self-motivated; must have good communication and interpersonal skills; must be flexible; must have good critical thinking / decision making skills and must have good understanding of systems and change processes. Must be able to: (1) perform a variety of duties often changing from one task to another of a different nature without loss of efficiency or composure; (2) accept responsibility for the direction, control and planning of an activity; (3) make evaluations and decision based on measurable or verifiable criteria: (4) work independently; (5) recognize the rights and responsibilities of patient confidentiality; (6) convey empathy and compassion to those experiencing pain, physical or emotional distress and/or grief; (7) relate to others in a manner which creates a sense of teamwork and cooperation; (8) communicate effectively with people from every socioeconomic, cultural and educational background; (9) exhibit flexibility and cope effectively in an ever-changing, fast-paced healthcare environment; (10) perform effectively when confronted with emergency, critical, unusual and/or dangerous situations; (11) demonstrate the quality work ethic of doing the right thing the right way; and (12) maintain a customer focus and strive to satisfy the customer's perceived needs.

G.   The 6 WEST STAFF NURSE will demonstrate the knowledge and skill necessary to provide care and services as defined in the job responsibilities and performance standards in this job description for the following AGE SPECIFIC PATIENT GROUPS:

☐	**Neonate**	**Birth to 1 Month**
☐	**Infant**	**2 months to 12 months**
☐	**Pediatric**	**1 Year to 12 Years**
☐	**Young Adult**	**13 – 17 Years**
☒	**Adult**	**18 – 64 Years**
☒	**Geriatric/Frail Elderly**	**65 Years and older**

H.   **WORKING CONDITIONS:** Primarily inside environment; usually protected from the weather but not necessarily temperature changes. Subject to frequent exposure to infection, contagious disease, combative patients, potentially hazardous materials and equipment. Variable noise levels. Also subject to rapid pace, multiple stimuli, unpredictable environment and critical situations. Frequent viewing of a video display terminal.   Occasional exposure to the outside environment and the weather.

I.   **PHYSICAL DEMANDS/TRAITS:** Must be able to: (1) perceive the nature of sounds by the ear; (2) express or exchange ideas by means of the spoken word; (3) perceive characteristics of objects through the eyes; (4) extend arms and hands in any direction; (5) seize, hold, grasp, turn or otherwise work with hands; (6) pick, pinch or otherwise work with fingers; (7) perceive such attributes of objects or materials as size, shape, temperature or texture; and (8) stoop, kneel, crouch and crawl. Must be able to lift 50 lbs. maximum with frequent lifting, carrying, pushing, pulling of objects weighing up to 25 lbs. Continuous walking and standing. Must be able to identify, match and distinguish colors. Physically able to comply with universal precautions and specific job duties in the specific care environment.

SECTION II
JOB RESPONSIBILITIES AND PERFORMANCE STANDARDS

PERFORMANCE RATING DEFINITIONS:

❖	**ROLE MODEL**	The associate's job performance and/or behavior can be held up as an example to others to follow.
❖	**COMMENDABLE**	This associate's job performance and/or behavior meets the high standards set by this organization.
❖	**UNACCEPTABLE**	This associate's job performance and/or behavior consistently fails to meet the standards required by this organization.

Note: Comments are required only for "Role Model" and "Unacceptable" ratings. Any overall ratings of "unacceptable" require the review & signature of the evaluator's immediate supervisor.

---

1. A SUCCESSFUL 6 WEST STAFF NURSE DEMONSTRATES THE ABILITY TO ASSESS ADULT AND GERIATRIC/FRAIL ELDERLY MEDICAL/SURGICAL PATIENTS' PHYSIOLOGICAL, PSYCHOSOCIAL, ENVIRONMENTAL AND SPIRITUAL NEEDS.	WT **10** x _____ % Achieved = _____ Points
– Completes the nursing admission assessment (including the history and physical assessment) and determines	SELF _____ LEADER

6 West   Staff Nurse

the patient's nursing needs within the specified time frame (NSP, B-102.5 and B-108.0) to serve as the baseline for the development of the patient's plan of care. – Monitors and interprets vital functions and clinical findings and correlates with patient condition. – Performs ongoing reassessments of the affected system(s) which are identified on admission or following a significant change in the patient's condition or diagnosis each shift to determine the patient's response to treatment and makes modifications in the plan of care, as appropriate. – Includes considerations of biophysical, psychosocial, spiritual, environmental, pain level, self-care, educational and discharge planning factors in the admission assessment and ongoing reassessments, as indicated. – Assesses the patient's continuing care needs in preparation for discharge and makes referrals for such care/interventions, as appropriate. – Assesses the patient's potential for skin breakdown and risk/safety concerns on admission and each shift. – Assesses the patient's pain level utilizing the numeric pain scale, demonstrating knowledge of pain management principles.	☐ Role Model ☐ ☐ Commendable ☐ ☐ Unacceptable ☐
2. A SUCCESSFUL 6 WEST STAFF NURSE ASSESSES THE NEEDS OF THE UNIT. – Makes sound, appropriate recommendations regarding unit policies, procedures and standards of care. – Assesses unit needs regarding drugs, supplies and equipment and provides input into budget preparation. – Is thoroughly familiar with unit standards of care. – Notifies the Charge Nurse of any problems with equipment/computer functioning and/or lack of availability of necessary supplies/equipment.	WT **5** x ____ % Achieved = ____ Points SELF LEADER ☐ Role Model ☐ ☐ Commendable ☐ ☐ Unacceptable ☐

3.   A SUCCESSFUL 6 WEST STAFF NURSE DEMONSTRATES THE ABILITY TO PLAN PATIENT CARE ACCORDING TO INDIVIDUAL, AGE-SPECIFIC PATIENT NEEDS AND ESTABLISHED STANDARDS OF CARE AND PRACTICE.
– Performs daily batch reporting for charge transactions; maintains and updates all charges in the system as they occur.
– Develops a documented, individualized plan of care evolving from needs identified on admission for the patient within the specified time frame to serve as the basis for the provision of nursing care. (Refer to NSP, B-102.5 and B-108.0)
– Integrates the information generated through the analysis of the assessment data to identify and prioritize the patient's need for treatment.
– Collaborates, as appropriate, with physicians and other clinical disciplines in making decisions regarding each patient's need for nursing care.
– Includes identified discharge and educational needs in the plan of care.
– Involves the patient and/or significant other in the patient's care, as appropriate.
– Demonstrates knowledge of the current condition as well as changes which have occurred in the past 24 hours and the plan of care for each patient.
– Reviews the multidisciplinary plan of care each shift and communicates with the RN assuming responsibility for patient management on the next shift to insure that outstanding interventions are accomplished, thereby promoting continuity of care.
– Assigns responsibility for the provision of various aspects of care which is reflective of the complexity of nursing care required and the competence of available staff; considers the following in making / revising patient care assignments:
   • The patient's status.
   • The environment in which nursing care is provided.
   • The competence of the nursing staff members who are to provide the care.
   • The degree of supervision required by and available to the associates.
   • The complexity of the assessment required by the patient.
   • The type of technology employed in providing nursing care.
   • Relevant infection control and safety issues.
	WT **10** x ____ % Achieved = ____ Points
	
	SELF LEADER
	☐ Role Model ☐
	☐ Commendable ☐
	☐ Unacceptable ☐

6 West   Staff Nurse

4. A SUCCESSFUL 6 WEST STAFF NURSE INTERVENES AS GUIDED BY THE PLAN OF CARE TO IMPLEMENT NURSING ACTIONS THAT PROMOTE, MAINTAIN, OR RESTORE PHYSICAL AND MENTAL HEALTH, PREVENT ILLNESS AND EFFECT REHABILITATION. – Provides compassionate nursing care with special attention to comfort and well-being of the patient, and his family/SO, acknowledging psychological and spiritual needs. – Bases patient care/treatment decisions on identified patient needs and treatment priorities. – Provides nursing care consistent with the therapies of other disciplines. – Demonstrates the necessary skill and knowledge to provide care for adult and geriatric/frail elderly patients in accordance with the Nursing Department and unit specific skills/competencies to contribute to positive patient outcomes. – Performs procedures/treatments in a timely manner and in accordance with physician orders and nursing policies and procedures. – Makes adequate preparation for patient admissions and discharges and for performance of procedures and/or treatments. – Functions promptly and effectively in codes, emergencies or other stressful patient situations. – Determines appropriate acuity level based on the care provided to the patient/SO. – Coordinates patient and family education, and the discharge process to promote continuity of care and optimal patient outcomes. – Demonstrates expertise in the referral process and use of community resources. – Practices safe nursing care daily in accordance with the Alabama Board of Nursing Nurse Practice Act. – Demonstrates knowledge of pain management principles in the delivery of patient care.	WT **10** x _____ % Achieved = _____ Points SELF ___ Role Model ___ LEADER ☐ Role Model ☐ ☐ Commendable ☐ ☐ Unacceptable ☐
5. A SUCCESSFUL 6 WEST STAFF NURSE DEMONSTRATES KNOWLEDGE OF DISCHARGE PLANNING, REHABILITATION MEASURES, AND COMMUNITY RESOURCES BY MAKING APPROPRIATE AND TIMELY REFERRALS TO PROMOTE CONTINUITY OF CARE AND OPTIMAL OUTCOMES FOR ADULT AND GERIATRIC/FRAIL ELDERLY MEDICAL/SURGICAL PATIENTS. – Analyzes system performance and gets appropriate personnel involved if necessary. – Completes the admission discharge screening assessment and reassessment and identifies potential / actual problems and needs. – Provides leadership and guidance to the multidisciplinary team in formulating and implementing an individualized plan of care for patients who require complex care management. – Assesses patient needs for discharge teaching and/or referral. – Participates in multidisciplinary team conferences to address specific patient's care management. – Demonstrates appropriate use of clinical resources such as case management nurse, dietician, social worker, clinical pharmacist, and home healthcare nurse; demonstrates collaboration and coordination with these resources in the planning / provision of patient care. – Initiates discharge teaching following the initial assessment. – Communicates by documenting in the chart and verbally with the multidisciplinary team to coordinate interventions and insure continuity of care. – Educates patients about accessing the health care system and their responsibilities. – Utilizes community resources to foster wellness, promote prevention of disease, and maximize care during acute, rehabilitative, and terminal stages of illness.	WT **10** x _____ % Achieved = _____ Points SELF ___ LEADER ☐ Role Model ☐ ☐ Commendable ☐ ☐ Unacceptable ☐
6. THE SUCCESSFUL 6 WEST STAFF NURSE DEMONSTRATES KNOWLEDGE AND UNDERSTANDING OF THE TEACHING / LEARNING PROCESS AND IMPLEMENTS PATIENT TEACHING TO MEET LEARNING NEEDS OF THE ADULT AND GERIATRIC/FRAIL ELDERLY MEDICAL/SURGICAL PATIENT/ SO AND PROMOTE OPTIMAL PATIENT OUTCOMES. – Stays current in new technology that may affect the system, its users and the hospital. – Identifies educational needs of patients at the time of admission. – Involves the patient / SO in setting learning goals. – Provides appropriate information, explanation, and in-depth teaching to the patient / SO. – Documents teaching and the patient's response. – Utilizes available educational resources (e.g., written materials, videos, patient education T.V. channel, Krames®, and/or Document Manager®) as components of the patient education process.	WT **10** x _____ % Achieved = _____ Points SELF ___ LEADER ☐ Role Model ☐ ☐ Commendable ☐ ☐ Unacceptable ☐
7. A SUCCESSFUL 6 WEST STAFF NURSE DEMONSTRATES KNOWLEDGE OF MEDICATIONS, ADMINISTRATION TO ADULT AND GERIATRIC/FRAIL ELDERLY MEDICAL PATIENTS, AND THOROUGHLY DOCUMENTS THE ADMINISTRATION OF MEDICATIONS. – Administers medications in accordance with hospital policies. – Demonstrates knowledge of normal dosages, actions and interactions with foods and other drugs, side effects and routes of administration. – Questions unusual dosages or routes of administration of medications.	WT **5** x _____ % Achieved = _____ Points SELF ___ LEADER ☐ Role Model ☐ ☐ Commendable ☐ ☐ Unacceptable ☐

6 West   Staff Nurse

– Withholds medications and notifies the physician when the patient's condition indicates that the medication may be harmful. – Documents the response for PRN medication administration. – Documents the administration of all medication on the Medication Administration Record and nurses notes, when indicated, to include time, date; site, when indicated; response, when indicated; and initials of person administering the drug. – Completes any appropriate follow-up documentation related to medication administration / events. – Demonstrates knowledge and practices patient focused pain management with regard to medication administration.	
8. A SUCCESSFUL 6 WEST STAFF NURSE DEMONSTRATES KNOWLEDGE OF INTRAVASCULAR FLUID AND BLOOD / BLOOD COMPONENT THERAPY, ADMINISTRATION TO ADULT AND GERIATRIC/FRAIL ELDERLY MEDICAL/SURGICAL PATIENTS, AND THOROUGHLY DOCUMENTS THE ADMINISTRATION OF INTRAVASCULAR FLUIDS / BLOOD / BLOOD COMPONENTS. – Administers intravascular fluid and blood / blood component therapy in accordance with hospital policies. – Demonstrates knowledge of fluid therapy administration. – Documents the administration of all types of intravascular therapy, to include site, condition of site, dressing and tubing changes, etc. – Demonstrates appropriate knowledge and management of vascular access devices. – Maintains the I.V. tubing and site in accordance with hospital policy; properly labels the I.V. bag.	WT **5** x _____ % Achieved = _____ Points SELF LEADER ☐ Role Model ☐ ☐ Commendable ☐ ☐ Unacceptable ☐
9. A SUCCESSFUL 6 WEST STAFF NURSE EVALUATES AND MODIFIES THE PLAN OF CARE BASED ON OBSERVABLE RESPONSES OF THE ADULT AND GERIATRIC/FRAIL ELDERLY MEDICAL/SURGICAL PATIENT, AND ATTAINMENT OF PATIENT OUTCOMES. – Makes rounds and assesses patients every two hours or more frequently if needed. – Documents the patient's pain scale rating following each pain management intervention. – Evaluates the effectiveness of care provided by the non-RN staff to achieve desired patient outcomes. – Assesses the effectiveness of medications administered to the patient each shift. – Assesses the effectiveness of comfort measures (including all PRN medications given) within at least 1 hour of the intervention. – Evaluates the patient's response to all procedures carried out both on a physical and psychological basis. – Assesses the patient's psychological response to hospitalization and diagnosis. – Evaluates the patient's / SO response to teaching / discharge planning. – Evaluates the patient's response to treatment (nursing care and/or medical orders). – Evaluates that the patient is properly positioned according to condition. – Evaluates that the drainage tubing and bag are patent, connected and positioned for maximal drainage and prevention of stasis, when applicable. – Evaluates that the equipment necessary for care of the patient is properly placed (e.g., personal articles, call light, O2, suction, etc.).	WT **10** x _____ % Achieved = _____ Points SELF LEADER ☐ Role Model ☐ ☐ Commendable ☐ ☐ Unacceptable ☐

10. THE SUCCESSFUL 6 WEST STAFF NURSE UNDERSTANDS THE IMPORTANCE OF AND PROMOTES THE MAINTENANCE OF A SAFE CLINICAL ENVIRONMENT FOR ADULT AND GERIATRIC/FRAIL ELDERLY MEDICAL/SURGICAL PATIENTS, AND STAFF.
 – Delivers care in accordance with policies and procedures regarding:
    • Patient safety.
    • Assistive devices.
    • Smoking.
    • Code Blue; Code 66; Code Pink; Code Yellow; Code Green; Code Orange.
    • Contingency plans (e.g., fire, disaster, bomb threats, hazardous weather, etc.).
    • Use of equipment and reporting of any malfunctioning equipment.
    • Electrical safety.
    • Obtaining, administering and maintaining inventory of narcotics.
    • Crash cart and defibrillator routine checks.
    • Disposal of needles and syringes.
    • Infection control.
    • Reportable incidents / accidents / events.
    • Use of restraints / protective measures.
    • Visitor control.
    • 7 plans related to the JCAHO Environment of Care standards.
    • Refrigerator temperature monitoring.
    • Infant security.
 – Maintains a clean and orderly patient and work environment at all times.
	WT **5** x _____ % Achieved =
	 _____ Points
	
	 SELF LEADER
	 ☐ Role Model ☐
	 ☐ Commendable ☐
	 ☐ Unacceptable ☐

6 West   Staff Nurse

11. A SUCCESSFUL 6 WEST STAFF NURSE FACILITATES AN EFFECTIVE COMMUNICATION PROCESS.
– Maintains a communication pattern that promotes collegiality among the associates within the unit.
– Identifies self and clarifies role to patient, family, staff, physicians, students, and other disciplines.
– Recognizes and responds appropriately to verbal and non-verbal cues.
– Communicates effectively with all members of the health care team in a timely manner by:
   • defending and supporting peer decision and actions;
   • asserting self with tact;
   • supporting collaboration;
   • maintaining open communication;
   • offering suggestions and criticisms constructively;
   • asking questions and sharing information during patient rounds and conferences;
   • using appropriate chain of command.
– Relates complete and pertinent information in verbal and written communication.
– Initiates and maintains open and effective communication with physicians, the multidisciplinary team members and other department associates as evidenced by improved patient outcomes.
– Demonstrates knowledge of new / revised hospital, department, and nursing policies.
– Demonstrates appropriate communication skills by sharing, clarifying, reflecting and interpreting.
– Communicates with the patient / family to elicit essential information with accuracy and timeliness to ensure safe patient care.
– Acts as a liaison to the patient / SO by providing accurate and timely information to ensure patient / SO participation in care.
– Verbalizes where patients are and the reason for their being off the unit or away from their room.
– Supports continuity of care through appropriate communication with other health care team members and physicians, especially during transfer / shift reports; shares accurate data / information gathered to includes patient condition, care to be given, patient response to care received, and any follow-up needed.
– Serves as a shift leader in the absence of the Charge Nurse, when requested.
	WT **10** x _____ % Achieved = _____ Points
	
	SELF LEADER
	☐ Role Model ☐
	☐ Commendable ☐
	☐ Unacceptable ☐

12. A SUCCESSFUL 6 WEST STAFF NURSE DEMONSTRATES UNDERSTANDING OF PATIENT RIGHTS AND DELIVERS CARE IN ACCORDANCE WITH POLICIES AND PROCEDURES REGARDING : – Patient confidentiality. – Organ / tissue donation. – Advance directives. – Informed consent. – Personal privacy. – Patient values and beliefs. – Resolution of patient complaints / dissatisfaction. – Addressing ethical issues. – Patient identification. – Restraints.	WT **10** x _____ % Achieved = _____ Points SELF LEADER ☐ Role Model ☐ ☐ Commendable ☐ ☐ Unacceptable ☐

6 West   Staff Nurse

SECTION III
KEY BEHAVIORS

A. MISSION, ETHICS, VALUES DRIVEN	WT 15 x _____ % Achieved =
Demonstrates the vision, mission, and philosophy of Ascension Health by showing a commitment to and actively displaying the core values through words and actions. *	_____ Points
	SELF LEADER
Understands the mission and exhibits compassion and service to all persons with special attention to those who are	☐ Role Model ☐
	☐ Commendable ☐
poor.	☐ Unacceptable ☐
Demonstrates reverence by showing respect for each individual and self.	
Demonstrates truth, honesty, and integrity in actions at all times.	
Demonstrates wisdom in providing high quality, cost-effective, compassionate care through the responsible use of	
talents and resources.	
Demonstrates commitment to continuous learning, creativity and innovation.	
Demonstrates dedication to spiritually centered, holistic care of all persons.	
Acts ethically in all interactions.	
Maintains, at all times, the confidentiality of information.	
Respects the principles and ethical teachings of the Catholic Church relative to health care issues.	
Treats people fairly and confronts prejudice and intolerant behavior.	
*For detailed discussion on living the core values at St. Vincent's, refer to the hospital publication **Our Core Values** available from Mission Services, Pastoral Care, and Leadership.	
B. CUSTOMER ORIENTED	WT 20 x _____ % Achieved =
	_____ Points
Consistently meets the Service Excellence standards.	SELF LEADER
Meets the needs or exceeds the expectations of our patients, physicians, associates, and others we serve.	☐ Role Model ☐
	☐ Commendable ☐
Builds loyal relationships based on communication and trust.	☐ Unacceptable ☐
Relates to all customers in a friendly, accommodating, respectful manner that creates good will.	
Seeks feedback about performance from customers and responds appropriately.	
C. ACCOUNTABLE	WT 15 x _____ % Achieved =
	_____ Points
Sets high personal standards of performance and accepts responsibility and accountability for all actions.	SELF LEADER
Demonstrates good judgment; recognizes and reports errors made in the course of one's performance.	☐ Role Model ☐
	☐ Commendable ☐
Accepts responsibility for "owning and solving" problems rather than "placing blame."	☐ Unacceptable ☐
Adheres to hospital/department policies and procedures.	
Makes effective use of time; reports to work on time and avoids unnecessary overtime; prioritizes work and achieves good results.	

6 West   Staff Nurse

D. COMMITTED TO PERFORMANCE IMPROVEMENT FOR POSITIVE CHANGE Looks for ways to continually improve processes in order to positively affect outcomes Customer satisfaction, clinical, financial, etc.). Demonstrates the quality work ethic of "doing the right thing in the right way." Is flexible and responsive to change. Appropriately challenges the way things have always been done. Approaches all situations with curiosity and open-mindedness in order to bring about positive change/improvements. Addresses problems early before they get out of hand.	WT 15 x _____ % Achieved = _____ Points SELF LEADER ☐ Role Model ☐ ☐ Commendable ☐ ☐ Unacceptable ☐
E. TEAM PLAYER Interacts with people openly, directly, tactfully and cooperatively; accepts criticism and is not defensive. Considers the impact of decisions on others and involves them. Shares information and resources with others. Works effectively with others to achieve a desired result' is patient; uses humor. Knows and utilizes appropriate channels of communication and chain of command. Listens carefully to others encourages them to express thier views and values their contribution.	WT 15 x _____ % Achieved = _____ Points SELF LEADER ☐ Role Model ☐ ☐ Commendable ☐ ☐ Unacceptable ☐
F. CONTINUOUS LEARNER Meets all mandatory education requirements with the specified timeframe. Assumes responsibility for personal and career development. Seeks opportunities for cross-training and new skill development.	WT 5 x _____ % Achieved = _____ Points SELF LEADER ☐ Role Model ☐ ☐ Commendable ☐ ☐ Unacceptable ☐
G. SAFETY MINDED Assumes responsibility for preventing incidents that could lead to injury. Promptly reports unsafe conditions that require actions from others. Promptly reports incidents and completes paperwork. Consistantly utilizes equipment properly.	WT 15 x _____ % Achieved = _____ Points SELF LEADER ☐ Role Model ☐ ☐ Commendable ☐ ☐ Unacceptable ☐

SECTION IV
GOALS AND OBJECTIVES

GOAL CATEGORIES:

A	**Voice for the Voiceless**
B	**Clinical Excellence**
C	**Well-Run Organization**
D	**Work–Life Community**
E	**Innovation**
F	**Other**

1. Category : A B C D E F (circle one)	WT _____ x _____ % Achieved = _____ Points SELF LEADER ☐ Role Model ☐ ☐ Commendable ☐ ☐ Unacceptable ☐
2. Category : A B C D E F (circle one)	WT _____ x _____ % Achieved =

6 West   Staff Nurse

	_____ Points
	SELF LEADER
	☐ Role Model ☐
	☐ Commendable ☐
	☐ Unacceptable ☐

3.   Category :   A   B   C   D   E   F   (circle one)

WT _____ x _____ % Achieved =
_____ Points
SELF   LEADER
☐   Role Model   ☐
☐   Commendable   ☐
☐   Unacceptable   ☐

4.   Category :   A   B   C   D   E   F   (circle one)

WT _____ x _____ % Achieved =
_____ Points
SELF   LEADER
☐   Role Model   ☐
☐   Commendable   ☐
☐   Unacceptable   ☐

5.   Category :   A   B   C   D   E   F   (circle one)

WT _____ x _____ % Achieved =
_____ Points
SELF   LEADER
☐   Role Model   ☐
☐   Commendable   ☐
☐   Unacceptable   ☐

6.   Category :   A   B   C   D   E   F   (circle one)

WT _____ x _____ % Achieved =
_____ Points
SELF   LEADER
☐   Role Model   ☐
☐   Commendable   ☐
☐   Unacceptable   ☐

ASSOCIATE'S OVERALL RATING

SECTION II	JOB RESPONSIBILITIES & PERFORMANCE STANDARDS	_____ %
SECTION III	KEY BEHAVIORS	_____ %
SECTION IV	GOALS AND OBJECTIVES	_____ %

ASSOCIATE COMMENTS:

6 West   Staff Nurse

EVALUATOR'S COACHING COMMENTS:

ACTION TAKEN:
____ None required – 6 month evaluation
____ Associate's Overall Rating in each section met or exceeded standards.
____ Placed on probation for 90 days due to "Unacceptable" rating in Section _____.
____ Probation begins _____ and continues until re-evaluation on _____.
____ **A Career Development form was completed by the associate, reviewed by me and forwarded to Personnel at some point earlier this year, or one is attached to this evaluation.**

RE-EVALUATION:

____ Termination of associate is recommended (Termination form attached).

____ Probationary status cleared.

---

*The associate's signature is required to indicate the evaluation has been reviewed prior to becoming part of the associate's personnel record. The associate's signature does not indicate agreement with the contents of the evaluation.

EVALUATOR:_____
                    (signature)   (title)   (date)

REVIEWER:_____
                    (signature)   (title)   (date)

ASSOCIATE:_____
                    (signature)   (title)   (date)

PERSONNEL:_____
                    (signature)   (title)   (date)

June 2001 6 West RN Job Description.doc

CHAPTER 6

RECRUITMENT AND SELECTION

Bruce J. Fried, Ph.D.

Learning Objectives

After completing this chapter, the reader should be able to:

- Understand the major decisions involved in designing and implementing a recruitment effort
- Describe the factors an individual considers when choosing to accept a job offer
- Design a recruitment effort for a particular job
- Discuss the advantages and disadvantages of internal and external recruitment
- Understand the concept of organizational fit and its relevance to recruitment and selection
- Discuss alternative selection tools and how they should be used in the selection process
- Understand the concept of validity in the use of selection tools

Introduction

In this chapter, attention turns to the processes of recruitment and selection. These processes are integrally related not only with each other but with other human resources management functions. For example, the development and stringency of criteria for selecting job applicants depends to a large degree on the success of the recruitment effort. An organization can be more selective when a relatively large supply of qualified applicants is available. Similarly, developing a recruitment plan for a particular position depends on the availability of an accurate, current, and comprehensive job description. As with human resources management functions, an organization must be cognizant of legal considerations when developing recruitment and selection procedures, and each of these functions must be addressed from both strategic and operational perspectives.

Recruitment and selection are key to employee retention. An important measure of the effectiveness of these functions is the extent to which the organization is able to attract committed employees who remain with the organization. While these functions are highly interdependent, for purposes of discussion, we address them separately and sequentially in this book.

In this chapter, we describe the most important steps involved in employee recruitment, define reliability and validity and their role in selection decisions, and enumerate the various elements of a selection interview and give guidelines on how to make selection interviews more valid and reliable.

Recruitment

Recruitment refers to the various processes an organization implements to attract a sufficient number of qualified individuals on a timely basis and to encourage them to apply for jobs in the organization

Recruitment refers to the various processes an organization implements to attract a sufficient number of qualified individuals on a timely basis and to encourage them to apply for jobs in the organization. When we think of recruitment strategies, our attention usually focuses on what the organization needs to do to recruit candidates. The organization has to consider a number of questions in developing recruitment strategies, including:

- Should the organization recruit and promote from within or should it focus on recruiting external applicants?
- Should the organization consider alternative approaches to filling jobs with full-time employees, such as outsourcing, flexible staffing, and hiring of part-time workers?
- How much emphasis should the organization give to finding applicants with precisely the right technical qualifications, rather than finding applicants who best fit the culture of the organization and utilizing training to improve their technical skills?

Prior to exploring these and other questions, we first explore recruitment from the perspective of potential employees. What factors influence an individual's decision to apply for and accept employment with a particular organization? An understanding of these factors is important because potential employees are actually the *customers* of the recruitment effort, and, as customers, an understanding of their needs and expectations is key to developing effective recruitment strategies.

Factors That Influence Job Choice

People consider a variety of factors when choosing to accept employment with an organization. While considerable research has been done on job choice (Schwab, Rynes, and Aldag 1987), the most important factors that affect job choice decisions are difficult to generalize. The relative importance of these factors varies depending on the individual, the job, and environmental factors such as the level of unemployment. The factors considered by a family physician to accept employment with a rural health center may be quite different from the factors that affect a nurse's decision to accept employment with an urban teaching hospital. One's life stage may also affect the salience of different factors in job choice decisions.

Although the relative importance of job choice factors does vary, understanding these factors is important so that they may be considered when developing recruitment strategies. A convenient way to think about the characteristics that affect job choice is to distinguish between vacancy characteristics and individual characteristics. **Vacancy characteristics** are those factors associated with the job, such as compensation, challenge and responsibility, advancement opportunities, job security, geographic location, and employee benefits. **Individual characteristics**, on the other hand, refer to personal circumstances or situations, such as family situation, age, and career status, that can change over time. The level of *compensation* is often considered, on face value, as a key element in an individual's decision to accept a position with an organization. The role of compensation, however, should not be overemphasized because even a relatively generous level of compensation can be outweighed by the presence or absence of other important factors, which are explained below.

The *challenge and responsibility* inherent in a particular job are frequently cited as important factors in an individual's job choice. This theory is likely even more salient in healthcare organizations where individuals with professional training seek out positions that maximize use of their professional knowledge and skills. Similarly, applicants may seek out jobs with substantial *advancement opportunities;* again, these types of opportunities are likely to be particularly important determinants of job choice for professionally trained individuals as well as individuals in management roles (London and Stumpf 1982). Advancement opportunities in healthcare are traditionally limited for clinically or technically trained individuals, given that in healthcare the only avenue to advancement frequently requires that the individual assume supervisory or management responsibilities. For many people, taking on these new responsibilities may lead to a loss of at least part of their professional identity. In healthcare and other industries, dual career-path systems have been established to enable highly talented clinicians to "move up" while not forcing them to abandon their clinical interests and expertise. Such systems provide specialists who are interested in pursuing a technical career with alternative career paths, other than that of management, while maintaining an adequate pool of talent within the organization in clinical and technical areas (Roth 1982).

Job security is clearly an important determinant of job choice. The current healthcare and general business environment is characterized by an unprecedented number of mergers and acquisitions, which lead to frequent

Vacancy characteristics are those factors associated with the job, such as compensation, challenge and responsibility, advancement opportunities, job security, geographic location, and employee benefits

Individual characteristics refer to personal circumstances or situations, such as family situation, age, and career status, that can change over time

downsizing and worker displacement. While this phenomenon was once limited largely to blue collar workers, professionals and employees in middle and senior management are clearly at risk in the current environment. An illustrative manifestation of the importance of job security is the current environment in union organizing and collective bargaining. Not too long ago, compensation and benefits were the most highly valued issues in labor relations; however, job security and restrictions on outsourcing have gained increasing importance in employees' decision to unionize (Caudron 1995). In fact, in many situations, unionized employees have made wage concessions in return for higher levels of job security (Henderson 1986).

Geographic location, along with other lifestyle concerns, is becoming increasingly important to individuals in job choice decisions. This issue is particularly acute for individuals in dual wage-earner families, where the employment of a spouse may be a significant determinant of job acceptance. In the healthcare environment, the issue becomes particularly acute when organizations attempt to recruit individuals to work in less desirable locations. The level and type of *employee benefits* continues to grow as an important determinant of job acceptance. Particularly in highly competitive industries, many companies have moved beyond providing traditional benefits, such as health insurance and vacation pay, into adopting more innovative approaches.

How do individual job applicants assess the relative importance of different features of a job? The reality is that individuals vary in the way they view the salience or importance of certain job features. Consider the three applicants depicted in Table 6.1. While the example oversimplifies the job choice process, it illustrates how different individuals value different aspects of the job depending on personal preferences and life circumstances. The first column provides a very brief description of each individual on the job market; the second column describes each individual's minimum standards for job acceptance along four dimensions: (1) pay, (2) benefits, (3) advancement opportunities, and (4) travel requirements. These minimum standards are sometimes referred to as **noncompensatory standards**, which are employee demands that have to be met because no other factor in the job can compensate for their lack. Thus, for Person 3, if a job requires substantial travel, then he or she cannot accept the job because it does not meet his or her noncompensatory standard of limited travelling. Similarly, for Person 2, at least 50 percent health insurance coverage is an absolute noncompensatory requirement for job acceptance. For Person 3, note that advancement opportunities are not a noncompensatory standard. The third column of the table includes very brief descriptions of each of the four dimensions.

Noncompensatory standards are employee demands that have to be met because no other factor in the job can compensate for their lack

This type of standard analysis is useful because it provides a way of narrowing down job choices. Assuming a job applicant has several job prospects that meet minimum requirements, he or she can engage in a more refined job choice process that allows for compensatory relationships among other job

TABLE 6.1

Three Hypothetical Job Applicants

Description of Person	Minimum Standards for Job Acceptance	Job Description
Person 1: Single	*Pay:* at least $40,000 *Benefits:* Health insurance covered at least 25% *Advancement Opportunities:* Very important *Travel Requirements:* Unimportant	*Job Title:* Insurance Company Provider Relations Coordinator *Pay:* $45,000 *Benefits:* Health insurance covered at 50% *Advancement Opportunities:* Recruitment done internally and externally *Travel Requirements:* Average 25% travel
Person 2: Sole wage earner for large family	*Pay:* at least $50,000 *Benefits:* Health insurance covered at least 50% *Advancement Opportunities:* Very important *Travel Requirements:* Cannot travel more than 25% of time	*Job Title:* Healthcare Consultant *Pay:* $55,000 *Benefits:* Health insurance covered at 50% *Advancement Opportunities:* Strong history of promotions within one year *Travel Requirements:* Average 50% travel
Person 3: Spouse of high-wage earner	*Pay:* at least $35,000 *Benefits:* Unimportant *Advancement Opportunities:* Unimportant *Travel Requirements:* Cannot travel more than 1 week per year	*Job Title:* Research Assistant in Academic Medical Center *Pay:* $37,000 *Benefits:* Health insurance covered at 50% *Advancement Opportunities:* Generally hires externally for higher-level positions *Travel Requirements:* Little or none

factors (Barber et al. 1994)—that is, using less important job choice factors, an individual can trade off one job dimension for another.

The Recruitment Process

The recruitment process uses as a foundation the organization's human resources plan. A human resources plan includes specific information such as the strategies being pursued by the organization, the types of individuals required to achieve organizational goals, an approach to how recruitment and hiring will be done, and a clear statement about how the human resources practices support the goals of the organization.

Those involved in recruitment and selection must have a thorough understanding of the nature and requirements of the position. A key step in the recruitment process naturally begins with a job analysis in which, at a minimum, the following questions are addressed:

- What are the tasks required for the job?
- What skills and knowledge are required?
- What qualifications are required of job applicants?

In addition to job-related information, the recruitment process also requires information about past recruitment efforts for this and similar positions. Is this a job that will require an international search or will the local labor market suffice? Optimally, a *human resources information system (HRIS)* will provide useful information in the recruitment process. While the sophistication of HRISs varies between organizations, many HRISs include some or all of the information described in Table 6.2, including an inventory of employee skills and knowledge. A *skills inventory* maintains information on every employee's skills, educational background, work history, and other important factors. This inventory can be very useful in identifying internal employees who have the attributes needed for a particular job.

Recruitment can be a very costly process, and information on cost is essential. In recruiting and hiring a new employee, organizations may incur

TABLE 6.2
Human
Resource
Information
System:
Recruitment
Data

HRIS Data	Uses in Recruitment
Skills and Knowledge Inventory	Identifies potential internal job candidates
Recruitment Source Information: • Yield ratios • Cost • Cost per applicant • Cost per hire	Helps analyze cost effectiveness of recruitment sources
Employee Performance Information	Provides information on the success of recruitment sources used in the past

a number of replacement costs. These costs, according to Fitz-Enz (1995), include:

- Source costs such as advertising and agency fees and referral bonuses
- Staff time cost for individuals involved in the recruitment and selection process
- Processing costs, including security checks, data entry, employment tests, medical exams, drug screening, orientation, and employment record verification
- Travel and relocation costs

Replacement costs vary, but a cost analysis does point to the importance of selecting cost-effective recruitment methods. Again, a good HRIS and cost-accounting system can help the organization to understand the major costs associated with recruitment and selection.

An early stage of recruitment also involves an assessment of the external environment, in particular the supply of potential job applicants and the relative competitiveness for a particular position. This analysis should also include an assessment of the compensation and benefits given to individuals who hold similar jobs in competing organizations. It may also include an assessment of external recruitment sources such as colleges, other organizations, and professional associations. This assessment should include information on past success with these external recruitment sources as well as information about logistical and timing concerns for particular professional groups; for example, certain positions may be easier to recruit for at particular times of year.

An initial question in the recruitment process is whether to recruit from within the organization through promotion or transfer or to seek applicants from outside the organization. Table 6.3 provides a summary of the advantages and disadvantages of internal and external recruitment. On the positive side of internal recruitment, internal applicants are generally a known entity; the organization has information about the applicant's past performance and future potential, so, basically, the organization knows what to expect. Internal applicants also tend to know the specific processes and procedures of the organization and may not require as much training and start-up time. However, recruiting from within may be viewed as a manifestation of the **Peter Principle**—a theory that argues that people are typically promoted one position above their level of competence. This principle is a particular problem and occurrence in healthcare organizations where individuals with clinical skills, but without leadership skills and training, are frequently promoted into supervisory and management roles.

An important advantage of external recruiting is that new ideas may be brought into the organization. The organization may also be able to more specifically target the skills it is looking for, rather than settle for an internal applicant who, while knowing the organization, may lack specific

Internal and External Recruitment

Peter Principle is a theory that argues that people are typically promoted one position above their level of competence

TABLE 6.3
Advantages and
Disadvantages
of Internal and
External
Recruitment

Advantages	Disadvantages
Recruiting Internal Candidates	
May improve employee morale	Possible morale problems among those not selected
Permits greater assessment of applicant abilities	May lead to inbreeding
May be faster and may lower cost for certain jobs	May lead to conflict among internal job applicants
Good motivator for employee performance	May require strong training and management development activities
Applicants have a good understanding of the organization	May manifest the "Peter Principle"
Recruiting External Candidates	
Brings new ideas into the organization	May identify candidate who has technical skills but does not "fit" the culture of the organization
May be less expensive than training internal candidates	May cause morale problems for internal candidates who were not selected
External candidates come without dysfunctional political problems	May require longer adjustment and socialization
May brings new ideas to the organization	Organization may be uncertain about skills and abilities

job-related skills and knowledge. External applicants may also be brought into difficult political environments, in which dysfunctional alliances and conflict may be present. An external applicant typically will be unencumbered by these political problems.

Related to this discussion is the question of organizational "fit." In the past, the question of fit often had a negative discriminatory connotation; for example, a woman in a management role would not fit because she would be out of place in a male-dominated corporate culture. In our discussion, we refer to a type of fit that focuses on the alignment between an applicant's values and those of the organization; this fit is important for both the employee and the organization. Fit between the applicant and the organization affects not only the willingness of an employer to make a job offer but also the willingness of a job applicant to accept a job with an organization (Bretz and Judge 1994).

Measuring potential fit is a challenge, but a good recommendation is for organizations to pay more attention to hiring individuals who fit the characteristics of the organization and not just the requirements of the job (Bowen, Ledford, and Nathan 1991). Generally, organizations know about the potential fit of internal applicants and less about the potential fit of external applicants. Of course, an organization may sometimes try to change its culture and may seek change-oriented job applicants who do not fit the current dysfunctional organizational culture. The choice between seeking internal or external applicants is not often clear, and organizations have been known to pursue simultaneously both internal and external applicants.

As a general rule, obtaining as many qualified job applicants as possible in a particular recruiting effort is a good idea. From the organization's perspective, having many applicants permits choice, and the appearance of many applicants who have additional skills sets that may be useful to the organization sometimes may even stimulate a rethinking of the design of the job; successful organizations are flexible enough to take advantage of these opportunities. Note also that recruitment efforts should be designed in a manner that yields job applicants who have at least the minimum job qualifications because processing unqualified applicants can be expensive as well as a waste of time for both the organization and the job applicant.

Internal and External Recruitment Sources

The most common sources of finding suitable candidates are:

- Current employees. Many organizations have a policy, termed **job posting**, of informing current employees about current job openings within the organization. Internal job postings may increase morale, motivation, and retention by illustrating that the organization provides career ladders within the organization for current employees. In some organizations and for certain positions, internal job posting is done prior to initiating external recruitment efforts. A skills inventory of current employees, which is stored in the HRIS, may help the organization to identify potential job applicants. Current employees typically move into new positions through promotion or transfer.

  Job posting is a system by which an organization notifies its current employees about current job openings within the organization

- Employee referrals. Many organizations use current employees to refer other individuals to the organization. The value of this approach is that current employees tend to have a good understanding of the needs and the culture of the organization, so in effect, employees act as an initial screen for applicants. This is a potentially powerful recruitment strategy, yielding employees who typically stay with the organization longer and who exhibit higher levels of loyalty and job satisfaction than employees recruited through other mechanisms (Rynes 1991; Taylor 1994).
- Former employees. Employees who may have left the organization for a number of noncontroversial reasons, including other employment opportunities, downsizing and restructuring, relocation, and personal reasons, are sometimes an excellent source of job applicants. Sometimes such employees may seek or be available for reemployment with the

organization, which is ideal because they are well known to the organization and vice versa.

- Former applicants. An organization can identify potential job applicants from its database of previous job applicants. These individuals may be employees of other organizations or may still be seeking employment.

External recruitment tends to be more costly than internal recruitment because of costs associated with advertising, applicant travel, and commissions paid to employment agencies. Particular sources used for recruitment are of course highly dependent on the job for which recruitment is taking place; these sources include:

- Professional and trade associations. Use of national, regional, and state professional associations is particularly common in healthcare organizations. Recruitment of this type is often done through advertising in academic and trade journals and attendance at professional meetings.
- Employment agencies and executive search firms. These firms include both state-sponsored as well as private agencies. Private agencies specialize in different types of searches and work either on a commission or on a flat-fee basis.
- Media. This recruitment source is very common, and it includes advertising in/on a range of newspapers, magazines, television, radio, billboards, and the Internet. Because of the wide circulation possible through use of the media, targeting the advertisement to the appropriate media outlet and being specific are particularly important.
- High schools, colleges and universities. Recruitment through educational institutions is common for virtually all levels of work.
- Competitor organizations. In many instances, the right candidate for a job may be found in a competing organization. In an era when commitment to one's current organization is on the decline, "raiding" other organizations is not at all unusual.

The Recruiting Message

An important objective of recruitment is to maximize the possibility that the right candidate will select the organization after it makes a job offer. The candidate must know all the pertinent information about the job from the recruiting message. What are the appropriate messages to include in recruitment messages? At its core, four types of information should be made available to job applicants:

1. Applicant qualifications: education, experience, required credentials, and any other preferences that the employer has within legal constraints.
2. The job: including job title, responsibilities, pay, benefits, location of the job, and other pertinent working conditions (e.g., night work, travel, or promotion potential).

3. The application process: deadlines, inclusion of resumes, cover letters, transcripts, application, references, and where and to whom to submit applications.
4. The organization and department: name and type of organization, a statement that it is an EEO employer, and other information of interest.

The Realistic Job Preview

One of the more innovative and effective tools for recruitment is the use of the **realistic job preview.** The goal of a realistic job preview is to present practical and actual information about job requirements, organizational expectations, and the work environment. This information would include negative as well as positive information about the job and the organization and may be presented to job applicants or to hired individuals prior to starting work in the organization. Evidence shows that the use of realistic job previews is related to higher performance and lower attrition, lower initial expectations, lower voluntary turnover, and lower turnover overall (Phillips 1998).

A realistic job preview provides applicants with an actual view of the job requirements, organizational expectations, and the work environment

A realistic job preview can be provided in a number of ways. Certainly the most straightforward approach is for the prospective or new employee to hold frank discussions with coworkers and supervisors. In addition, the new employee could observe the work setting and perhaps shadow an employee who performs a similar job. Regardless of the approach used, the central element to a realistic job preview is to avoid surprises and to provide the employee with an honest assessment of the job and work environment.

Evaluating the Recruitment Function

As for all HR functions, the effectiveness and efficiency of recruitment efforts must be assessed. Such an evaluation process is dependent on the existence of reliable and comprehensive data on applicants, the quality of applicants, their disposition, and recruitment costs. Some common measures of the success of recruitment include:

- Quantity and quality of applicants. A recruitment effort should not only generate sufficient numbers of job applicants, but it should also bring applicants who have the appropriate qualifications.
- EEO and diversity goals. Assuming one of the goals of a recruitment program is to enable the organization to identify and hire qualified candidates who represent the diversity of the population, the organization must examine the mix of applicants that have been identified through the recruitment process.
- Cost per applicant. A recruitment initiative may yield many applicants, but the effort may be at a cost that is unacceptable to the organization. In addition to looking at overall costs per applicant, costs associated with different recruiting methods and sources must also be examined. This cost

analysis reveals the need to consider the cost effectiveness of alternative recruitment methods.

- Time required to fill jobs. Time factor is often the most important criterion used in evaluating recruitment efforts. The costs associated with not hiring, or use of part-time and temporary staff, may be quite substantial.

Selection

Employee selection is the process of collecting and evaluating information about job applicants to find the right individual to whom to extend an offer of employment

Employee selection is the process of collecting and evaluating information about job applicants to find the right individual to whom to extend an offer of employment. The entire selection process is to a great extent a matter of prediction regarding which among a set of applicants for a position is likely to achieve "success in the job." Of course, the definition of success in the job is not always straightforward. Job performance may be defined in terms of technical proficiency, but the definition may also include longevity in the position or "fit" with the goals of the organization. Thus, evaluating the effectiveness of selection processes may include not only the time taken to fill the position but the hired individual's performance, length of service in the organization, and other factors.

The selection process must be distinguished from a simple hiring (Gatewood and Feild 1998). In selection, a careful analysis is performed of applicants' knowledge, skills, and abilities (KSAs) as well as applicants' attitudes and other relevant factors; the applicant who scores highest on these factors is then extended an offer of employment. Sometimes, however, offers are made with little or no systematic collection and analysis of job-related information; a common example of which is hiring individuals based on political considerations or their relationship with owners or managers in the organization (e.g., family members). In such instances, these non-job-related factors take precedence over objective measures of job suitability.

In circumstances where a position has to be filled in a short period of time, or when labor shortages in a particular area is present, an organization may simply hire whoever is available, assuming the individual possesses the minimum level of qualifications. This scenario is a frequent occurrence in and challenge to staffing health centers in remote or otherwise undesirable locations. Applicant availability, rather than the comparative competence of the applicant, is key in these situations.

Understanding the Job

Selection tools refer to any procedures used to obtain job-related information on job applicants

If the goal of selection is to identify who should be offered employment among a group of applicants, then tools are needed to evaluate applicants' KSAs. **Selection tools** refer to any procedures used to obtain job-related information on job applicants, such as the job application form, standardized tests, personal interviews, simulations, and references. Each of these (as well as others) tools elicits pertinent information about applicants' job-related KSAs.

Prior to designing and utilizing selection tools, those involved in the selection process should at a minimum have a thorough understanding of (1) the technical requirements of the job and its required qualifications such as education, credentials, and experience, and (2) the informal and less technical aspects of job performance such as interpersonal skills, attitudes, judgment, values, fit, ability to work in teams, and management skills. Hiring someone with the technical skills to do the job but who lacks the ability to perform effectively would be an unfortunate consequence to not having a thorough understanding. Understanding all of the job requirements ensures that selection tools can be designed to capture applicants' KSAs. Among the most common methods for understanding the requirements of a job are:

- conducting a job analysis;
- seeking out the views of individuals currently in the position or in similar positions;
- obtaining the perspectives of supervisors and coworkers; and
- conducting a critical incidents analysis.

A **critical incidents analysis** is very useful in discovering the "hidden" or less formal aspects of job performance. This process is designed to generate a list of good and poor examples of job performance exhibited by current or potential job holders. Once these behaviors are collected, they are grouped into job dimensions. Measures are then developed for each of these job dimensions, which involves the following steps:

*A **critical incidents analysis** is useful in discovering the "hidden" or less formal aspects of job performance*

1. *Identify job experts and select methods for collecting critical incidents.* Incidents can be obtained from the job incumbent, coworkers, subordinates, customers, and supervisors. Generation of critical incidents can be done in a group setting, in individual interviews, or through administration of a questionnaire. Note that different job experts may view the job differently and may identify different aspects of job performance, which is the strength of this method.
2. *Generate critical incidents.* Job experts should be asked to reflect on the job and identify examples of good and poor performance. Each critical incident should be structured such that:

   - it is specific and pertains to a specific behavior;
   - it focuses on observable behaviors that have been, or could be, exhibited on the job;
   - it describes, in summary form, the context in which the behavior occurred; and
   - it indicates the positive or negative consequences of the behavior (Bowns and Bernardin 1988).

3. *Define job dimensions.* Job dimensions are defined by analyzing the critical incidents and extracting common themes.

Table 6.4 provides examples of three critical incidents and the job dimensions that result from each incident. The result of this exercise is a thorough understanding of the technical requirements; formal qualifications (e.g., training, credentials); and the informal, though critical, aspects of successful job performance. Not only does this understanding provide a strong foundation for selection, it also provides strong protection against charges of unfair hiring practices by specifically identifying job-related aspects of performance.

Designing Selection Tools

As noted earlier, selection tools include any method used to distinguish among job applicants along job-related dimensions. At the most fundamental level, selection tools should elicit information that is predictive of job performance. Applicants who "score" better on selection instruments should exhibit higher levels of job performance than individuals who score at lower levels. To be useful, selection tools should be both reliable and valid.

Reliability is the degree of the tool's dependability, consistency, or stability. A selection tool is reliable if when administered to an individual the tool yields the same findings, regardless of who administered the tool and the context (such as time of day or version of the tool) in which the tool was used. Consider the employment interview, which is a notoriously unreliable selection tool because a job applicant may be evaluated very differently by different interviewers. For example, one interviewer may be particularly struck by an applicant's impressive management skills, which in fact may be unrelated to job performance; similarly, if an interviewer has recently interviewed several very strong candidates, a particular candidate may appear mediocre by comparison, and the reverse may also hold.

Time pressures may also constrain an interviewer's ability to obtain information from an applicant. A number of techniques may be used to increase the reliability of interviews, including the use of multiple interviewers. A word processing test is among the more reliable selection tools. Assuming the same computer and word processing program is used, and the test is administered in roughly the same physical environment, an individual's score likely will not vary significantly between different administrations of the test.

The reliability of measuring different types of traits varies considerably. Personal characteristics, such as height, weight, vision, and hearing, can be assessed very reliably. Attitudes and skills, such as mathematical ability, mechanical aptitude, and intelligence, are less reliably measured, although standard tools are available to assess these qualities. Traits that are the most difficult to measure reliably, and often among the most important for selection purposes, are personality traits such as sociability, cooperativeness, tolerance, and emotional stability. A "snapshot" obtained by one interviewer may provide misleading information about an applicant (Albright, Glennon, and Smith 1963; Gatewood and Feild 1998). Use of multiple interviewers and discussion among interviewers may increase the reliability of measuring such

TABLE 6.4

Critical Incidents Approach to Defining Job Dimensions

Job	Critical Incident	Job Dimensions
Physician, Public Health Department	An administrative staff meeting was being held to review plans for coming year. This physician exhibited strongly condescending and rude behavior toward other team members.	• Ability to work in teams • Respect for other professionals
Nurse, Emergency Room	After a school bus accident, the emergency department was overwhelmed with patients and frightened parents. This nurse effectively and appropriately managed communication with parents and successfully obtained further assistance from elsewhere in the hospital.	• Creativity and resourcefulness • Leadership • Ability to work effectively under crisis conditions • Strong interpersonal skills
Medical Director, Local Public Health Department	An outbreak of salmonella was reported in the local media. One child was hospitalized in serious condition as a result. The outbreak was traced to a fast-food restaurant that was inspected by health department personnel less than one week ago. The health department was blamed for not preventing the outbreak. The health director conducted a thorough internal investigation and found that this was an isolated incident in which food was mishandled on a single occasion. She communicated effectively at a press conference, defending the department and assuring the public of the safety of local eating establishments.	• Effective crisis manager • Strong communication and media skills • Strong sense of public accountability

characteristics. Further, discussing these applicant characteristics with former employers and co-workers can also provide important and valuable insights.

The validity of selection tools must also be considered. *Validity* refers to the extent to which a selection tool actually corresponds to job performance—that is, does a particular predictor of future job performance actually predict performance? Three types of validity are commonly considered with selection tools: (1) criterion-related validity, (2) content validity, and (3) construct validity.

Criterion-related validity is the extent to which a selection tool is associated with job performance, where job performance is measured through an objective measure

1. **Criterion-related validity** is the extent to which a selection tool is associated with job performance, where job performance is measured through an objective measure; this validity can be demonstrated through two strategies: (1) concurrent validity and (2) predictive validity. *Concurrent validity* involves administering the selection tool to a current group of employees and then correlating their scores with actual job performance. For the selection tool to be deemed concurrently valid, a correlation has to exist between scores on the selection tool and actual job performance.

   Predictive validity involves administering a selection tool to a group of job applicants and, because the selection tool has not yet been validated, making actual selection decisions on the basis of other measures and criteria. Over time, data are obtained on actual job performance and the two sets of scores—those from the selection tool under study and those from actual performance measures—are correlated and examined for possible relationships.

Content validity is the extent to which a selection tool representatively samples the content of the job for which the measure will be used

2. **Content validity** is the extent to which a selection tool representatively samples the content of the job for which the measure will be used. Using this strategy, a selection tool is considered valid if it includes a sufficient amount of actual job-related content. Expert judgment, rather than statistical analysis, is typically used to assess content validity. One might look to content validity in designing a knowledge-based selection tool for laboratory technicians. A test that requires applicants to describe procedures associated with the most common laboratory tests would likely be judged to have content validity.

Construct validity refers to the extent to which a selection tool actually measures the construct it is intended to measure

3. **Construct validity** refers to the extent to which a selection tool actually measures the construct it is intended to measure. Assume that a selection committee has determined that a particular job requires the employee to exhibit strong time-management skills. The selection committee has designed a simulation exercise that is expected to assess this construct of time management. To determine if this selection tool actually predicts an individual's time-management skills, the exercise might be evaluated on the basis of a criterion-related validation study between the time management simulation and actual measures of the individual's time-management skills exhibited on the job. Construct validity studies

are most useful for determining whether selection tools actually measure the constructs that we hope they measure.

Reliability and Validity of Specific Selection Tools

Most organizations employ a range of selection tools but pay little or no attention to their reliability and validity. Below we examine the reliability and validity of some of the more common selection tools.

Reference Letters

In the few studies that assess the reliability of reference letters, researchers have sought to determine the level of agreement (inter-rater reliability) among different individuals who provide a reference for the same prospective employee. Reliability estimates for reference letters are typically poor, at a level of .40 or less; this low level may be explained by a number of factors including the reluctance of many referees to provide negative feedback and the real possibility that different raters may be evaluating different aspects of job performance. In studies of validity, it has been found that references have low to moderate predictive validity. Several explanations have been suggested for the poor predictive power of reference letters, including:

- Many measures used in reference checks have low reliability; where reliability is low, validity must be low as well.
- Individuals who provide references frequently only use a restricted range of scores—typically in the high range—in evaluating job applicants. Even if virtually all reference letters are positive, they likely will not predict success for all individuals.
- In many instances, job applicants preselect the individuals who will provide the reference, and applicants are likely to only select those who will provide a positive reference.

How can the validity of reference letters be improved? Research in this area (Gatewood and Feild 1998) concludes that:

- the most recent employer tends to provide the most accurate evaluation of an individual's work;
- prediction improves when the reference giver has had adequate time to observe the applicant and when the applicant is the same gender, ethnicity, and nationality as the reference giver; and
- the old and new jobs are similar in content.

Reference letters have an intuitive appeal and are well institutionalized in virtually all selection processes. The usefulness of references, however, is becoming even more problematic as many organizations are advising their employees to provide only skeletal information on former employees, such as job title and dates of employment. This is being done to reduce the liability of the referring organization to lawsuits by both the hiring organization through charges of negligent hiring and the prospective employee who might claim defamation of character.

Reference checks should be used to validate or expand on information provided by the applicant. Ideally, several standards should be followed during the process, including:

- Do not ask for information that would not be allowed in a job interview
- Permission should be obtained from job applicants prior to checking references
- Individuals who check references should be trained on the legal issues associated with the process
- Reference information should be recorded in writing

Interviews   The job interview is the most common selection technique and is very often given the greatest weight in hiring decisions. It is used for virtually all positions largely because those involved in hiring simply wish to find out more about applicants than can be obtained from written information about the applicant, references, and other sources of information. The fundamental problems with job interviews, however, are that they typically have low reliability and validity, they are often unfair to applicants, and they may be at least partially illegal. With respect to reliability, questions asked in an interview may vary from interviewer to interviewer, and two applicants applying for the same position may be asked very different questions. Similarly, the manner in which answers to interview questions are interpreted and scored by interviewers may also vary substantially.

The validity of the job interview—whether a positive interview actually predicts job success—has also been questioned. The questions asked in an interview are often not planned in advance and may bear little relationship with future job success. All of these factors make many interviews unfair to job applicants because they are not given the opportunity to present their abilities and they may be treated inequitably. Finally, untrained interviewers may ask questions of applicants that violate the law or compromise ethical principles.

Notwithstanding these problems, the job interview provides employers an opportunity to recruit good applicants. If conducted properly, the interview can be an effective tool in obtaining information and assessing whether the applicant is a good match for the organization.

Considered at the broadest level, those involved in selection can choose between unstructured and structured interview techniques. *Unstructured interviews* require few constraints regarding how interviewers go about gathering information and evaluating applicants. As a result, unstructured interviews may be very subjective and thus tend to be less reliable than structured interviews. However, because unstructured interviews give free reign to interviewers, they may be more effective than structured interviews in screening out unsuitable applicants.

The basic premise of a *structured interview* is that interview questions are clearly job related and based on the results of a thorough job analysis. In highly structured interviews, the "correctness" of answers are predetermined, and scores allocated to different answers prior to the interview. In an ideal situation, interviewers are not given ancillary information about applicants that might have a positive or negative impact on their evaluation of the information provided in a job interview. The most common types of questions asked in a structured interview are situational questions, experience-based questions, job-knowledge questions, and worker-requirements questions.

A *situational question* asks applicants to describe how they might handle a hypothetical job-related situation, while an *experience-based question* asks how the applicant previously handled a situation similar to the type of situation he or she may face on the job. Following are examples of each type of question for the position of office manager in a pediatric group practice. The constructs being assessed are handling stressful situations, dealing with the public, and professionalism.

> *Situation:* This medical practice has seven pediatricians who are very busy. The waiting room is overcrowded, and two of the pediatricians have unexpectedly been called away from the office—one for a personal situation and the other to attend to a patient in the hospital. Several patients and their parents will have to wait up to two hours to see the doctor, and the level of anger and frustration is increasing in the waiting room. They are taking out their anger on you.
>
> *Situational questions:* How would you handle this situation? What and how would you communicate with the remaining physicians about this situation?
>
> *Experience-based questions:* Think about a job-related situation in which you were faced with a situation where you had to deal with angry and upset patients or customers. What was the situation? What did you do? What was the outcome?

With situational questions, the question designers should decide a priori how alternative responses will be evaluated or scored. If an interview panel is used in which two or more interviewers are in the same room with the applicant, the interviewers can confirm answers and their meaning.

Job-knowledge questions simply assess whether job applicants have the knowledge to do the job. These questions are asked in a structured interview, where questions and follow-up probes are predetermined and based on the job description. Similarly, *worker-requirements questions* seek to determine if the applicant is able and willing to work under the conditions of the job. For example, applicants for a consulting position may be asked if they are able and willing to travel for a designated portion of their work. Whatever form of interview is used, the guidelines in Figure 6.1 would ensure that the interview is productive.

FIGURE 6.1

Guidelines for
Conducting
Job Interviews

1. Be prepared for the interview. For an unstructured interview, be clear that you understand the KSAs required. For a structured interview, become familiar with the questions to be asked. Finally, review materials about the applicant.
2. Prepare the physical environment for the interview.
3. Describe the job and invite questions about the job.
4. Put applicants at ease and convey interest in the applicant. The idea of a purposefully stressful interview is rarely desirable; there are other more reliable and ethical ways to assess an individual's ability to handle stress. Further, a stressful interview reflects poorly on the organization.
5. Don't come to premature conclusions (positive or negative) about an applicant, which is particularly important in unstructured interviews.
6. Listen carefully and ask for clarity if an individual's responses are not clear.
7. Observe the applicant and take notes on relevant aspects of dress, mannerisms, and affect.
8. Provide an opportunity for the applicant to ask questions.
9. Do not talk excessively. Remember that this is an opportunity to hear from the applicant.
10. Do not ask questions that are unethical or that put the organization in a legally vulnerable position.
11. Explain the next step in the selection process.
12. Evaluate the applicant as soon as possible after the interview.

Application Forms and Resumes

Application forms and resumes potentially contain very useful information about job applicants. The major drawback to relying on these documents is that they may simply be inaccurate or exaggerate an applicant's qualifications. One method that can improve the usefulness of application forms is to have specific information requirements for different jobs; in this way, specific KSAs can be targeted for different jobs. In addition, include a statement on the application form, to be signed by the job applicant, that states "all information reported is accurate," which ideally will encourage the applicant to be truthful. Ensure that only job-related information is requested on the application form and that information that is illegal to use in selection decisions (such as marital status, height, and weight) is *not* included.

Following are general items to exclude on job application materials and to avoid during an interview (Kahn, Brown, Lanzarone 1995; Gomez-Mejia, Balking, and Cardy 1998):

- Children (number of, plans to have, or childcare arrangements)
- Age, height, or weight

- Physical or mental disability or illness (e.g., whether the candidate has AIDS or is HIV positive). Asking whether the applicant can do the job is permissible, but inquiries about disability status can only be made after the job offer.
- Marital status and maiden names
- Citizenship status
- Religion, race, or nationality
- Arrest record, although asking about convictions is permissible
- Membership in organizations or clubs

Ability and Aptitude Tests

A variety of ability and aptitude tests are available, many of which have demonstrated reliability and validity. The list of tests is massive and includes tests of personality, honesty, integrity, cognitive reasoning, and fine motor coordination; a number of firms specialize in the production and assessment of these tests.[1] Although some debate continues about the issue of *situational validity*—the notion that the nature of job performance differs across work settings and that the validity of tests may vary according to work setting—in general, studies have tended to conclude that most basic abilities are generalizable across work settings, assuming that the test itself is valid and reliable. The key is to ensure that such tests are actually representative of the work of a particular job.

Assessment Centers

The use of assessment centers is an increasingly popular method of assessing job applicants. Assessment centers may be an actual physical location where testing is done, but they may also refer to a series of assessment procedures that are administered on job applicants, professionally scored, and reported to hiring personnel. Assessment centers have traditionally been used to assess individuals for management skills, but they are now used for a variety of hiring situations. Tests typically used in assessment centers include paper-and-pencil tests, intelligence tests, personality tests, interest measures, work task simulations, in-basket exercises, interviews, and situational exercises. Evidence indicates that assessment centers have positive statistical relationships with job performance (Gaugler et al. 1997).

Conclusion

Recruiting and selecting employees continues to be important as healthcare organizations struggle to be competitive and respond to pressures for effectiveness, efficiency, and consumer responsiveness. The challenges that face recruiters are enormous; they seek individuals who (1) have specialized skills yet are flexible, (2) bring new expertise to the organization yet are able to work effectively in groups, (3) are strongly motivated yet are comfortable with relatively flat organizational structures where traditional upward mobility may be difficult, and (4) bring diversity to the organization yet also fit into the organizational culture. With strong human resources management practices and positive organizational cultures, these challenges may be surmountable.

Discussion Questions

1. Given two apparently equally qualified job applicants—one from inside and one from outside the organization—how would you go about deciding which one to hire?
2. What advice would you give a public health department that seeks to hire nurses but whose wage structure is not competitive with that of area hospitals and other healthcare organizations?
3. How could the reliability of selection interviews be improved?
4. What methods could be used to verify the information contained in a job application or resume?
5. Given that a realistic job preview seeks to communicate both the positive and negative aspects of a job, should the job preview be structured such that the positive aspects of the job outweigh the negatives? Why or why not?

Note

1. See for example, the web site for Walden Personnel Testing and Consulting: http://www.waldentesting.com.

References

Albright, L. E., J. R., Glennon, and W. J. Smith. 1963. *The Use of Psychological Tests in Industry*, p. 40. Cleveland, OH: Howard Allen.

Barber, A. E., C. L. Daly, C. M. Giannantonio, and J. M. Phillips. 1994. "Job Search Activities: An Examination of Changes Over Time." *Personnel Psychology* 47: 739–66.

Bowen, D. E., G. E. Ledford, and B. R. Nathan. 1991. "Hiring for the Organization, Not the Job." *Academy of Management Executive* 5 (4): 35–51.

Bowns, D. A., and H. J. Bernardin. 1988. "Critical Incident Technique." In *The Job Analysis Handbook for Business, Industry, and Government*, edited by S. Gael, pp. 1120–37. New York: Wiley.

Bretz, R. D., and T. A. Judge. 1994. "The Role of HR Systems in Job Applicant Decision Processes." *Journal of Management* 20: 531–51.

Caudron, S. 1995. "The Changing Union Agenda." *Personnel Journal* (March): 42–9.

Fitz-Enz, J. 1995. *How to Measure Human Resources Management, Second Edition.* New York: McGraw-Hill.

Gatewood, R. D., and H. S. Feild. 1998. *Human Resource Selection, Fourth Edition.* Fort Worth, TX: Dryden.

Gaugler, B. B., D. B. Rosenthal, G. C. Thornton, and C. Bentson. 1997. "Meta-analysis of Assessment Center Validity." *Journal of Applied Psychology Monograph* 72: 493–511.

Gomez-Mejia, L. R., D. B. Balking, and R. L. Cardy. 1998. *Managing Human Resources, Second Edition.* Upper Saddle River, NJ: Prentice Hall.

Henderson, R. 1986. "Contract Concessions: Is the Past Prologue?" *Compensation and Benefits Review* 18: 17–30.

Kahn, S., B. Brown, and M. Lanzarone. 1995. *Legal Guide to Human Resources.* Boston: Warren, Gorham, and Lamont.

London, M., and S. A. Stumpf. 1982. *Managing Careers.* Reading, MA: Addison-Wesley.

Phillips, J. M. 1998. "Effects of Realistic Job Previews on Multiple Organizational Outcomes." *Academy of Management Journal* 41: 673–90.

Roth, L. M. 1982. *A Critical Examination of the Dual Ladder Approach to Career Advancement.* New York: Center for Research in Career Development, Columbia University Graduate School of Business.

Rynes, S. L. 1991. "Recruitment, Job Choice, and Post-Hire Consequences: A Call for New Research Directions." In *Handbook of Industrial and Organizational Psychology, Second Edition,* edited by M. D. Dunnette and L. M. Hough, pp. 399–444. Palo Alto, CA: Consulting Psychologists Press.

Schwab, D. P., S. L. Rynes, and R. J. Aldag. 1987. "Theories and Research on Job Search and Choice." In *Research in Personnel and Human Resources Management,* edited by G. Ferris and T. R. Mitchell. Greenwich, CT: JAI Press.

Taylor, G. S. 1994. "The Relationship Between Sources of New Employees and Attitudes Toward the Job." *Journal of Social Psychology* 134: 99–111.

PERFORMANCE MANAGEMENT

Bruce J. Fried, Ph.D.

Learning Objectives

After completing this chapter, the reader should be able to:

- Define performance management, and describe the purposes of a performance management system
- Discuss the reasons that organizations engage in performance management
- Identify the characteristics of good rating criteria for performance appraisal
- Describe various sources of job information, including managers, subordinates, team members, and the employee
- Define methods of assessing performance, and discuss whether each meets an administrative or a developmental purpose
- Define the common formats of performance appraisals, and discuss the strengths and shortcomings of each
- Identify and discuss the three types of information revealed by a performance appraisal
- Distinguish between rating errors and political factors as sources of distortion in performance appraisal
- Conduct a performance management interview with an employee using key points to make the interview successful

Introduction

Healthcare organizations are labor intensive, so they depend on high levels of employee performance. Measuring and improving employee performance is among the most highly examined aspects of management, both in the scholarly academic works and in the popular press. It is also one of the areas of management most prone to popular passing fads, which have been widely adopted in the popular management literature and by countless consulting firms that seek to identify and promote the quick fix to improving employee productivity and performance.

Every manager seeks to have employees who are highly motivated and productive, which is a challenging goal for a number of reasons. First, employee motivation is in itself a complex phenomenon and is influenced by many things outside of the manager's control. Second, the types of managerial interventions that are effective in motivating employee performance are still unclear; clearly, compensation is a motivator for most employees, but even money is not completely effective or, for that matter, available in adequate supply for managers to use as a motivational tool. Third, employee performance is often difficult to observe and measure in a reliable manner. In light of these complex factors, organizations have developed performance management systems.

*A **performance management system** monitors, measures, reports, improves, and rewards employee performance*

A **performance management system** monitors, measures, reports, improves, and rewards employee performance. Such a system does more than measure performance (as in the traditional idea of performance appraisal), but it also provides performance information or feedback to employees, which is helpful in training and developing employees toward higher levels of performance. As with all HR functions, performance management activities are carried out within a legal context in which employment law, equal employment opportunity law, and labor-relations law affect performance management procedures.

In this chapter, we describe the essential components of performance management. To the extent possible, we avoid the jargon and fashions that come and go and maintain a focus on those structures and processes most likely to lead to improved employee performance. In addition, we discuss the advantages and disadvantages of common formats and methods of assessing performance; describe common sources of errors and other problems in performance appraisal; and provide guidelines on conducting effective performance management and feedback interviews.

Purpose of Performance Management

As illustrated in Table 7.1, performance management is highly interrelated with other HR activities. Performance management activities affect and are affected by all other HR activities in the organization, so for a performance management system to be effective, it must be integrated with other HR functions.

Organizations engage in performance management for a number of reasons, including:

1. to give employees the opportunity to discuss performance and performance standards regularly with supervisors and managers;
2. to provide managers the opportunity to identify strengths and weaknesses of employees;

TABLE 7.1

Relationship of Performance Management to Other Human Resources Functions

HR Function	Affected by Performance Management	Influences Performance Management
Job Analysis	Information on performance may lead to redesign of jobs.	Accurate information about jobs is key to develop criteria for performance appraisal.
Recruitment and Selection	Performance information provides managers with information on the effectiveness of alternative sources of recruitment and the effectiveness of their selection criteria and procedures.	Ability to recruit and select employees may affect the types of criteria and standards developed for performance appraisal.
Training and Development	Performance management systems provide information on employees' training and development needs. Information on the performance appraisal systems assesses the effectiveness of training.	Performance appraisal tools may be designed to assess the impact of training programs.
Compensation	Compensation systems may be designed such that performance appraisal information has an impact on employee compensation.	A fair and equitable compensation system may lead to higher levels of employee performance.

3. to provide a venue for managers to identify and recommend strategies for employees to improve performance;
4. to provide a basis for personnel decisions such as compensation, promotion, and termination; and
5. to comply with regulatory requirements.

The Joint Commission on Accreditation of Healthcare Organizations (JCAHO) requires, as a condition of accreditation, healthcare organizations to assess, track, and improve the competence of all employees (Joint Commission 1997; Decker, Strader, and Wise 1997). Thus, the Joint Commission actually requires a performance management system from each organization.

Performance appraisal is a formal system of periodic review and evaluation of an individual's or team's performance

A key element of a performance management system is performance appraisal. **Performance appraisal** is a formal system of periodic review and evaluation of an individual's or team's performance. Although our focus is on the appraisal aspect of performance management, note that appraisal is only one, albeit important, aspect of a performance management system.

Performance appraisal is used for two general purposes: administrative and developmental. The administrative purpose commonly includes using performance appraisal information to make decisions about promotion and termination as well as compensation. To defend against charges of discrimination, organizations also attempt to maintain accurate and current performance appraisal information on employees. The developmental purpose of appraisal typically relates to attempts to improve performance by identifying employee strengths and weaknesses and developing strategies for improvement. Organizations can, of course, use appraisals for both administrative and developmental purposes. However, the debate continues on whether a manager can seriously conduct an honest developmental appraisal of an employee who is concerned with the impact of the appraisal on his or her income, promotion potential, and other bread-and-butter issues. This concern relates directly to the debate on pay-for-performance issues and on whether linking pay with the performance appraisal has an adverse impact on coaching and employee development.

The traditional assumption about performance appraisal is that above a certain organizational level, performance appraisal is no longer necessary and may even be demeaning. Evidence indicates that as an individual moves up the organization, he or she is in fact less likely to receive performance appraisal information. When performance appraisals are done at higher levels, the process tends to be poorly conducted or haphazard. However, strong evidence also suggests that individuals at the executive level have a strong desire to receive assessment of their performance (Longenecker and Gioia 1992). The bottom line is that performance appraisal and performance management is for everyone in the organization, although the types of performance information obtained may vary according to one's level and role in the organization.

Criteria for Performance Appraisal

As with so many HR activities, an effective performance management system must begin with clear job expectations and performance standards. Managers and employees must agree on and understand the content of the job description and job expectations. Afterward, employees and managers must develop **performance criteria**, which are measurable standards used for assessing employee performance; naturally, these criteria need to be job related and relevant to the needs of the organization. The development of criteria is a challenging task; therefore these criteria must be agreed upon well in advance of a formal performance appraisal interview.

Performance criteria are measurable standards used for assessing employee performance

How should performance criteria be defined, and what are useful criteria? First, criteria should have strategic relevance to the organization as a whole; for example, if patient satisfaction is an important organizational concern, then including patient-relations criteria makes sense for employees who interact with patients or clients. Criteria for individual performance appraisal are in many ways an extension of criteria used to evaluate organizational performance.

Second, criteria should be comprehensive and take into consideration the full range of an employee's functions as defined in the job description, including those that are hard to measure; but the criteria should exclude factors that are outside the employee's control. **Criterion deficiency** occurs when the performance appraisal focuses on a single criterion and excludes other important but less quantifiable performance dimensions (Barrett 1995; Sherman, Bohlander, and Snell 1998). For example, counting the number of visits made by a home care nurse is certainly simpler than assessing the quality of care provided during those visits. However, the latter criterion should not be undermined and excluded from the standards because it is more important, although it is more difficult to measure.

Criterion deficiency occurs when the performance appraisal focuses on a single criterion and excludes other important but less quantifiable performance dimensions

Third, criteria should be free from contamination. **Criterion contamination** occurs when factors out of the employee's control influence his or her performance. This contamination is a particular problem in healthcare because of the complexity of patient care and the interdependence of the many factors that affect patient care and clinical outcomes. Clinicians, for example, may have little control over patient volume or the speed that laboratory test results are reported; therefore, clinicians should not be penalized for their inability to provide care at a slower or faster pace.

Criterion contamination occurs when factors out of the employee's control influence his or her performance appraisal

Fourth, criteria should be reliable and valid. **Reliability** is the consistency of a manager's ratings in successive employee performance appraisals and assuming consistent employee performance or the consistency of the rating when two or more managers with comparable information perform the appraisal. The reliability of criteria can increase by selecting objective criteria and by training managers in applying the criteria. For example, measuring items such as sales or number of patients seen in a given interval is relatively simple,

Reliability is the consistency of a manager's ratings in successive employee performance appraisals and assuming consistent employee performance or the consistency of the rating when two or more managers with comparable information perform the appraisal

although of course extraneous factors may exist outside of the employee's control that affect—positively or negatively—employee performance. However, if we are interested in measuring employee behaviors such as teamwork or courtesy, different managers may interpret these criteria differently and focus on different behaviors. Thus, developing consistent operational measures of criteria, training managers in the use of these measures, and communicating how criteria will be measured can improve the reliability of a performance appraisal system.

Validity is the extent to which appraisal criteria actually measure the performance dimension of interest

Validity is the extent to which appraisal criteria actually measure the performance dimension of interest. For example, if we are interested in measuring a nurse's ability to carry out the nursing role during emergency medical procedures, is assessing knowledge of the role a more sufficient criterion than evaluating performance under real emergency conditions? Questions of validity are also difficult when measuring attitudes deemed important for a particular job.

Sources and Methods of Performance Appraisal

A traditional performance appraisal typically involves the manager or supervisor observing the employee's performance through the use of whatever appraisal format the organization has designed (which are described later in this chapter) and recording the appraisal information. Given the complexity of many jobs, however, the task of accurately evaluating and describing each employee's performance has become impossible for only one individual to do. In recent years, a variety of alternative approaches to appraising job performance has surfaced, including self-appraisal, subordinate appraisal, team-based appraisal, and 360-degree appraisal. These approaches use various sources, including managers, subordinates, team members, and the employee.

A self-appraisal is a performance appraisal done by the employee and is generally done in parallel with the manager's appraisal

A **self-appraisal** is a performance appraisal done by the employee and is generally done in conjunction with the manager's appraisal. This approach is very effective when a manager is seeking to obtain the involvement of the employee in the appraisal process. Because of the obvious potential for bias on the part of the employee, self-appraisals are almost always done for developmental rather than administrative purposes. Managers occasionally become concerned with their own performance, particularly with respect to their subordinates' perceptions of their performance, so they seek out their employees' opinions. A **subordinate appraisal** is an appraisal conducted by an employee on his or her boss, and it is conducted for developmental purposes. The potential benefits of doing subordinate appraisal include, most notably, identifying the "blind spots" that many managers have about their performance and improving their performance as managers. From the subordinate's perspective, this type of appraisal has obvious risks. Employees may fear retribution from the manager for making unfavorable or critical comments, or they may simply feel that negative comments may tarnish the relationship with the manager and possibly jeopardize compensation increases or the chance for

A subordinate appraisal is an appraisal conducted by an employee on his or her boss; it is conducted for developmental purposes

promotion. Employees may feel that honest subordinate appraisals are just not worth the risk. For this type of appraisal to be workable, a high level of trust must exists within the organization and such appraisals should be done anonymously; if this is not possible, the subordinate appraisal is unlikely to yield reliable results.

Another form of appraisal is team-based appraisal. **Team-based appraisal** is a method of assessment in which the work of a team, rather than the work of individual employees, is evaluated. This approach is most appropriate when individuals have common objectives, work in close collaboration with each other, and are dependent on each other for team performance (Gomez-Mejia 1998). Team-based appraisals may be linked with financial incentives. The major benefit of this approach is that it explicitly encourages teamwork, which is important in the healthcare environment where there is great dependency on well-functioning teams. A major drawback is that some individuals may perceive this appraisal as unfair because of the "free-rider" theory, in which one (or more) team members benefit from team rewards without putting forth corresponding effort. One may also involve team members in the appraisal of other team members as a method of identifying problems in team functioning. As with other forms of appraisal, these problems are exacerbated when rewards are linked with the appraisal process. Perhaps the most potentially useful form of appraisal is one that takes advantage of multiple sources of information about employee performance. Termed **360-degree appraisal** (or multirater assessment), this approach recognizes the fact that for many jobs, relying on one sources of performance data is inadequate; therefore, a comprehensive assessment of performance may be necessary to obtain the perspectives of individuals from multiple layers of the organization, including the manager or supervisor, peers, subordinates, clients, and even individuals external to the organization. This type of appraisal is typically done for developmental purposes, but it must be designed and administered with great care. The 360-degree appraisal can certainly be combined with other methods, and the benefits to the individual and organization are numerous (see Figure 7.1).

Team-based appraisal is a method of assessment in which the work of a team, rather than the work of individual employees, is evaluated

360-degree appraisal or multirater assessment recognizes the fact that for many jobs, relying on one sources of performance data is inadequate and that obtaining a comprehensive assessment of performance may be necessary

Common Formats of Performance Appraisal

Regardless of how performance appraisal information is obtained, a performance appraisal yields three types of information: (1) traits, (2) behaviors, and (3) results or outcomes. The common formats of performance appraisal listed below measure these three types of information. Each format has strengths and shortcomings and is useful for particular types of jobs and circumstances.

A *graphic rating scale refers to* any rating scale that utilizes points along a continuum to measure specific performance dimension; this scale may be used to measure traits or behaviors (Cascui 1991). Graphic rating scales are the most common format used to assess performance largely because they are easy to construct and may be used for many different types of employees in an

Graphic Rating Scales

FIGURE 7.1

Ten Reasons
to Use
360-Degree
Feedback

1. Defines corporate competencies
2. Increases the focus on customer service
3. Supports team initiatives
4. Creates a high-involvement workforce
5. Decreases hierarchies and promotes streamlining
6. Detects barriers to success
7. Assesses developmental needs
8. Avoids discrimination and bias
9. Identifies performance thresholds
10. Easy to implement

Source: Hoffman, R. 1995. "Ten Reasons You Should Be Using 360-degree Feedback." *HR Magazine* (April): 82–5. Reprinted with the permission of *HR Magazine* published by the Society for Human Resource Management, Alexandria, Virginia.

organization. The scale lists a series of measurable dimensions on one column and a range of ratings on the opposite column that indicates different levels of effectiveness; Figure 7.2 is an illustration of part of a graphic rating scale. In this example, both traits and behaviors are assessed, but note that many of these dimensions are prone to subjective judgment (for example, flexibility). One of the drawbacks of graphic rating scales is that they are quite general and often do not include specific behaviors that could illustrate positive or negative aspects of performance. Information on how to change is frequently lacking because behaviors or traits are stated in general form. Because of this subjectivity, raters may be uncomfortable using this method, particularly when ratings are linked with compensation. Graphic rating scales can be improved by including specific behaviors associated with each scale.

Perhaps the most important drawback of graphic rating scales is that they typically do not weigh behaviors and traits according to their importance to a particular job; in Figure 7.2, for example, pace of work may be extremely important for one group of employees but relatively unimportant for others. Another problem arises when an organization simply imports a graphic rating scale from another organization without considering the scale's relevance to the organization or to particular jobs.

Ranking

Ranking is a method by which a manager ranks employees from worst to best on an overall criterion of employee performance. This method is typically done for administrative purposes, usually for making personnel decisions such as promotions and layoffs. The major advantage of this ranking is that it forces supervisors to distinguish among employees, which allows them to avoid many of the problems associated with other methods. Among the disadvantages of ranking are:

- It focuses only on a single dimension of work effectiveness and may not take into account the complexity of work situations.
- It becomes cumbersome with large numbers of employees and may force appraisers to artificially distinguish among employees.
- It simply lists employees in order of their performance, but it does not indicate the relative differences between employees' effectiveness.
- It provides no guidance on specific deficiencies in employee performance and therefore is not useful in helping employees improve.

Ranking appears to be a rather crude method of appraising performance. Interestingly, a number of notable companies, such as Microsoft, Ford Motor, General Electric, and Conoco, use ranking methods to help determine pay and sometimes termination. At General Electric, supervisors identify the top 20 percent and the bottom 10 percent of managerial and professional employees every year; the bottom 10 percent are unlikely to stay (Abelson 2001). Ranking employees for termination purpose is not performance management as we tend to think of it; rather, it is a method of forcing managers to distinguish among employees at times when terminations are necessary for

FIGURE 7.2

Example of a Graphic Rating Scale

Please rate the following dimension about this employee: _____

Name of Employee

Performance Dimension	Scale
1. Rate this person's pace of work	1 2 3 4 5 6 slow fast
2. Assess this person's level of effort	1 2 3 4 5 6 below capacity full capacity
3. What is the quality of this person's work?	1 2 3 4 5 6 poor good
4. How flexible is this person?	1 2 3 4 5 6 rigid flexible
5. How open is this person to new ideas?	1 2 3 4 5 6 closed open
6. How much supervision does this person need?	1 2 3 4 5 6 a lot little
7. How readily does this person offer to help out by doing work outside his or her normal scope of work?	1 2 3 4 5 6 seldom often
8. How well does this person get along with peers?	1 2 3 4 5 6 not well very well

financial reasons. Several companies have faced lawsuits based on the claim that ranking systems discriminate against specific demographic groups.

Behavioral Anchored Rating Scale

Behavioral anchored rating scale (BARS) are a significant improvement over traditional graphic rating scales. BARS includes specific behavioral descriptions of different levels of performance dimension, which can be rated as unacceptable, poor, good, and so forth. Figure 7.3 provides an illustration of a BARS measuring the performance dimension "patient relations" for a nurse. Note that instead of a manager simply rating the employee's performance as "unacceptable" or "average," the scale provides specific behavioral description of the employee's level of performance, and it explicitly states the expectations for improved performance.

Among the advantages of BARS are:

- It reduces rating errors because job dimensions are clearly defined for the rater and are relevant to the job being performed.
- It clearly defines the response categories available to the rater.
- It is more reliable, valid, meaningful, and complete.
- It receives a higher degree of acceptance and commitment by employees and supervisors.

FIGURE 7.3

A Behavioral Anchored Rating Scale for Performance Dimension: Patient Relations

Rating	Behavioral Description
Excellent	1. Employee always treats patients with dignity and cheerfulness, respecting their individual needs while performing professional duties. Employee receives frequent favorable comments from patients under his or her care.
Good	2. Employee treats patients with dignity and respect without becoming involved in their individual problems. Employee receives occasional favorable comments from patients.
Average	3. Employee is impersonal with patients, tending their medical needs but avoiding personal interaction. Employee is the subject of few comments by patients.
Poor	4. Employee becomes impatient with patients and is concerned more about performing his or her tasks than being of assistance to patient's nonmedical needs. Employee generates some complaints from patients.
Unacceptable	5. Employee is antagonistic toward patients, treating them as obstacles or annoyances rather than individuals. Employee generates frequent complaints from patients and causes them to be considerably upset.

- It reduces defensiveness and conflict because individuals are appraised on the basis of observable behavior.
- It improves ability to identify areas for training and development.

Developing a BARS for each job dimension for a particular job is not a trivial task, given that among its disadvantages is the amount of time, effort, and expense involved in its development. Use of BARS is most justifiable when there is a large number of job holders for a position for which the BARS is being developed. Finally, the use of BARS is most appropriate for jobs whose major components consist of physically observable behaviors.

A variation of BARS is a *behavioral observation scale (BOS)*. With this approach, highly desirable employee behaviors are identified, and the rater is asked to indicate the frequency that the employee exhibits those behaviors. Desirable behaviors are identified through the job analysis and discussions with managers and supervisors. Figure 7.4 provides an illustration of a BOS for a manager for the performance dimension "overcoming resistance to change." Note that six desirable behaviors are associated with this performance dimension, and the supervisor (or other raters) rates the frequency that each behavior is likely to be observed. As with BARS, the employee has a clear understanding of the types of behaviors expected.

Behavioral Observation Scales

The *critical incident* technique is a process in which the manager maintains a record of unusually favorable or unfavorable occurrences in an employee's work. A major strength of this method is that it provides a factual record of

Critical Incidents

Item	Scale				
	Almost Never				Almost Always
1. Describes the details of change to subordinates	1	2	3	4	5
2. Explains why the change is necessary	1	2	3	4	5
3. Discusses how the change will affect the employee	1	2	3	4	5
4. Listens to the employee's concerns	1	2	3	4	5
5. Asks the employee for help in making the change work	1	2	3	4	5
6. If necessary, specifies the date for a follow-up meeting to respond to the employee's concerns	1	2	3	4	5

FIGURE 7.4
A Behavioral Observation Scale for Performance Dimension: Overcoming Resistance to Change

an employee's performance and can be very useful in subsequent discussions with the employee. The approach does require that the manager closely and continuously monitor employee performance, which is not always feasible, although linking a critical incident method with 360-degree feedback raises the possibility that incidents may be observed and recorded by a number of different individuals in the organization. Documentation of critical incidents need not be very long but should be tied to an important performance dimension. Below is an example of a critical incident for a mental health case manager; this incident illustrates the employee's creativity and negotiations skills, which is an important performance dimension:

> In speaking with her client, an individual with a severe mental disorder, it was discovered that the client was about to be evicted from her apartment for nonpayment of rent. She (the mental health case manager) was able to work with the client and landlord to work out a payment plan and to negotiate successfully with the landlord to have much-needed repairs done in the apartment. She followed up with the client weekly on payment to the landlord and the repairs, and positive outcomes have been achieved in both areas.

Management by Objectives

Management by Objectives (MBO) refers to a specific technique that has enjoyed substantial popularity. The basic premise of MBO is that the organization first defines its strategic goals for the year; these goals are then dispersed to multiple layers in the organization. Each individual in the organization defines her goals for the year based on the goals established by the organization. Achievement of these goals then becomes the standard by which each individual's performance is assessed (Carroll and Tosi 1973).

MBO has three key characteristics (Odiorne 1986):

1. The establishment of specific and objectively measurable goals for employees.
2. The establishment of goals in collaboration with the employee.
3. Provision by the manager of objective feedback and coaching to improve performance.

As with most managerial practices, MBO has been found to be most effective when support and commitment is given by senior management. MBO also requires managers to have substantial training in goal setting, giving feedback, and coaching. While goal setting is central to MBO, the process by which goals are set is of great importance.

MBO is in fact only one of several methods of results-based performance management. Depending on the position, organizations may use a variety of results-oriented methods; such methods are most useful when objectively measurable outcomes exist. The MBO approach is most commonly used in positions in which objectively measurable bottom line concerns may be paramount, such as senior executive, sales, and certainly sports teams and individual athletes. MBO may, of course, be combined with other performance appraisal methods, particularly for jobs in which both the manner in which work is done and the outcomes are important and measurable.

Cynicism About Performance Appraisal

Most managers and employees are quite cynical about performance appraisal. This cynicism grows out of a belief that nobody likes performance appraisals: managers are uncomfortable sitting down and discussing issues with employees, and employees may resent the paternalism and condescension that often accompanies performance appraisals. This cynicism is clearly based in the reality that performance appraisals are traditionally punitive in nature, and they can be highly emotional particularly when tightly tied to employee compensation.

Regardless of the type of data used in performance appraisal, rating errors persist. **Rating errors** refer to positive or negative distortions in performance appraisal ratings that reduce the accuracy of appraisals; the most common rating errors are:

Rating errors refer to positive or negative distortions in performance appraisal ratings that reduce the accuracy of appraisals

- *Distributional errors:* the tendency of raters to use only a small part of the rating scale; these errors come in three forms:

  1. Leniency: the tendency of some raters to be overly generous in their ratings, thereby avoiding conflict and confrontation.
  2. Strictness: the tendency of some raters to be overly critical in their ratings, leading to unfair comparisons with employees in the same position who may be rated by managers without this tendency.
  3. Central tendency: the predisposition of some raters to rate all employees as more-or-less average, thereby avoiding conflict.

- *Halo effect*: the tendency of some raters to rate employees high (or low) on all evaluation criteria without distinguishing between different aspects of the employee's work; this leads to evaluations that may be overly critical or overly generous.
- *Personal bias*: the tendency of some raters to simply rate employees higher or lower than is deserved based on personal like or dislike of the employee (Wexley and Nemeroff 1974).
- *"Similar to me" bias*: the tendency, well developed in the literature, to judge those who are similar to the rater more highly than those who are not. Research shows that the strongest impact of similarity occurs when manager and employee share demographic characteristics (Noe et al. 1996).
- *Contrast effect*: the tendency of raters to compare employees with each other rather than using an objective standard; this points to the importance of having clear standards for job performance.

The most important strategy for overcoming these rating errors is training. Training typically helps to increase managers' familiarity with the rating scales and the specific level of performance associated with different points on these scales. The objective is to increase each individual's consistency in using rating scales and to improve inter-rater reliability among managers. Training also typically focuses on minimizing managers' error rate. At a minimum, managers need to be aware of potential rating errors in performance appraisal. Strategies may be offered to help managers both identify when they may be making errors and develop strategies to avoid making errors in appraisal. For example, managers may avoid distributional errors by improving their awareness of the appraisal tool and by being knowledgeable about the objective standards used to evaluate performance. Of course, the success of training efforts is contingent on the existence of valid and reliable assessment instruments and clear performance standards.

Even with extensive training and well-tested appraisal tools, a set of problems persists with performance appraisal, which may be summed up as the "politics of performance appraisal" (Longenecker, Sims, and Gioia 1987). All managers are aware that political considerations affect the appraisals given to particular employees. For example, managers are well aware that after an appraisal is completed, they must in most cases continue to live with their employees; therefore, a common perception among managers is that a negative appraisal will tarnish their relationship and perhaps hurt team dynamics and productivity. Managers may also feel that a negative appraisal results in a negative impact on an employee's career (as the excerpt below demonstrates) or, more immediately, on the employee's finances.

> The mere fact that you have to write out your assessment and create a permanent record will cause people not to be as honest or as accurate as they should be. . . . We soften the language because our ratings go in the guy's file downstairs [the Personnel Department] and it will follow him around his whole career (Longenecker, Sims, and Gioia 1987).

As a result of these and other pressures, managers may artificially inflate or deflate an employee's appraisal. Table 7.2 provides a summary of the political reasons managers may distort an employee's true performance. Note that these problems with performance appraisal accuracy are more difficult to deal with than the errors discussed earlier because these problems are deeply rooted in the organizations and in the relationship between manager and employee.

Conducting Effective Performance Management Interviews

As noted earlier in this chapter, the ultimate objective of a performance management system is to improve employee performance. Because performance management has historically focused on the evaluation or measurement

Managers May Inflate an Appraisal to:	Managers May Deflate an Appraisal to:
Maximize merit increases for an employee, particularly when the merit ceiling is considered low.	Shock an employee back on to a higher performance track.
Avoid hanging dirty laundry out in public if the appraisal information is viewed by outsiders.	Teach a rebellious employee a lesson.
Avoid creating a written record of poor performance that would become a permanent part of the individual's personnel file.	Send a message to an employee that he or she should think about leaving the organization.
Avoid confrontation with an employee with whom the manager had recently had difficulties.	Build a strongly documented record of poor performance that could speed up the termination process.
Give a break to a subordinate who had improved.	
Promote an undesirable employee "up and out" of the organization.	

TABLE 7.2
Why Managers
Inflate and
Deflate
Performance
Appraisals

Source: Academy of Management Executive by C. O. Longenecker, H. P. Sims, and D. A. Gioia. Copyright 1987 by Academy of Management. Reproduced with permission of the Academy of Management via Copyright Clearance Center.

aspects of performance management, relatively little attention has been given to the improvement aspects of performance management.

A key step in the improvement process is providing performance information or feedback to the employee. Many managers are, of course, reluctant to provide feedback because of the fear of confrontation and conflict, which are real concerns for both managers and employees, given most employees' negative experiences with performance management. In informal surveys with our students, we typically find that the great majority of them either rarely have a performance evaluation or have had poorly done evaluation. Finding someone who has had a well-implemented appraisal is rare.

Following are points that may be helpful in conducting performance feedback for employees:

1. *Do appraisals on an ongoing basis.* Make performance an ongoing process that does not just occur during the formal appraisal process; giving continuous feedback is, after all, a key element in a manager's role. By using ongoing feedback, surprises at the formal appraisal are also avoided.

   A common question asked about performance appraisals is how often they should be held on a formal basis; the answer is that it depends on the employee. For a high-performing employee, an annual appraisal (as well as ongoing informal feedback) may be sufficient. These appraisals will usually be done for developmental purposes to reward and reinforce existing levels of performance. For the average employee, for whom performance improvement may be an important goal, more frequent appraisals may be useful. Finally, for marginal or low-performing employees, for whom remediation is a central goal, formal appraisals may need to be held monthly or perhaps more often.

2. *Prepare.* The manager who gives formal performance feedback should be equipped with data, have a strategy for presenting performance information, be prepared for employee reactions, and be prepared to engage in problem solving and planning with the employee. An appropriate physical location should be found, and relevant supporting information should be available.

3. *Encourage participation.* The employee should believe that the performance management process is something that will be beneficial to him or her. The literature refers to two traditional modes of presenting performance information: (1) the tell-and-sell and (2) the tell-and-listen methods. The "tell-and-sell" method involves the manager presenting (telling) performance ratings and then justifying (selling) the ratings and encouraging the employee to use a recommended strategy for improvement. This type of strategy may be useful in situations where the manager must be very clear about expectations or with young employees who may not yet be prepared to engage in self-evaluation (Downs, Smeyak, and Martin 1980). It may also be useful with very loyal employees who are strongly committed to the organization.

   The "tell-and-listen" approach involves presenting (telling) performance information and then hearing (listening) the employee's side of the story and the employee's ideas for improvement. This type of approach is most useful for employees with a strong need to participate in their jobs, for employees who are close in status to the interviewer, and for highly educated employees (Downs, Smeyak, and Martin 1980).

   The most promising approach to participation is the problem-solving approach, in which the goal of the interview is to help the employee develop a plan for improvement. This involves a partnership between manager and employee and requires an atmosphere of respect and support. This approach is supported by strong empirical evidence that indicates that employees are consistently satisfied with this approach (Cederblom 1982) and that participation in feedback and problem solving is a key predictor of job satisfaction (Giles and Mossholder 1990; Noe et al. 1996).

4. *Focus on future performance and problem solving.* While reviewing past performance is important, the emphasis should be on setting goals for the future and on generating specific strategies for meeting those goals. In many cases, the employee will identify factors outside of his or her control that may contribute to lower-than-expected levels of performance, which

are certainly appropriate factors to discuss during performance feedback sessions. Follow-up sessions should also be scheduled as appropriate.

5. *Focus on behavior or results, not on the employee or her personality.* In almost all cases, the purpose of performance feedback is to help the employee improve, not to change as a person. The performance feedback interview is not the time to change an employee's values, personality, motivation, or fit with the organization; if these are true problems, they should have been considered during the selection process. The manager should focus on behaviors and outcomes and not on the value of the person. Condescending criticism and reciting a litany of employee problems are rarely useful and are more likely to generate defensiveness and resentment.

6. *Reinforce positive performance.* Performance appraisal interviews have gained the reputation for being punitive and negative. One of the most effective ways to ally oneself with an employee is to ensure that the interview focuses on all aspects of performance, not just the negative. Reinforcing positive performance is essential.

7. *Ensure that performance management is supported by senior managers of the organization.* The best way to destroy any effort at implementing a performance management system is for word to get out that senior management is either unsupportive of or ambivalent about the process. Senior management must assertively communicate that performance management is important to meeting organizational goals and that it needs to be done at all levels of the organization. If this message is absent or weak, the performance management system will either fade away or become a meaningless bureaucratic exercise.

Conclusion

In the past ten years, performance appraisal has transformed into performance management. Historically, performance appraisal focused primarily on judging employee behavior, and that process was viewed as negative and punitive in nature and generally avoided by both managers and employees. Performance management implies an improvement-focused process in which efforts are made to not only assess performance but also to develop specific collaborative strategies to improve performance. Recognizing that employee performance results from an employee's skills, motivation, and facilitative factors in the work environment, improvement strategies may include training, work-process redesign, and other changes that are both internal and external to the employee.

Discussion Questions

1. Distinguish between performance appraisal and performance management.

2. Why does the Joint Commission now require hospitals and other healthcare organizations to have performance management systems?

3. What is the relationship between performance management and continuous quality improvement?

4. What are the advantages and disadvantages of including discussions of compensation during a performance management interview?

5. Distinguish between performance appraisal rating errors and political factors that influence the accuracy of performance appraisal information.

6. How does a manager decide how often to conduct formal performance management interviews?

7. Why is employee participation in the performance management process important? Under what circumstances is employee participation not necessarily important?

References

Abelson, R. 2001. "Companies Turn to Grades, and Employees Go to Court." *The New York Times* (March 19): A1, A12.

Barrett, R. S. 1995. "Employee Selection with the Performance Priority Survey." *Personnel Psychology* 48: 653–63.

Carroll, S., and H. Tosi. 1973. *Management by Objectives.* New York: Macmillan.

Cascui, W. F. 1991. *Applied Psychology in Personnel Management.* Reston, VA: Reston Press.

Cederblom, D. 1982. "The Performance Appraisal Interview: A Review, Implications, and Suggestions." *Academy of Management Review* 7: 219–27.

Decker, P. J., M. K. Strader, and R. J. Wise. 1997. "Beyond JCAHO: Using Competency Models to Change Healthcare Organizations. Part 2: Developing Competence Assessment Systems." *Hospital Topics* 75 (2): 10–17.

Downs, C. W., G. P. Smeyak, and E. Martin. 1980. *Professional Interviewing.* New York: Harper and Row.

Giles, W., and K. Mossholder. 1990. "Employee Reactions to Contextual and Session Components on Performance Appraisal." *Journal of Applied Psychology* 75: 371–7.

Gomez-Mejia, L. R. 1998. "Team-based Incentives." In *Encyclopedic Dictionary of Human Resource Management,* by L. H. Peters, C. R. Greer, and S. A. Youngblood. Malden, MA: Blackwell Publishers, Inc.

Joint Commission for the Accreditation of Healthcare Organizations. 1997. *Comprehensive Accreditation Manual for Hospitals.* Oak Brook, IL: JCAHO.

Longenecker, C. O., H. P. Sims, and D. A. Gioia. 1987. "Behind the Mask: The Politics of Employee Appraisal." *The Academy of Management Executive* 1 (3): 183–93.

Longenecker, C. O., and D. Gioia. 1992. "The Executive Appraisal Paradox." *Academy of Management Executive* 6 (2): 18–28.

Noe, R. A., J. R. Hollenbeck, B. Gerhart, and P. M. Wright. 1996. *Human Resource Management: Gaining a Competitive Advantage, Second Edition.* Boston: Irwin McGraw-Hill.

Odiorne, G. 1986. *MBO: II: A System of Managerial Leadership for the 80s.* Belmont, CA: Fearon Pitman Publishers.

Sherman, A., G. Bohlander, and S. Snell. 1998. *Managing Human Resources, Eleventh Edition.* Cincinnati, OH: Southwestern College Publishing.

Wexley, K., and W. Nemeroff. 1974. "Effects of Racial Prejudice, Race of Applicants, and Biographical Similarity on Interview Evaluations of Job Applicants." *Journal of Social and Behavioral Sciences* 20: 66–78.

TRAINING AND DEVELOPMENT

James A. Johnson, Ph.D.

Learning Objectives

After completing this chapter, the reader should be able to:

- Distinguish the difference between training, development, and education
- Describe techniques for designing, evaluating, and implementing training
- Discuss the learning environment and the adult learning process
- Define organizational development
- Understand fundamentals and utility of training and development in the organizational setting

Introduction

As described by Kilpatrick and Johnson (1999), the healthcare industry is in an era of major social and cultural change, which compels us in the industry to manage our healthcare organizations with greater efficiency, effectiveness, and value; many observers even believe that we are engaged in the refinement of the best healthcare system in the world. If this theory is so, then we need new knowledge, tools, skills, and particularly perspectives. With exponential increases in information, technological breakthroughs, and scientific discovery we must make a solid commitment to lifelong learning.

Healthcare organizations are fundamentally dependent on personnel to help them accomplish their organizational tasks and goals. Fried (1999) described healthcare personnel as individuals, ranging from those with little formal training and education to highly skilled and educated professionals, who are engaged in very complex tasks and decision making. This dependence on personnel has led to a point where having strong human resource competencies has become a critical strategic value to any healthcare organization (Friesen and Johnson 1996) and where the pace and intensity of training and development has increased dramatically (Blanchard and Thacker 1999). Training and development is essential to continuous quality improvement (Johnson and Omachanu 1999) and to strategic management (McIlwain and

Johnson 1999); it is also the bedrock for creating a capacity for change and organizational learning (Senge 1990; Friesen and Johnson 1996; Tobin 1998). According to the Robert Wood Johnson Foundation, one of the most salient approaches to improving our health delivery systems is "investing in people" (Isaacs and Knickman 2001).

Healthcare at its most fundamental level is about people caring for people. Increasing our knowledge and skill and coupling that with compassion and a commitment to continuous learning will lead to an even better system of care. In this chapter, we explore the unique aspects and place for training in healthcare organizations.

Training

Training is typically a function of the human resources department and is the main vehicle for human resource development (HRD). Blanchard and Thacker (1999) describe the role of the HRD function as improving the organization's effectiveness by providing employees with the learning needed to improve their current or future job performance. Training primarily focuses on the acquisition of knowledge, skills, and abilities, which are often referred to as KSAs. Focusing on areas that do not meet the needs of the organization, nor providing training that fails to be seen as relevant and important by employees, will not be effective. The most effective approaches to training simultaneously meet the needs of the organization and the employee.

KSAs required in various health professions are extremely varied. For example, a nurse needs to be skilled in taking blood pressure, while a radiology technician needs to know how to operate imaging equipment. Administrative positions also require different KSAs, such as knowledge of compliance issues, skills in interacting with internal and external customers, or ability to generate a flow chart.

Although knowledge, skill, and ability seem the same in that each involves learning, each is distinctive in that each warrants a different approach to the learning process. *Knowledge* is a byproduct of both remembering and understanding information. *Skills*, on the other hand, are general capacities to perform a task or set of tasks; these capacities are usually gained from training or experience. *Abilities* are capabilities to perform based on experience, social or physical conditioning, or heredity. Many training methods are effective in improving KSAs.

Training is different from education. While training focuses on enhancement of a given job or role, education tends to be more global in its purpose. Education is the development of general knowledge related to a profession, but education is not necessarily designed for a specific position within that profession. For example, acquiring a Master of Health Administration degree entails getting a comprehensive education on organizational management, but that education is not targeted to learning specific roles that a healthcare administrator encounters or becomes interested in later in his or her career; that role would necessitate additional training. Similarly, a Doctor of Medicine degree is designed to teach basic concepts, but if a doctor wants to pursue a more specific branch of medicine or a specialty, he or she needs further training or education.

Training Cycle

Training typically follows a systematic design or cycle, starting from an analysis or identification of needs through the phases of method selection, implementation, and evaluation (see diagram below). This design helps to ensure that the training process is under control so that organizational goals can be accomplished. Without a systematic design, training has been shown to be only modestly effective and wasteful of time and resources.

Gordon, Morgan, and Ponticell (1995) and Blanchard and Thacker (1999) advises the trainer or training department to consider nine principles before and during any training initiative:

1. Identify the types of individual learning strengths and problems and tailor the training around them
2. Align learning objectives to organizational goals
3. Clearly define program goals and objectives at the start
4. Actively engage the trainee to maximize attention, expectations, and memory
5. Use a systematic, logically connected sequencing of learning activities so that trainees can master lower levels of learning before moving onto higher levels
6. Use a variety of training methods
7. Use realistic job- or life-relevant training material
8. Allow trainees to work together and share experiences

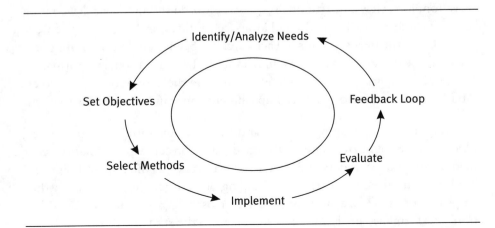

9. Provide constant feedback and reinforcement while encouraging self-assessment

The discussion on the training cycle below supports these nine principles.

Needs Identification/ Analysis

The primary purpose of training is to improve the performance of both the employee and the organization; thus, identifying and analyzing needs is essential prior to developing a training program. This phase involves organizational analysis, operational analysis, and employee analysis to determine ways to bring up performance to an expected or ideal level. Sometimes the analysis may reveal the employee lacks the necessary KSAs to do the job effectively, while at other times the analysis may identify barriers in the organization or its climate, which both warrant organization development intervention. A needs analysis may also disclose elements of a given job or task that need to be redesigned or altered. Most importantly, a needs analysis ensures that the right training and development are provided to the right people in the organization.

An *organizational analysis* involves an assessment of the strategic objectives, resources, and internal environment of the organization. Data about these aspects of the organization are taken from the strategic plan, labor and skill inventories, interviews with leaders and workers, organizational climate surveys, and customer service data. *Operational analysis,* on the other hand, involves an examination of the tasks needed to do a specific job or closely aligned set of jobs, the level of the job, and the KSAs needed for effective performance. Data sources include job descriptions, performance standards and appraisals, observation of the job, literature on the job, job holder and supervisor, and quality control data. A *person analysis* identifies individuals who are not meeting the desired performance requirements or goals. The comparison of expected performance to actual performance may reveal a discrepancy from which the training intervention can be designed. Data sources for the person analysis include supervisor ratings, performance appraisals, observation, interviews, questionnaires, tests, attitude surveys, checklists, rating scales, in-basket exercises and simulations, self-ratings, and assessment centers.

Once the needs analysis at each level has been complete a training program can be designed to improve individual and organizational performance. Developing a training program entails identifying the desired outcome and establishing conditions for goal accomplishment and standards of measurement.

Objective Setting

The importance of training analysis and the determination of clear learning objectives cannot be overstated. Objectives based on actual performance needs help (1) the trainee understand what is expected and (2) the trainer design and implement more effective training. Training objectives, whether for individual employee or entire organization, must be closely aligned with the organization's performance goals and must be linked to the strategic direction. In addition, objectives should always be written and stated clearly in terms that are easy to understand, and each objective should have a behavioral component that describes a desired outcome.

Selection of Methods

Many methods are already used in the facilitation of learning, and still many more are being developed constantly. The American Society of Training and Development and other training-focused organizations monitor, distribute, and provide training tools and technologies for continuing education. The most widely used methods of training are lectures and discussions, which can be done live, through video, or video conferencing. Another commonly used method is computer-based training and programmed instruction. In addition, games and simulations, in-basket exercises, case studies, role playing, and on-the-job training can be used either as a complementary or a primary method, although each of these methods has its strengths and weaknesses. Depending on the desired learning objective, the tasks involved, and the audience, a trainer may select any or all of the methods.

Implementation

For training or any other improvement effort to be effectively implemented, the organization must be a *learning environment,* in which continuous learning is central to the organization's definition of itself. According to Tobin (1998), a positive learning environment is where:

- all employees recognize the need for continuous learning to improve their own performance and that of the organization overall;
- the organizational culture facilitates and encourages learning and open sharing of knowledge and ideas; and
- opportunities and means for a wide variety of learning activities are present, such as coaching and reinforcement of newly acquired knowledge and skills.

In addition, the learning environment is where active listening takes place and where people are not intimidated to ask questions. Trainees, and people in general, are more apt to remember concepts, terms, skills, etc., if they:

- learned most recently;
- heard or saw more than once;
- were able to practice;
- can implement in their own setting and right away; and
- are encouraged or rewarded for using or trying the method.

The *trainer* also has a big role in successful implementation, which necessitates the understanding of the adult learning process. A trainer should always keep in mind that the trainees are adults and thus have certain expectations. The adult learner generally wants to learn and views the training as a key to better performance and career success, so the trainer must make them see that the content is relevant to their situation and setting. Many adult learners also wish to be challenged and to be actively involved in the learning process, which can be done by allowing open communication, asking questions, encouraging skills to be practiced in a risk-free environment, and providing feedback and validation.

The trainer must also have a set of training-related KSAs. Many books, resources, and programs are available to "train the trainer" or to enhance the trainer's abilities. Because training is focused on the facilitation of learning, the trainer must have a good understanding of human behavior and learning theory, which are important especially when dealing with the adult learner as discussed earlier. Specifically, the trainer must be highly skilled at interpersonal communication, listening, questioning, and providing feedback; however, the trainer must also be aware of nonverbal communication. Because the credibility of the trainer is paramount to the trainees willingness to learn, the trainer should have a strong knowledge base of the subject matter and ideally some experience in a similar setting. Having good organizational skills, the ability to present materials effectively and clearly, and know-how in using various media are also important.

Many times an organization will utilize outside consultants for their training programs. Some advantages to this approach are that outside consultants can provide a fresh perspective for employees, responsiveness to meet tight deadlines, training expertise in specialized areas, and skills or programs not made available by in-house trainers. However, using outside consultants could have some disadvantages as well, such as less commitment to long-term goals of the organization, higher fees and training cost, and no in-depth appreciation of the organization's culture.

Evaluation   As Bramley (1996) points out, the common view of evaluation is that it completes the training cycle. However, he suggests that evaluation is an integral part of the cycle and has a key role in quality improvement and control in that it provides feedback on:

- the effectiveness of the methods being used;
- the achievement of the objectives set by both trainers and trainees; and
- whether the needs originally identified, both at organizational and individual level, have been met.

Goldstein (1993) defines evaluation as "the systematic collection of descriptive and judgmental information necessary to make effective decisions related to selection, adoption, value, and modification of various instructional activities."

Two broad categories of assessment are evaluated: process and outcome. *Process analysis* examines how the training was designed and conducted, whereas *outcome evaluation* determines how well the training accomplished its objectives. Process data come from two sources: (1) the process before the training, including setting behavioral objectives, and (2) the instructional design features. Outcome data typically looks at various outcomes such as reactions, learning, job behavior, and organizational results. These data come from questionnaires, interviews, focus groups, records, observation, and skill testing.

In addition to evaluating the process of training and its outcomes, cost is another factor that must be evaluated. A *cost benefit analysis* can be used to compare the cost of the training to the benefits to the organization, although many of these benefits, such as improved attitude or better interpersonal relations, are hard to measure but are important outcomes to the organization. Training can also be assessed according to cost effectiveness; a *cost savings analysis* determines just what the organization saved, which may come in the form of reduced absenteeism or reduced malpractice claims or bad debt.

Once training is implemented and evaluated, a feedback loop about the outcomes of the effort must be reported to the original sponsors and designers. This feedback should help to inform the need for future training and development in the organization.

Development

Organization development (OD) is the preferred approach, among a growing number of organizations, to dealing with change. The processes of OD are designed to improve the ability of an organization to deal with external and internal changes in a way that is effective and meets the needs of its employees. OD utilizes planned interventions (Bennis 1969; Johnson 1996) that include force filed analysis, survey feedback, confrontation meetings, and coaching. These approaches tend to be diagnostic in nature but also provide solution-oriented intervention.

OD, more than most approaches, has demonstrated considerable success in working through the natural resistance to change that we see in organizations. This success is in part a result of OD's philosophy of participation and mutuality and its belief in the value of knowledge at all levels of the organization. OD empowers participants in the change process by involving them in the process and by encouraging their commitment to the desired change. This commitment to change is the core of any OD effort, and it occurs because of the following reasons (Blanchard and Thacker 1999):

- Participants are intimately familiar with the current system and can make valuable contributions to the change effort, which increases its chances of success.
- Participants become knowledgeable about what will happen as a result of the change, which reduces fear of the unknown.
- Participants support the change because they are a part of the process, which makes their beliefs about the change become more positive.

An excellent source of further information on OD is the Organization Development Institute, which has an international network of OD practitioners.[1]

Conclusion

As new methods of training and development are created, the range of options will increase, which will provide trainers and training departments with even more tools. However, until our full appreciation of human learning and the importance of learning environments are inculcated into the organization, these tools and techniques will have only marginal benefit. Ultimately, learning organizations are those that "liberate the human spirit' (Bickham 1996) to achieve and accomplish creatively. When the organization's goals are in alignment with the individual's goals, they can work in unison to improve performance and growth and learning become a continuous process that is rewarded and recognized for their value. Training and development then become vehicles designed to enhance the individual, the organization, and the communities that are served.

Discussion Questions

1. How would you go about designing a training program for a new group of nurse supervisors? Identify the steps involved at each phase of the training cycle.
2. Describe how training, development, and education are used in your organization.
3. What are the prime characteristics of the ideal learning environment? Why is it so important to adult learning?

Note

1. The address for the Organization Development Institute is O.D. Institute, 11234 Walnut Ridge Road, Chesterland, Ohio, 44026-1299.

References

Bennis, W. 1969. *Organization Development*. Reading, MA: Addison-Wesley.

Bickham, W. 1996. *Liberating the Human Spirit in the Workplace*. Chicago: Irwin.

Blanchard, P. N., and J. W. Thacker. 1999. *Effective Training Systems, Strategies, and Practices*. Upper Saddle River, NJ: Prentice Hall.

Bramley, P. 1996. *Evaluating Training Effectiveness*. New York: McGraw-Hill.

Fried, B. 1999. "Human Resources Management." In *Handbook of Health Administration and Policy*, edited by A. Kilpatrick and J. Johnson. New York: Marcel Dekker.

Friesen, M., and J. A. Johnson. 1996. *The Success Paradigm: Creating Organizational Effectiveness Through Quality and Strategy*. Westport, CT: Quorum Books.

Goldstein, I. L. 1993. *Training in Organizations*. Pacific Grove, CA: Brooks/Cole.

Gordon, E., E. Morgan, and J. Ponticell. 1995. "The Individualized Training Alternative." *Training and Development* (September): 52–60

Isaacs, S. L., and J. R. Knickman. 2001. *To Improve Health and Health Care 2001*. San Francisco: Jossey-Bass.

Johnson, J. A. 1996. "Organization Development in Health Care Organizations." *Organization Development Journal*.

Johnson, J. A., and V. Omachanu. 1999. "Total Quality Management as Health Care Strategy." In *Handbook of Health Administration and Policy*, edited by A. Kilpatrick and J. Johnson. New York: Marcel Dekker.

Kilpatrick, A. O., and J. A. Johnson. 1999. *Handbook of Health Administration and Policy*. New York: Marcel Dekker.

McIlwain, T., and J. Johnson. 1999. "Strategy: Planning, Management and Critical Success Factors." In *Handbook of Health Administration and Policy*, edited by A. Kilpatrick and J. Johnson. New York: Marcel Dekker.

Senge, P. 1990. *The Fifth Discipline: The Art and Practice of the Learning Organization*. New York: Doubleday.

Tobin, D. R. 1998. *The Knowledge-Enabled Organization*. New York: American Management Association.

COMPENSATION

John Crisafulli, M.B.A., M.H.A., and *Bruce J. Fried, Ph.D.*

Learning Objectives

After completing this chapter, the reader should be able to:

- Describe the purposes of compensation and compensation policy in healthcare organizations
- Distinguish between extrinsic and intrinsic rewards and the value of each to employees
- Understand the concepts of balancing internal equity and external competitiveness in compensation
- Describe the objectives of job evaluation and discuss the merits of alternative approaches to job evaluation
- Discuss the concept of broadbanding
- Discuss alternative types of incentive plans
- Articulate the challenges and problems faced in designing and implementing pay-for-performance plans

Introduction

People work for a number of different reasons, and the motivation behind work has been studied for many years. Findings from both research and practice conclude that a number of factors are related to job satisfaction and performance, including interest in work, competent supervision, and personal reward. While "money isn't everything," it is a significant motivator and a universal measure of the value we place on jobs and individuals. People assess their own value in terms of the amount of money they receive for their work and in terms of how their pay compares with others'. The way people are paid also sends a message to employees about what is valued in the organization. Employees must see that their compensation compares favorably to market rates and that equitable treatment among employees exists in the organization. The basic objective of compensation is to ensure that compensation is externally competitive and internally equitable. Consistent with the balanced scorecard perspective, achieving alignment between what the organization values and how it rewards its employees is important (Kaplan and Norton 1996).

In this chapter, we review the strategic role of compensation as well as the operational issues involved in determining individual compensation, discuss the need for organizations to have a process that places a monetary value on jobs, describe the most common forms of job evaluation, and describe different types of incentive compensation and the challenges encountered in developing and implementing such approaches.

Strategic Role of a Compensation Policy

Although the healthcare environment is stressful, a general belief presumes that healthcare workers/professionals work in the industry primarily because of the intrinsic value of that type of work. While most healthcare professionals do work because of the satisfaction they derive from their work, financial rewards are also a great factor in their performance and in their drive to contribute to achieving organizational goals. This finding has been validated in numerous studies (see, for example, Figure 9.1 for a summary of such a study).

FIGURE 9.1

Compensation is Important in Healthcare

A research study regarding nursing shortages conducted by William M. Mercer, one of the world's largest human resources consulting firms, gathered the opinions of executives at 185 healthcare organizations (93 percent of which were hospitals). The results are as follows:

- 30 percent of respondents said RN turnover was a "significant problem"
- 63 percent said RN turnover was "somewhat of a problem"
- Only 7 percent said RN turnover was not a problem
- The biggest reason given for turnover problems was "increased market demand"

"The results of a study appearing in the American Journal of Nursing (AJN) confirms . . . (the) belief that more than money is needed to retain good nurses. The study found that (hospitals retaining more nurses) have fewer patients in their workload, better support services, greater control over their practices, greater participation in policy decisions, and more powerful chief nurse executives. In addition, they were less apt to burn out and twice as likely to rate their hospitals as providing excellent care."

Source: Egger, E. 2000. "Nurse Shortage Worse than You Think, but Sensitivity May Help Retain Nurses." *Healthcare Strategic Management* 18 (5): 16–8.

Compensation should enhance employee motivation and growth while aligning employees' efforts with the objectives, philosophies, and culture of the organization. A strategic compensation policy typically includes the following set of goals:

1. to reward employee performance;
2. to achieve internal equity within the organization;
3. to remain externally competitive in relevant labor markets;
4. to align employee performance with organizational goals;
5. to attract and retain employees;
6. to maintain the compensation budget within organizational financial constraints; and
7. to maintain a compensation program that abides by legal constraints.

These goals come into conflict in certain situations. In attempting to recruit various types of employees, offering compensation levels to certain employees that appear internally inequitable may be necessary. In most cases, the discrepancy between an employee's worth, relative to other employees in the organization, and the amount that employee is paid is related to supply-and-demand factors. For example, to recruit physical therapists, who are in short supply in many parts of the United States, offering compensation packages that may be out of line with organizational pay schemes may be necessary. In fact, the conflict between the goal of internal equity and external competitiveness is one of the major challenges of a compensation policy; this conflict is particularly acute in healthcare because of periodic shortages of particular professionals.

Organizations face a number of other decisions in developing a compensation policy, which in turn may affect the goals of the compensation program. First, organizations must establish a general policy on whether to pay above, below, or at prevailing rates. This decision may be made explicitly or implicitly; in either event, organizations typically get a reputation for the amount it pays its employees. Second, organizations must decide exactly what will be rewarded. This decision may seem trivial at first, but the factors chosen to be rewarded usually signal what the organization values. For example, annual raises that are not explicitly tied to performance would tend to reward longevity and seniority in the organization. Again, whether this is the intended effect of the policy is not relevant. Employees generally respond to the incentives that they are presented. Alternatively, if an organization adopts a pay-for-performance approach, it faces a multitude of decisions about performance criteria to be used in determining compensation as well as the unanticipated consequences of rewarding certain aspects of performance.

Organizations will also face a multitude of other concerns in implementing a compensation program. These include determining the worth of individual jobs, assessing the additional value of employees' education and experience, and formulating a policy on pay secrecy.

Intrinsic Versus Extrinsic Rewards

Intrinsic compensation is intangible and may include rewards such as praise from a supervisor for completing an assignment or meeting established performance objectives or having feelings of accomplishment, recognition, or belonging in the organization

Compensation is but one part of the reward structure of an organization. Rewards can be intrinsic (internal) or extrinsic (external). **Intrinsic compensation** is intangible and may include rewards such as praise from a supervisor for completing an assignment or meeting established performance objectives or having feelings of accomplishment, recognition, or belonging in the organization. **Extrinsic compensation** is tangible and may include both monetary and nonmonetary rewards such as monetary compensation, benefits, good working conditions, and stock options.

Determining which type of reward motivates each individual employee is difficult; in most instances, employees are motivated by a combination of intrinsic and extrinsic rewards. In one early approach to reward systems, Herzberg, Mausner, and Snyderman (1959) suggested that employees need to have basic "hygiene" factors, which specifically refer to extrinsic rewards such as adequate pay and working conditions. However, he suggested that for employees to be *motivated and satisfied,* intrinsic motivating factors needed to be present, such as feelings of accomplishment. Thus, extrinsic rewards (most notably monetary compensation) are necessary, but insufficient, tools for promoting job satisfaction and motivation. Furthermore, the presence of extrinsic rewards may prevent dissatisfaction but do not necessarily lead to satisfaction. This perspective is similar to Maslow's (1970) view that individuals must have their basic needs met (biological and safety) before they are able to achieve higher-level goals. A good manager, therefore, should not ignore either type of reward. Nonprofit healthcare organizations with limited budgets should be especially mindful of the potential for using intrinsic rewards to supplement limited extrinsic rewards. Regardless of the forms of rewards an organization uses, employees must value the specific rewards for them to be effective.

Extrinsic compensation is tangible and may include both monetary and nonmonetary rewards such as monetary compensation, benefits, good working conditions, and stock options

Internal Equity Versus External Competitiveness

Every organization must maintain a delicate balance between internal equity and external competitiveness. Equity theory (Homans 1961; Adams 1963) provides a useful and well-tested framework for understanding the impact of perceived equity on individual performance. **Equity** is the perceived fairness of the relationship between what a person contributes to the organization (input) and what that person receives in return (outcome). Inputs refer to such things as an individual's education, seniority, skills, effort, loyalty, and experience. Outcomes, on the other hand, refer to pay, benefits, job satisfaction, opportunities for growth, and recognition. According to equity theory, employees constantly assess the ratio between their outcomes and inputs and,

Equity is the perceived fairness of the relationship between what a person contributes to the organization (input) and what that person receives in return (outcome)

more importantly, compare their own ratio to the ratio of others in the organization and, in some cases, to employees in other organizations. For example, an operating room nurse in a hospital will likely compare his ratio with other operating room nurses in the same hospital, with other individuals in the organization (to determine the comparability of their outcomes in relation to their inputs), and with individuals who perform similar work in other organizations. When employees find that their ratio is *smaller* than others', their motivation and performance are expected to decline.

This "comparing" feature of equity theory is pervasive in all organizations. Consider, for example, the interest generated when the salaries of senior executives are publicized in the media. Of course, the comparative judgments made by employees may be highly subjective and based on limited and inaccurate information. Regardless of how subjective we think these assessments are, managers must contend with these perceptions because those very perceptions in the end affect motivation and performance. Thus, managers must be aware not only of what they as managers perceive as the fairness of the reward system but also employees' assessments of equity.

When employees perceive inequity, they may attempt to remedy the situation by restoring a feeling of equity. They may increase their ratio in two ways: (1) by increasing their outcomes or (2) by decreasing their inputs. Employees may increase their outcomes by working harder and perhaps obtaining additional compensation or a promotion (note that working harder may also increase the "inputs" side of the ratio); by organizing other employees, possibly in the form of unionization; and by engaging in illegal activities such as theft. Similarly, employees may decrease their inputs by working fewer hours (through coming in late, leaving early, or being absent) and putting forth less effort. Employees may also attempt to restore a sense of equity by changing their perceptions of the inputs or outcomes of others, saying "That other employee really does have more experience than me"; "I may receive less pay in the health department than my coworkers in the hospital, but I have much better working relationships." In other instances, employees may change the person with whom they compare themselves.

While organizations seek to ensure equity, they must also be competitive externally to recruit staff. To be externally competitive, organizations must provide compensation that is perceived to be equitable in relation to compensation provided to employees who perform similar jobs in other organizations. If an organization is not externally competitive, it is likely to face problems of turnover and staff shortages, particularly in geographic areas where the supply of particular professionals may be scarce. Employers in healthcare and other fields currently find that attracting and retaining employees with specialized skills is difficult.

In the face of a tight labor market, organizations should have specifically stated policies that indicate what strategies can be used to position themselves in the labor market. These positioning policies generally use the quartile strategy, and most employers position themselves in the second quartile— in the middle of the market—based on compensation survey data of other employers' compensation plans. By choosing this position, organizations attempt to balance employer cost pressures and the need to attract and retain employees.

An employer that uses a first-quartile strategy, on the other hand, is choosing to pay below-market compensation; an employer might take this position for several reasons. First, shortage of funds or an inability to pay more may coincide with the need to continue to meet strategic objectives. Second, if a large number of applicants with lower skills are available in the labor market, this strategy can be used to attract sufficient workers at a lower cost. A major disadvantage of using a first-quartile strategy is high turnover, and, if the labor supply tightens, the organization may have difficulty attracting and retaining workers.

A third-quartile strategy, in which employees are paid above-market value, is more aggressive. This strategy may be used to ensure that a sufficient number of workers with the required capabilities are attracted and retained; it also allows the organization to be more selective. However, the expectation in most organizations is that those employees paid above-market rates must be more productive.

Determining the Monetary Value of Jobs

Job evaluation refers to one of several formal processes for determining the value of jobs in monetary terms. The development of a wage and salary system starts with a job analysis, which initiates the establishment of accurate job descriptions and job specifications for each position. This information is then used to perform a job evaluation and to conduct pay surveys. These activities are designed to ensure that the pay system is both internally equitable and externally competitive. The data gathered in the job evaluation and pay surveys are then used to design pay structures, including pay grades and pay ranges.

In a job evaluation, every job in an organization is examined and ultimately priced according to the job's relative importance to the organization; the knowledge, skills, and abilities the job requires; and the difficulty of the job. The employees' perception of the appropriateness of their pay in relation to the pay for other jobs is very important. To conduct a job evaluation, *Benchmark jobs* benchmark jobs are identified. **Benchmark jobs** are jobs that require similar *provide a basis on* knowledge, skills, and abilities and are performed by individuals who have *which other unique* similar duties; these benchmark jobs are used to provide a basis on which *jobs can be* other unique jobs can be evaluated. Job evaluation methods that are used to *evaluated* develop a wage and salary system for the organization are listed in the next section.

Methods of Job Value Evaluation

The *ranking method* is one of the simplest job value evaluation methods in that it ranks jobs based simply on their value to the organization. The entire job, rather than the individual components of the job, is considered in this method. This method is extremely subjective, and, therefore, managers find difficulty in explaining why a specific position is ranked higher. In addition, this method becomes very cumbersome in organizations that have a large number of jobs; therefore, it is more appropriate in small organizations with relatively few jobs.

Ranking Method

The *classification method* places each job in the organization into a grade, based on the job class that it most closely matches; as a result, this method suffers considerable subjectivity and manipulation. The classification method also relies heavily on job titles and duties and assumes that these are similar among different organizations. Comparison of pay rates among organizations may be inaccurate because the same job title may have very different responsibilities in different settings.

Classification Method

Broadbanding is an alternative pay structure that uses fewer pay grades with broader ranges than traditional pay structures. A broadband is a single, large salary range that spans the pay opportunities formerly covered by several separate small salary ranges. Broadbanding allows an organization to classify jobs into a few wide bands, rather than into narrowly defined salary ranges. A major advantage of broadbanding is that it provides more discretion to individual managers to shift employees within a particular pay range without concern for changing job titles. Employees may be rewarded within a broad pay grade for taking on new responsibilities or obtaining new skills.

Broadbanding

Broadbanding is an alternative pay structure that uses fewer pay grades with broader ranges than traditional pay structures

Broadbanding has become more popular. A 1996 survey of 380 large companies by Buck Consultants in New York found that 29 percent of these companies were using or implementing broadbanding, up from 16.7 percent in 1994. In addition, 27 percent of the respondents indicated they were considering making the change (Jacobs 1997). In fact, a growing number of organizations are in the midst of transformational changes and are looking for alternative pay structures to fit their new organizational structures. Broadbanding fits these new structures because it is more consistent with the current trend toward flatter, less hierarchical organizations. It is also more applicable to the current trend of having employees work in cross-functional positions, allowing the organization to respond more quickly to competitive pressures and environmental changes. With broadbanding, employees can shift responsibilities as the market and organizational requirements change.

Broadbanding provides many other advantages. For example, it enables companies to base compensation decisions on characteristics of the person who performs the job and not just on the job itself. With broadbanding, the authority for a larger number of compensation decisions is decentralized to the operating managers. Therefore, managers no longer need special approval for changes in compensation because broadbanding allows managers to reward their employees without having to promote them. In addition, the wider spread between pay grades gives managers more flexibility to recognize and reward different levels of individual contribution.

Another advantage of broadbanding is that it utilizes fewer pay groupings. Job evaluation is potentially simpler because organizations no longer need complex job evaluation schemes. Managers can encourage employees to move into other job areas that may broaden the employee's knowledge, skills, and abilities. Finally, broadbanding allows employees to evaluate their own skill acquisition and cross-training opportunities in terms of their own professional development and personal growth rather than to focus on pay grades. However, broadbanding is not appropriate for every organization and organizational culture. The narrow range spread of the traditional pay system may serve as an automatic cost-control mechanism to keep compensation expenses in check. With broadbanding, all employees may potentially float to the maximum pay level within their band, resulting in higher-than-market compensation for many or most employees.

The most difficult part of implementing broadbanding is getting employees to think differently about how they are paid. Pay grades have long been used to determine status, titles, and eligibility for perquisites, and employees have difficulty letting go of these preconceptions. The organization may also be seen as having fewer upward promotion opportunities. With fewer bands, employees recognize that promotions to a higher grade level will occur less frequently than before. Also, because the broadbands are typically further apart than traditional salary ranges, employees recognize that they must assume significantly greater job responsibilities to warrant placement in a higher band (Jacobs 1997).

Point Method

The *point method* is the most widely used job evaluation method. A basic assumption behind this method is that organizations do not pay for jobs but for aspects of these jobs, known as compensable factors. Examples of **compensable factors** include knowledge and skill requirements, experience needed, accountability, supervisory responsibilities, and working conditions. Through job analysis, jobs are broken down into compensable factors, and values or weights are assigned to these factors. Jobs are evaluated and points are assigned to each job based on the extent to which each compensable factor is present. Compensation levels and pay ranges are linked to the points assigned to each job. The point system provides a level of compensation based solely on job analysis, although actual compensation for a particular job may vary based on market and other factors.

Compensable factors are aspects of the job that can be compensated; these include knowledge and skill requirements, experience needed, accountability, supervisory responsibilities, and working conditions

Numerous challenges are posed by using a point system, including the following:

- Compensable factors must be acceptable to all parties.
- Compensable factors must validly distinguish among jobs.
- Compensable factors must be relevant to the jobs under analysis.
- Jobs must vary on the compensable factors selected so that meaningful differences in jobs can be identified.
- Compensable factors must be measurable.
- Compensable factors must be independent of each other (Hills, Bergmann, and Scarpello 1994).

Job evaluation based on a point system can indicate whether certain jobs are under or overpaid. Compensation decisions for particular jobs may have been based on salary survey data, which may be at odds with an organization's priorities as expressed in its choice of compensable factors. The choice of compensable factors, and the weights assigned to each factor, is of utmost importance. This point method is popular because it is relatively simple; is based on job analysis; may be used for many jobs; and, once established, is relatively easy to implement. However, this method does have several drawbacks, including the amount of time needed to develop the system, and may also reinforce traditional organizational structures and job rigidity.

The *factor comparison method* is a combination of the ranking and point methods. It differs from the point system in that the compensable factors for a job are evaluated against compensable factors in benchmark jobs in the organization. Using this method, the organization first determines the appropriate benchmark jobs. Benchmark jobs, in addition to the definition given above, are jobs that (1) are important to employees and the organization; (2) vary in their job requirements; (3) have relatively stable job content; and (4) are used in salary surveys for wage determination.

Factor Comparison Method

The benchmark jobs are evaluated against five compensable factors: skill, mental effort, physical effort, responsibilities, and working conditions. Monetary rates of pay are assigned to each compensable factor for each benchmark job. For example, the job of emergency room (ER) nurse may be identified as a benchmark job. Our analysis may determine that of the $17 hourly wage paid to an ER nurse, $5 is paid for mental effort, $3 for responsibility, and so forth. Similarly, we may use a hospital medical technologist's job as a benchmark, and we may decide that of the $15 hourly wage paid to this individual, $4 is paid for mental effort, $2.50 for responsibility, and so forth. A factor comparison scale may then be developed to evaluate other jobs in the organization. Thus, if we are attempting to evaluate the job of recreational therapist, we would compare the mental effort (and other factors) with that of the nurse and the medical technologist.

In sum, benchmark jobs are used to classify other jobs in the organization according to their compensable factors. A key advantage of a factor comparison approach is that it is tailored to one organization. It also indicates which jobs are worth more and how much more, so factor values can be more easily converted into monetary wages. Disadvantages of this method are that it is complex, time consuming to establish, and difficult to explain to employees.

Variable Compensation

Pay for Performance

Pay-for-performance systems are built on the principles that good work deserves to be rewarded and that pay based on good performance produces more good performance. In a pay-for-performance system, managers evaluate the work of their employees based on preestablished goals and standards or company values. Based on this judgment, the employee is given variable or contingent financial rewards. Linking compensation directly to individual contributions that are consistent with the organization's mission suggests that an organization can maintain the highest caliber of workers regardless of their particular role or specialty (Grib and O'Donnell 1995). In an incentive-based compensation system, pay is tied to specific goals that are established with employees prior to the time that they are being evaluated. The focus here is on specific actions that the employee has performed in pursuit of these pre-established goals (see Figure 9.2 for example).

Many writers, researchers, and management consultants argue that pay-for-performance systems decreased focus on customer needs, caused loss of accurate information about defects and improvement opportunities, led to avoidance of stretch goals, and decreased innovation. They argue that pay-for-performance systems make the supervisor the most important customer. Therefore, these systems divert energy away from the true customers and turn people inward. It also deprives the organization of essential information because managers learn less about defects and changes that need to be made. Employees under a pay-for-performance plan may be reluctant to report problems because of the impact on their compensation. When goals are set in advance, employees may also be more likely to argue for lower goals than for stretch goals to ensure that they receive performance-related rewards. In addition, pay-for-performance systems may hamper change; this is especially detrimental in healthcare because constant breakthroughs in performance require substantial changes in the way employees do their work (Berwick 1995; Pfeffer 1998). Figure 9.3 summarizes the most compelling arguments against pay for performance.

Incentive plans discourage risk taking and reduce creativity because the fear of not getting the reward makes people less inclined to take risks or explore other possibilities. Thus, the effectiveness of incentive plans is a topic of considerable debate. Those who support incentive plans point to the fact that most of us are, in reality, motivated by money. In other words, most people would rather have more money than less money. Therefore, money can be used to change employee behavior. Supporters of incentive compensation

FIGURE 9.2
Case Study:
Bassett Health
System

Bassett Health System employs 170 physicians, owns three hospitals with 248 beds, and operates a managed care plan, Community Health Plan, which handles 30,000 lives. Bassett also trains medical students through its affiliation with Columbia University in New York City. The Bassett Health System also consists of 19 primary care clinics in a ten-county area of 500,000 people.

Bassett administrators discovered in 1995 that Bassett physicians were not the lowest-cost physicians partnering within their own Community Health Plan; therefore, the physicians were not practicing the most efficient medicine. This discovery caused concern because these administrators realized if physicians did not practice the most efficient medicine, Bassett would not receive insurers' best rates.

The administrators decided to try to solve this problem through compensation, which at the time was mostly salary based, and they wanted to expand variable compensation so that it was 20 percent to 30 percent of the physicians' salary. The administrators decided that salary should remain the predominant means of compensation at Bassett because of the need to reward excellent teachers.

Maximum and minimum salaries were set for primary care physicians and specialists based on national surveys. The balance of the physicians' compensation would come from the new incentive system, which had three components:

1. Community Health Plan performance: Bassett would split the operating loss/gain 50–50 with the Community Health Plan and share half of its operating gain with the physicians. The share each physician gets would depend on the size of his or her subscription base and utilization rates and on subjective measures. The physician must adhere to an established norm for the number of office visits per subscribing patient per year, inpatient utilization rates, and the number of emergency department visits.
2. Departmental performance: This measure is tied to the financial performance of the physician's department. If an operating gain was achieved, 10 percent to 50 percent would be distributed among the doctors in that department.
3. Institutional performance: Bassett sets aside 25 percent of its operating gain for the year for the doctors. The amount a physician gets from this bucket depends on his or her contribution toward meeting Bassett's institutional goals.

Because of this change in physician compensation, Bassett has found that utilization rates, as well as admission rates and lengths of stay, are lower. Bassett administrators, however, do not expect the incentives themselves to manage physicians' behavior directly. They are hoping that by defining the health system's expectations they are beginning to build incentives in the compensation system to move doctors toward becoming more cost efficient.

Source: Coddington, D. C., C. R. Chapman, and K. M. Pokoski. 1996. *Making Integrated Health Care Work: Case Studies.* Englewood, CO: Medical Group Management Association. Used with permission from the Medical Group Management Association Center for Research, 104 Inverness Terrace East, Engelwood, Colorado 80112-5306; 303-799-1111. www.mgma.com. Copyright 1996.

FIGURE 9.3

Arguments
Against Pay-for-
Performance
Method

- Incentive plans produce only temporary improvements in performance and are ineffective in producing long-term change.
- Pay for performance poisons the role of manager as coach and mentor by injecting financial concerns into the supervisory relationship.
- The performance appraisal process is negatively affected because employees become overly concerned with money at the expense of growth and improvement.
- Incentives do not alter the underlying attitudes that determine behavior.
- Pay-for-performance systems operate under the assumption that employees are only motivated by extrinsic rewards (e.g., compensation), thus undermining intrinsic rewards (e.g., satisfaction derived from the work itself) as a motivational force.
- Although inadequate compensation can irritate and demotivate employees, this does not imply that more money will create increased satisfaction and motivation.
- Pay-for-performance plans are manipulative and may even reduce the possibility for cooperation, and therefore organizational excellence, by forcing people to compete against each other for rewards, recognition, or rankings.
- Relying on incentives does not address possible underlying problems or bring about meaningful change.
- Incentive systems are often used as a substitute for providing employees with the proper resources to do their jobs.

also assert that behaviors that are rewarded are repeated and behaviors that are punished are eliminated. People tend to set aside behaviors for which they are not rewarded. When rewarding behaviors, however, organizations must ensure that all relevant aspects of behavior are measured. Incomplete measurement and rewards may result in incomplete performance, with employees only doing those tasks or exhibiting those behaviors that are rewarded. Rewards also provide an opportunity for management to demonstrate to employees its values. Numerous studies suggest that financial incentives do improve work quantity. Too few studies exist, however, to determine their effect on performance quality (Gupta and Shaw 1998).

Under the new dynamics of managed care, pay for performance is being increasingly adopted in the healthcare sector. For physicians to be compensated at or near traditional levels, they must practice more efficiently. In other words, physicians must practice according to the rules of managed care. Because of these changes, physicians must now be more attuned to production targets, quality and outcomes measurements, and critical pathways (Clements 1996).

Team-Based Compensation

Healthcare and other industries have seen a pronounced emphasis toward the use of work teams. This emphasis on teams has stimulated the development of compensation systems that reward team performance. Team-based compensation systems can be difficult to implement because of the continued requirement to reward individual performance. Organizations interested in rewarding team performance need to strike a balance between individual and team rewards. Paying the same amount for everyone on the team regardless of his or her competencies or contributions is unacceptable in most organizations because it creates pay-equity problems.

Organizations that use team-based pay typically use team incentives as variable pay added to base pay. For base pay, employees are compensated using traditional job evaluation methods. On top of this base pay, variable pay is used based on business entity performance. These rewards are then distributed at the team level. In this way, organizations can reward the team for performance above a satisfactory level. This approach to team-based pay makes the compensation system relatively simple and easy to understand.

Skills-Based Pay

In a skills-based compensation system, employees are paid based on their personal skills and competencies relatively independent of the competencies required in their current position. The reward structure of this approach is based on the range, depth, and types of skills that individual employees are capable of using. To determine compensation levels, organizations must measure employees' competencies directly. Pay only increases after the employee demonstrates an ability to perform specific skills. This approach to compensation supports the notion that employees with more skills are more valuable to the organization.

Conclusion

In an effort to achieve greater levels of effectiveness and efficiency, we will likely continue to witness a variety of new compensation arrangements in healthcare. Compensation is perhaps the most sensitive topic for employees, and tampering with compensation arrangements can have disastrous effects if we do not consider the anticipated and unanticipated consequences of new compensation arrangements. What may look good on paper as an innovation in compensation can have effects of which we are unaware. Perhaps the most important lesson in the area of compensation, and incentive compensation in particular, is to involve employees at all organizational levels in the design and implementation of compensation plans. In this way, we can plan more effectively and implement compensation plans with a broader and more accurate understanding of the likely effects of a plan.

Discussion Questions

1. In seeking to motivate employees in a low-budget healthcare operation (such as a local health department), how would you recruit and motivate employees when the competition (for example, area hospitals) are able to pay staff 30 to 40 percent higher wages?

2. Assume that you are working as a staff nurse in a hospital and you are working under an incentive system. Do you have an obligation to disclose the nature of the compensation arrangement to patients? If so, how should this information be communicated and by whom?

3. Regardless of your personal feelings about pay for performance, what cautions would you communicate to a team that is designing an incentive system in a healthcare organization?

4. How would you design a team-based compensation system such that free riders (or "loafers") could not take advantage of the system?

5. How can job evaluation procedures be used to determine if a healthcare organization is undercompensating women?

References

Adams, J. S. 1963. "Toward an Understanding of Inequity." *Journal of Applied and Social Psychology* 67: 422–24.

Berwick, D. M. 1995. Toxicity of Pay for Performance. *Quality Management in Health Care* 4 (1): 27–33.

Clements, B. 1996. "Pay for Performance." *American Medical News* (August 12).

Grib, G., and S. O'Donnell. 1995. "Pay Plans that Reward Employee Achievement." *HR Magazine* (July): 49–50.

Gupta, N., and J. D. Shaw. 1998. "Let the Evidence Speak: Financial Incentives Are Effective." *Compensation and Benefits Review* 26 (March/April): 28–32.

Herzberg, F., B. Mausner, and B. Snyderman. 1959. *The Motivation to Work.* New York: John Wiley.

Hills, F. S., T. J. Bergmann, and V. G. Scarpello. 1994. *Compensation Decision Making, Second Edition.* Forth Worth, TX: Dryden.

Homans, G. C. 1961. *Social Behavior: Its Elementary Forms.* New York: Harcourt, Brace and World.

Jacobs, K. 1997. "The Broad View." *The Wall Street Journal* (April 10), Eastern Edition: R10.

Kaplan, R. S., and D. P. Norton. 1996. *The Balanced Scorecard.* Boston: Harvard Business School Press.

Maslow, A. 1970. *Motivation and Personality, Second Edition.* New York: Harper & Row.

Pfeffer, J. 1998. "Six Dangerous Myths About Pay." *Harvard Business Review* (May/June): 108–19.

PHYSICIAN COMPENSATION

Derek van Amerongen, M.D., M.S.

Learning Objectives

After completing this chapter, the reader should be able to:

- Understand the impact of third-party payment on physician compensation
- Understand how compensation came to be seen as a means of changing physician behavior
- Describe how different practice settings affect physician income
- Understand the conflicts that can arise in different compensation models
- Understand possible future directions for physician compensation models

Introduction

Any compensation system must accomplish several basic objectives. First, it must fairly reward the individual for the labor performed and expertise exhibited. Second, it must align the incentives of the worker with those of the organization that provides the reimbursement. Third, it should reduce or eliminate undesirable behavior—that is, activities that prevent the successful achievement of required tasks. Fourth, it should prepare the way for the future evolution of the job or industry, particularly for someone involved in a highly technical, complicated field. These goals must apply to the medical practitioner as well.

American medicine is unique among other professions, and among medical professions in other countries, in the way it has developed in the past fifty years. Prior to World War II, most physicians were general practitioners who made a tolerable living for the time, receiving payment on a piece-meal basis (Starr 1982). Indeed, medicine was considered one of the more successful cottage industries, but that success did not prevent some physicians from becoming destitute during the Depression; in fact, several "homes" for penniless physicians were established in the 1930s. This situation changed radically after the war with the explosion in the medical subspecialties brought on by battlefield needs, the rise of care within hospitals instead of the home, and the advent of employer-based medical insurance. Employer-based medical insurance is the factor that generated many of the cost and appropriateness of medical care issues with which we are now struggling. Once the consumer of care (the patient) was no longer responsible directly for the cost, the payer of the service (the employer or government) did not receive the service, and the deliverer of care (the physician) was no longer obliged to justify the utility of treatments or the costs to the patient, the constraints that typically exist in any economic interaction (recognizing that medical care has other important dimensions as well) were lost. The result was a system that paid physicians whatever they requested, without attempting to validate the appropriateness of those services. This series of events, in short, led to the managed care movement that has marked the last few years.

In this chapter, we review the most critical current and future issues in physician compensation. Specifically, we describe the effect of a third-party payment system on physician income; define capitation and discuss how it has been used as a tool for modifying how physicians practice; differentiate among various practice settings and discuss how they determine physician reimbursement; discuss the differences between independent and employed physicians; illustrate how compensation models address physician productivity; and discuss potential innovations for the future.

Failure of Current Compensation Schemes

With the development of managed care, attention turned to using payment mechanisms to modify physician behavior. Analysts identified several problems with the way doctors practice in the United States. A key concern has been that medical evidence is infrequently used in treatment decisions (Winslow 2000); for example, two patients with the same condition may receive vastly different therapies, or two patients with very different diseases may be treated exactly the same. Allowing for the so-called "art of medicine" still does not explain the lack of implementation of well-documented treatment guidelines that have been shown to improve outcomes. In addition, variation in practice is widespread and is not linked to medical differences in populations. Two adjacent communities, with similar populations and demographics, may have dramatically different rates of surgery or use of certain modalities. Scientific justification of such differences is often impossible to find, resulting in the conclusion that such discrepancies in care come from physician choice and habit, not medical data.

Capitation is a system that pays a physician a certain amount for each patient assigned to his or her panel or list of patients

A key objective of health policy advocates in the early 1990s was to leverage reimbursement mechanisms to address these problems; however, the track record for reducing practice discrepancies or improving practice behaviors in the last ten years has been disappointing. Modifying physician behavior using various forms of reimbursement has been a notable failure. One common alternative was **capitation**—a system that pays a physician a certain amount for each patient assigned to his or her panel or list of patients; the fee was meant to cover the services needed to care for the patient, as spelled out in the certificate of insurance coverage. The challenge for the practitioner was to provide these services within the limits of the capitated payment, but the incentive was that any money left over would revert to the physician as revenue. Capitation was initially seen as a solution to the problem of physicians having the incentive, under a fee-for-service system, to perform more services whether they were needed or not and to neglect preventive measures. The logic was that by giving the physician a set amount per patient (a capitated payment), the physician would be encouraged to do as much as possible to keep patients healthy so they would not need expensive services. This ideal reflects the health maintenance goal of the original HMOs, which was seen in the late 1970s as an altruistic alternative to the traditional system. (In my career, I have seen the common perception of the HMO move from the "socialist plot" of the 1970s to the "robber-baron plot" of the 1990s.)

The Achilles' heel of capitation was that it put the physician at risk for the care of the patients in his or her panel and it rendered physicians responsible for patients whom they may never have seen. Juggling the care of patients who may or may not want to visit the office, and doing so in a longitudinal manner that stretched far beyond the examination room, was too much of a risk for most doctors. While many physician groups initially were enthusiastic about accepting risk payment, mainly because of the increased payments it brought, they usually failed to understand the full implications of being responsible for a population versus caring for an individual patient. Bankruptcies of medical groups were not uncommon because of their inability to manage the very problems with physician behavior that capitation was supposed to solve. As a result, risk payment method has become increasingly unpopular as a payment option. Because of capitation's inability to change practice patterns (Grumbach et al. 1999; *Managed Care Outlook* 1999) and its adverse impact on both physician group viability and the willingness of groups to participate in such plans, other approaches are now taking precedence.

An important element that affects the ability of new compensation models to change behaviors is the continued growth in physician income. In the early 1990s, the general belief was that by putting the brakes on the rise in salaries, physicians could be brought in line with the directions that health plans and employers wanted them to go; this concept is frequently referred to as *aligning incentives*. However, numerous studies (Thompson 2000; Kilborn 1999) have demonstrated the surprising talent of physicians to continue to increase their incomes, albeit at lower rates than in the 1980s. Nevertheless, with most specialists making well over $200,000 per year, using income as a tool for change has become difficult. The unique ability to increase volume even as the cost per unit decreases has largely protected most physicians from experiencing radical shifts in income. Furthermore, unlike other professions, increased supply of physicians has actually led to higher levels of health spending. Competition has had a minimal impact on total costs, unlike other industries in which more suppliers typically result in lower overall costs and revenues.

An additional issue is the backlash against managed care that has gained force recently. This backlash includes how doctors are paid. Risk structures have generated intense controversy, as MCOs and medical groups have both been accused of skimping on patient care to increase revenues. Numerous lawsuits have been initiated against managed care companies, some of which are led by the same lawyers who were responsible for suing the tobacco industry. Although the Supreme Court rejected the case of *Pegram v. Herdrich* in June 2000, giving the managed care industry continued protection against one form of liability (Mariner 2000), more suits are likely in the future. An important issue for Congress in the next few years will be to decide on the level of liability appropriate for MCOs. Regardless of the action Congress takes, recent history suggests that creative lawsuits will continue to be filed against MCOs. Consequently, any new compensation model must anticipate the potential for legal action. This undercuts the willingness of employers, who ultimately pay most of the costs for medical care, to aggressively promote such models.

Employment Setting

Most variation in how doctors are paid derives from the setting in which they practice or are employed. Each one has its benefits and drawbacks, depending on the goals of the different types of practice.

Office-Based Practices

Office-based physician practice is the classic practice model in which two or more physicians work together in an office setting. The degree of affiliation between the physicians can range from tight to very loose; a closely knit group would have the physicians seeking to practice with a common philosophy and approach. This closeness might extend to the business functions of the practice as well as the medical ones. A loosely connected group may find physicians sharing some common office services, such as clerical and billing, but practicing independently in all other regards.

An independent practice association (IPA) usually consists of a collection of practices that may include both solo and group practitioners who come together to take advantage of economies of scale for contracting, business services, or ancillary services

Three broad categories of office practice are solo, group, and **independent practice association (IPA)**. The solo practitioner practices alone, and the group practice may be arranged as noted in the previous paragraph. The IPA usually consists of a larger collection of practices that may include both solo and group practitioners who come together to take advantage of economies of scale for contracting, business services, or ancillary services (such as laboratory). The IPA may negotiate on behalf of the members and have signature authority to arrange contracts and distribute reimbursements.

For the solo and group physicians, the dominant reimbursement mode is pure *fee for service (FFS)*. The fee schedules used in determining payments have been significantly reduced in recent years, reductions which have come from both private payers and the government. An unintended, but not unexpected, consequence has been an increase in utilization of services, so that even as the price of each unit has declined, the number of units provided has increased. This increase in service has further resulted, as noted previously, in higher incomes for many specialties even as fee schedules were driven lower.

Despite this incongruity, the discounted FFS model is not likely to change in the foreseeable future. Solo physicians and smaller groups are not good candidates to accept risk structures. Rather than set such practices up to fail, leading to network disruption and the dissatisfaction of patient, physician, and employer, most payers will continue to reserve risk contracts for the few large, highly integrated groups that can handle them. Discounted FFS is simple and straightforward in contrast to risk models, and it is also easier for most health plans to administer, even for multispecialty groups.

IPAs may well decide to ask for risk contracts from a payer, particularly if the IPA is large and well integrated. This implies a shared philosophy of care among the physicians, with a high degree of self-discipline. Such groups will actively monitor utilization internally, usually comparing it to national standards and scientifically validated treatment guidelines. Physicians who deviate significantly from these norms are either re-educated by their peers or are asked to leave the group. Frequently, a relatively sophisticated information-gathering system is in place within the group to facilitate monitoring of outcomes and utilization. The product of this attention is a group that knows what its costs are and where opportunities exist to maximize efficiency, which creates a climate that is ready to accept risk and one in which the physicians feel comfortable being part of a larger team.

Few IPAs are developed to the extent that they are free to take on a risk project and make it work. More typical is the IPA that is paid from a discounted FFS schedule but also has some sort of incentive program to add dollars to the total reimbursement for the group. Such incentive plans may award a portion of any savings realized if the group achieves targeted utilization in areas such as use of pharmaceuticals or lab tests. Such incentives may be simply a bonus, or they may be more complicated. A pool of money may be put aside to be shared if targets are met, or a percentage increase in the fee schedule may occur if the group successfully manages its patients. The key point is that incentives are designed to encourage the group to perform at a higher level, but regardless of the success in reaching these goals, the physicians are still paid for each service provided.

Staff Model Groups

Some medical groups or HMOs employ physicians on a *straight salary basis* or staff model—a model common in the late 1970s and early 1980s. Many early HMOs, such as Prudential and Humana, formulated the staff model as their primary method of caring for their members. The staff model concept is simple: A physician employed by an organization will not be distracted by concerns of generating revenue to cover practice expenses and will be able to focus on practicing medicine. The drawback to this approach is the difficulty in recruiting physicians who want to be employees, because many people go into medicine to be independent. Furthermore, the ability of the employer to control an employee who is a highly trained professional turned out to be far more difficult than many would have expected. Despite having an employed group of doctors who theoretically had their personal goals aligned with the organization, many HMOs found utilization by their physicians to be as high and as variable as physicians in private practice. The work ethic of employed physicians also came into play; many medical directors of staff-model HMOs have been frustrated by the difficulty in getting salaried physicians to extend themselves beyond the prescribed hours and tasks. As a result, the staff model has withered in the last ten years. However, the model is still a force in California because of the strong presence of the Permanente group, the staff model organization that serves Kaiser HMO. Elsewhere in the country, isolated staff model groups remain as relics of the past, supported primarily by a loyal base of long-time patients. However, the era of the salary-based physician practice has probably come and gone.

Hospital-Based Physicians

A large core of physicians—pathologists, radiologists, and anesthesiologists, among others—practice almost exclusively within the confines of the nonacademic hospital. In the past, many were directly employed by the hospital and received a straight salary. Recently, however, they have formed professional corporations that contract with the hospital for services, often on an exclusive basis. For instance, a hospital may arrange to have services provided by a group of emergency medicine physicians. This group will staff the emergency room, be paid on a contractual basis, and may even take over the administration of the unit. The basis for the contract is typically some formula that represents the billings the unit generates, with an additional amount included for such items as administration, participation on hospital committees, etc. The same model can apply to other specialties as well. The key interaction from a reimbursement perspective occurs between the administrators of the hospital and the physicians' organization. The doctors function as independent contractors within the hospital; they are "in it" but not "of it."

The scenario changes somewhat for physicians in the academic, tertiary care medical center. Several unique aspects of these institutions must be considered. A large percentage of the physicians in this setting are in training as residents or fellows. Their salaries are paid in large measure from Medicare reimbursements received by the medical center for the purpose of supporting graduate medical education. Thus, their salaries are not linked to their clinical performance, number of patients seen, rate of procedures performed, or other measures of productivity or quality. For staff or faculty physicians, salary is also the rule (because typically these physicians receive a straight salary that is not based on productivity) although the role of clinical activity is often figured into it. The mission of the academic physician may be summarized as combining teaching, research, and patient care. With decreased reimbursements to hospitals, the need for these physicians to perform more clinical work has grown. This may or may not be accompanied by an increase in salary and often depends on whether a "faculty practice plan," essentially a group practice that consists of the faculty of the medical center, exists. Such a group is created as a way to leverage the billings generated by the faculty into some sort of shared distributions, or at least a higher salary for those physicians who produce high clinical volumes. The amount of additional income that flows from the faculty practice plan is usually not great; the principle source of income for an academic physician remains the salary from the institution. These salaries are invariably lower than those in the private practice sector and reflect the typical differential for salaries between the academic and commercial environments. Some physicians within the academic setting may see no patients at all but focus entirely on research. Many of them will derive the bulk of their salaries from the grants they are able to secure from outside agencies; the remainder may come from the university. As a result, the longevity of a researcher in this environment may well depend on his or her skill at preparing grant applications and performing research that is deemed worthy of outside support.

Physicians in Management and Administration

One interesting trend over the last decade has been the rise in the number of physicians who are employed full time as medical directors, consultants, and administrators. Aside from those working for MCOs, health insurers, and large provider groups, many are now working for large employers who want to better understand and control the resources devoted to healthcare benefits. These physicians fill critical roles as internal experts on medical care and health policy. They help benefits coordinators and human resources administrators address the complex issues that arise for their company's employees by functioning as internal experts attuned to the unique problems of their employer. They also serve as liaisons between the benefits and human resources personnel of the company and external vendors such as health plans, large provider groups, and ancillary providers. Medical directors are also increasingly found in important roles in state and federal agencies for the same reasons. As healthcare costs continue to escalate, this trend will likely continue. As employees of the organization, medical directors are salaried and given the same sorts of benefits and incentives offered to an executive in most companies.

Difficulties and Conflicts

For the salaried physician, whether in an academic medical center, a large provider group, or large employer, the most likely issues to arise are the same ones that might involve any employee: benefits, perks, and the salary amount. The most difficult area in which to fairly determine physician pay is in assessing the parameters that factor into any compensation model based on productivity. Even for a medical group of two physicians the potential exists for disagreements over what constitutes productivity levels. The following examples illustrate the complexity of resolving these arguments:

- If a patient new to the practice is "counted" at a higher value than a returning patient, what defines a new patient? Someone who has never been seen before? Someone who has not been seen within a given time frame? Someone who has not been seen for a nonacute visit?
- For a procedure-based specialty such as gastroenterology, does the physician who performs the procedure get full credit for it, or should partial credit go the physician who has seen the patient most frequently over the past year?
- For an obstetric practice, should the physician who performs more vaginal deliveries (which represent more time at the bedside) receive more credit than a physician who has a higher rate of cesarean section operations (which produce a higher fee for the practice)?

A myriad of complicating factors can make a straightforward determination of productivity extremely difficult. Such fine points may seem unimportant until one understands that each element can be linked to a dollar value to the practice, which can make a significant difference in overall compensation for the physician. Add to this such elements as seniority in the group, the number of call days taken, or outside activities such as service on hospital or medical society committees, and one can appreciate the dilemma many practices face in dividing up the practice revenues.

Many groups have attempted to address these problems by designing formulae to incorporate the multiple contributing factors they wish to consider when calculating compensation. By their nature, these formulae can become extremely complex as they try to account for a number of unrelated items, often items that are difficult to accurately measure. For example, surgical groups may try to include the number of cases seen with various weightings based on the severity of illness of the patient as well as a factor for covering the emergency room, teaching residents at the medical school, and the number of holiday calls taken. Ironically such projects take an inordinate amount of time to devise and typically end up affecting a small fraction of the total income of the physician. A further problem is the inability of any scheme so complicated to either reinforce behavior desired by the practice or extinguish undesirable behavior.

While the employed physician in a large medical group may not be directly affected by such productivity questions, the group itself is. For many groups that went on a hiring binge in the mid-1990s, as well as hospitals that bought practices to lock in patient referrals, the assumption was frequently made that employed physicians would maintain the same high productivity rates they achieved when self-employed. However, many such physicians sold their practices to reduce their workload, leading to a dramatic drop in patient volumes. As a result, many employers of physicians have been faced with large deficits from their employed providers, leading to severe financial strains.

Future Directions

The current framework of compensation for physicians has not substantially changed how medical practice is performed. The advent of capitation and the use of incentives were assumed to be the beginning of a revolution in how physicians would treat patients as well as how they would be paid. After a decade of change in the healthcare industry, the vast majority of practicing physicians continue to be paid on some sort of FFS basis. Rather than this number decreasing as a result of the expansion of managed care, it is actually growing as more health plans move away from risk-based contracts in a tacit acknowledgment of their failure to substantially modify physician behavior (*Managed Care Outlook* 1999). As such, new methods are necessary if the goal of changing the patterns of medical practice is to be achieved. Changes in how medical care is delivered cannot be entirely successful unless physicians support them. This support depends very much on making sure physicians are fairly and adequately compensated.

During the next few years, more opportunities for innovation will be created as the healthcare industry searches for new paths to follow. Some of the possibilities are listed below:

- Physicians will be more creative in their fee and payment structures. The leaders in this area have been cosmetic surgeons, who have always been paid out-of-pocket for the bulk of the work they do. They were among the first physicians to make payment for services with credit cards possible and to set up payment schedules in advance of surgery. While these payment options are commonplace in the rest of the economy, in medicine they were revolutionary.

    Another specialty that has taken on the challenge of making patient access to high-cost services easier is infertility treatment by reproductive endocrinologists. Some groups are now asking for a fee up-front, say $30,000, to cover three cycles of in vitro fertilization. If the patient does not conceive at the end of the third cycle, the money is refunded except for a small amount to cover costs. The patient is thus provided with a sort of money-back guarantee. By seeking flexibility in payment and recognizing that their services are expensive and must be made more accessible to those without insurance coverage, these specialists have found new ways to secure their revenue stream.

- Americans spend more than $13 billion per year on complementary and alternative medicine modalities, such as acupuncture, massage therapy, homeopathy, and biofeedback. Almost 100 percent of this alternative medicine expenditure is not typically covered by insurance. The public seems to have an insatiable demand for these kinds of therapies, and physicians will seek to capture some of this huge volume of care by offering more options to receive alternative medicine within the context of their (traditional) medical practices. Because this care occurs outside of a fee schedule negotiated with a payer, it may well come to represent a large portion of some doctors' incomes in the future.

- For physicians who are still paid primarily by third-party payers, reimbursement will be tied to performance. As tools for assessing outcomes of care improve and are tied to such parameters as patient satisfaction and use of various treatments, report cards on doctors' practice and performance will be widely available. Just as consumers now go to a variety of sources, especially the Internet, to research the purchase of a new car or house, in the near future they will be able to do the same for selecting their physicians and hospitals. Once chosen, the level of reimbursement for that provider will be related to their reported performance. Those providers who perform at a high level will be paid at a higher level than those who do not perform well. An ever-increasing differentiation between the "good" doctors and the "poor" ones will develop, with the factors being the scorecard results and the reimbursement levels that follow.

- Employers are nearing the end of their 50-year run as the source for most Americans' health insurance. In the next few years, a sea of change will occur, with more and more employers divesting themselves of this responsibility and returning it to the individual. The patient-consumer will then be accountable for making the kind of healthcare choices currently left up to the benefits manager at work. Having this freedom to choose will require that consumers become more educated in managing their own health, which will be facilitated by the thousands of web sites devoted to medical topics on the Internet. In turn, physicians will see their patients become more informed and discriminating consumers. They will need to provide their patients with the type of service and quality that will lure them back for a second visit and will represent value to them as the ultimate payer. Price will certainly be part of this value equation, and physicians will need to respond to price in ways they have never contemplated.

Conclusion

Note that all the options discussed above still revolve around some variation of the FFS model. This will continue to be the primary method for paying for medical services, although the context will continue to evolve. After an intense decade of experimentation with novel methods of reimbursement, ironically we return to the time-tested FFS structure. Yet important differences exist between the models represented by FFS in 2001 and 1985. FFS payment levels will no longer be dictated by "usual and customary" rates that were established by a de facto agreement of the practicing physicians in a community. They will instead be based on a market formulation that more directly relates to the value of the service as perceived by the patient-customer. Therefore, those physicians and groups who can demonstrate a higher value will command a higher price for their services. This will remake the FFS system into one that more closely resembles the compensation mechanisms we are familiar with in other sectors of the economy.

Discussion Questions

1. Why was the healthcare sector compelled to try to change how physicians practice medicine?
2. What effect has the managed care "backlash" had on designing physician compensation models?
3. What are the likely roles for capitation and fee-for-service reimbursement in the future?
4. For a four-person surgical group, what kind of formula might be devised to fairly and consistently measure and reward productivity? What changes might be needed if one surgeon decides to perform more office work and less surgery?

References

Grumbach, K., J. V. Selby, C. Damberg, A. B. Bindman, C. Quesenberry, A. Truman, and C. Uratsu. 1999. "Solving the Gatekeeper Conundrum: What Patients Value in Primary Care and Referrals to Specialists." *Journal of the American Medical Association* 282: 261–6.

Kilborn, P. T. 1999. "Doctors' Incomes Rising Again Despite HMOs." *Cincinnati Enquirer* (April 22): A2.

Managed Care Outlook. 1999. "Florida Blues Ditch Capitation in Favor of Fee-for-Service." *Managed Care Outlook* (May 21): 5.

Mariner, W. K. 2000. "What Recourse? Liability for Managed-Care Decisions and the Employee Retirement Income Security Act." *New England Journal of Medicine* 343: 592–6.

Starr, P. 1982. *The Social Transformation of American Medicine,* pp. 198–235. New York: Basic Books.

Thompson, E. 2000. "Physician Compensation Report: Docs' Income Growth Stabilizes." *Modern Healthcare* (August 7): 37–41.

Winslow, R. 2000. "A Type of Heart Drug Wins Wide Use Owing to Small Firm's Efforts." *The Wall Street Journal* (November 17): A1.

CREATING AND MAINTAINING A SAFE AND HEALTHY WORKPLACE

Michael T. Ryan, Ph.D., CHP, and
Anne Osborne Kilpatrick, D.P.A.

Learning Objectives

After completing this chapter, the reader should be able to:

- Understand the factors associated with safe and healthy workplaces
- Describe key steps in improving the safety and health of a workplace
- Know the seven principles that form the foundation of workplace health and safety programs
- Discuss the elements contained in a safety program
- Discuss the concept of "toxins," which may interfere with organizational effectiveness

Introduction

All organizations are concerned with creating and maintaining a safe and healthy workplace. As illustrated in the following brief scenarios, the issue has particular importance in healthcare organizations. In each case, consider what the regulatory requirements are and what course of action management should follow.

- An employee attends a scheduled after-hours function at which attendance is mandatory. Alcoholic beverages are served without charge. The employee is involved in a fatal automobile accident while driving home from the event. Is this fatality a job-related injury?
- A radiological technician who is pregnant does not declare her pregnancy to her employer. Upon later notification of the pregnancy, the supervisor wants to restrict the employee to "low-exposure-potential" assignments, which place the technician at a lower pay level.
- A nurse's aide tests positive for HIV and claims it is the result of an unreported needle stick.

- A nurse assigned to care for tuberculosis (TB) patients tests positive for TB during routine, periodic testing. The nurse claims that she contracted the disease as a result of improper ventilation maintenance in the TB care area.

Healthcare managers could find themselves addressing worker health and safety cases such as the ones briefly described above or other issues that involve regulatory requirements related to workplace safety and health. The most successful programs, however, avert problems proactively. While low rates of recordable injuries are often used as a measure of safety excellence, or improvement, this is not the best way to measure safety program success. Proactive, rather than reactive, responses to problems are key responsibilities of healthcare managers. This chapter presents practical steps and guidelines to follow in creating safe and healthy workplaces that result in improved, cost-effective performance. In addition, we provide further information on safety and healthy issues and resources in Appendix B.

Safety in the Workplace

Maintaining a safe workplace and conforming to federal, state, and local regulations require a comprehensive safety compliance program (American Society for Healthcare Services 1997; Chaff 1994). Such a program must include the essential elements of careful planning, preparation, implementation, performance tracking, and process improvement. Using a disciplined approach by adhering to the following seven key principles can facilitate this process.

1. *Develop and maintain a positive safety culture.* This is best established with a strong, visible commitment and program participation from executive management.
2. *Understand the requirements for safety compliance and the regulations under which your activities will be governed.* Document all work practices and assess all tasks regarding safety and related regulatory requirements (Government Institutes, Inc. 1997; Wilson 1998).
3. *Review carefully all rules and regulations that apply to your activities.* Pay particular attention to overlapping and seemingly conflicting requirements under different rules or regulations (Moeller 1997).
4. *Develop formal, written communications that explain safety policies and instructions to workers regarding how to perform tasks in a safe manner.* Instructions should include specific requirements for documentation of routine activities. Methods of reporting incidents, accidents, or other unexpected circumstances should also be included in written procedures.
5. *Conduct formal training and retraining to routinely inform employees regarding safety issues.* This training can include initial and refresher training on program basics, special issue training following an incident or accident, or new developments that occur as a result of facility work practice changes or changes in regulatory requirements.

6. *Develop a plan to ensure buy-in throughout all levels of the organization.* Executive management must set the standard by participating in program development and safety training and recognizing safety performance. Throughout the organization positive safety practices must be reinforced and poor safety practices must be replaced.

7. *Investigate incidents and accidents in a proactive, not punitive, fashion.* Be responsive to the facts. For incidents that do occur, such as some of those listed above, a pre-established investigation team, including legal and technical experts, should thoroughly investigate. These investigations should be done for purposes of fact finding, prevention of recurrence, and satisfactory resolution of the incident at hand.

Management Leadership Regarding Safety

Management commitment should be visible in two ways. First, active leadership and participation in safety program activities such as key meetings, training, and celebration events are important. Setting the safety example is key to establishing a positive safety culture. Second, direct and indirect financial commitment to the safety program and its implementation are essential. If safety programs are to be an important part of a facility's activities, the allocation of resources is a visible way to confirm this commitment. Safety programs should be managed using the same cost, schedule, and control approaches as any other important programs within a facility. Safety should not be viewed as an add-on to someone's responsibilities or fit into the schedule of other activities; however, in smaller facilities, assigning safety responsibilities as part of a manager's overall responsibilities may be necessary. Care should be taken to ensure that safety receives due attention.

Safety Program Elements

The first step in developing a safety program is to define, clearly and completely, all activities that occur in all parts of the facility. A realistic approach is needed to accomplish this. Program requirements will be dictated by what activities are formally identified and included in the program, and both overemphasis and underemphasis regarding safety requirements will result in ineffective programs. Being unrealistic will result in safety (and perhaps other) permit requirements being set inappropriately and may create regulatory obligations that could be underprotective or overprotective for some activities. Defining all safety activities clearly and accurately is in the facility's best interest.

The successful development of safety programs relies on five elements:

1. *Safety program policies must be well written.* Procedures must clearly convey what work is to be done, how to do it safely, and what documentation is required.

2. *The safety program must meet all the regulatory requirements associated with those activities.* Regulatory agencies will include but are not limited

to the Occupational Health and Safety Administration (OSHA), the U.S. Environmental Protection Agency (EPA), the Centers for Disease Control and Prevention (CDC), and the U.S. Nuclear Regulatory Commission (NRC). In some cases these federal agency responsibilities may be delegated to state agencies.

3. *Information from recommending bodies will also be helpful.* The recommending bodies include but are not limited to the Joint Commission on Accreditation of Healthcare Organizations, the National Fire Protection Association (NFPA), the National Institute of Standards and Technology (NIST), the Compressed Gas Association (CGA), and other state and local agencies.

4. *The safety program must be a living program that can accommodate change and improvement without starting over for each change.*

5. *The safety program must guide activities in a positive fashion both when things are going well and when incidental, accidental, and off-normal circumstances occur.*

Safety Program Implementation

If management sets a positive attitude, safety program implementation is much easier. Successful implementation of safety programs rests on conveying program requirements throughout the workforce with a focus on the positive benefits of avoiding on-the-job injury and illness. Four key elements to successful implementation of safety programs are as follows:

1. *Under the Joint Commission requirements, the CEO of a healthcare institution must appoint a qualified safety director.* Specific implementation of this requirement may vary according to the size of the facility. An effective safety director sets program direction and goals, leads the safety committee and safety activities at the facility, and responds to success or failure in safety performance with recognition or process improvement.

2. *The facility safety committee must be an active group that helps implement program requirements, changes, and improvements in an ongoing way.* This committee should reach into every department and activity within the facility on matters of safety. The committee should also be involved in setting, measuring, and evaluating safety measures; reporting results; and suggesting improvements to the safety director and facility executive management.

3. *Individual groups and departments throughout the facility must be involved in implementing safety in a meaningful way for their specific activities.* Tailoring program requirements in a way that is sensible for each area is important. In the laundry, where material handling and heat stress may be key issues, safety program emphasis may be different from patient care areas. If safety requirements do not seem reasonable and practical, workers will have a tendency to view safety requirements as something

that must be done to meet requirements instead of something that should be done to ensure safety.

4. *Cost effectiveness and balance between the use of work practice modification and engineering controls in combination will help establish an effective safety program.* Individuals in departments can often provide the safety committee and executive management with excellent suggestions regarding safety improvements. A combination of changing the way things are done and the facilities, tools, and environments in which they are done will likely reduce injury and illness on the job.

Safety Program Measurements

Safety program measurement should be tailored to a facility's specific activities. All measurements should be aimed at identifying safety performance with an eye toward improvement, and they should not be punitive. The safety director and the safety committee must lead the establishment of measures that provide effective feedback on safety performance and direction for safety improvement. Three key points must be considered:

1. *Measures of program performance should be derived directly from program requirements.* If certain documentation is required, that documentation should be reviewed as a first step in program evaluation.
2. *Incidents and accidents should be evaluated as keys for process improvements.* Additional evaluation tools include announced inspections, unannounced inspections, topical inspections (fire, ventilation, or other systems), and inspection reports provided by regulatory agencies, facility insurance carriers, and so on.
3. *Measurements should not be limited to numerical measures or documentation; they should include observation of work practices, practical factor demonstrations, and drills.* If safety measurement becomes just a "numbers game," program effectiveness will suffer.

Continuous Improvement

One method to ensure a safe workplace is to make safety an expectation and requirement of every employee's performance. To avoid the perception of a punitive environment, establishment of a CQI program is the ideal approach. (A more detailed discussion of continuous quality improvement appears elsewhere in this book.) CQI describes an organizational culture based on a data-based approach to improving processes and systems, involving high employee ownership and participation. Safety assessment, hazard analysis, and accident prevention are logical processes to include in a CQI program.

The Healthy Work Environment

A safe workplace is necessary, but this fact alone will not guarantee a healthy work environment (Kilpatrick 2000). Classic health and safety issues do not

cover the broad spectrum of healthy workplace issues that involve both analytical measures of safety and managerial issues of team dynamics. Success
in safety is as much a matter of cooperation, collaboration, and participation
among all work group members. Safety programs that focus only on analytical
measures but do not pay attention to workplace and workgroup dynamics
may fail to discover the development of toxic workplace conditions or toxins.
Without effective identification and management of toxins in the workplace,
effective safety management is less likely to develop or flourish. A partial list of
work environment toxins is presented in Figure 11.1. Several characteristics
of healthy workplaces and organizations are listed in Figure 11.2.

   Some of the most important toxins to identify and correct are:

- unrealistic goals that make safe performance seem unachievable;
- poor supervision that leads to fragmentation within workgroups;

FIGURE 11.1
Partial List
of Toxins

Fear	Discrimination and harassment
Unfair conflict	Threats/intimidation
Violence	Inequity
Excessive stress	Privacy
Poor communication	Physical hazards
Poor supervisory skills	Excessive hours worked
Ownership	Cutbacks
Unreasonable goals/punishment	Insecurity
Supervision by intimidation	
Power imbalances: abuse of power	

Source: Kilpatrick, A. O. 1995. "Organizational Ecology: Managing the Attitudes and Behaviors That Poison the
Workplace Environment." Presented at the Southeastern Conference for Public Administration (July).

FIGURE 11.2
Characteristics
of Healthy
Workplaces

Efficiency and effectiveness	Few grievances and disciplinary actions
Low rates of absenteeism and turnover	Accountability, responsibility, and authority
High, positive, and creative energy	Synergy (one plus one = three, four, more)
Collaboration	
Jobs that stretch and test	Conflict is over issues, not personalities
Participatory democracy	Enthusiasm
Positive communication	Moderate noise level
Tolerance	Respect
High productivity	Healthy competition
Negotiation is present	Trust
Empowered employees; high ownership	

Source: Kilpatrick, A. O. 1995. "Organizational Ecology: Managing the Attitudes and Behaviors That Poison the
Workplace Environment." Presented at the Southeastern Conference for Public Administration (July).

- poor communication that reinforces negative processes and practices; and
- unrealistic workloads that result from downsizing, cutbacks, or excessive work hours.

Conversely, the most important dynamics to encourage in healthy work environments are:

- positive communication without fear of retribution;
- freedom to identify safety issues;
- fair, accountable, and responsible participation by management in safety issues; and
- issue-focused resolution not individual-focused problem identification.

Safety program achieve best results when fairness, equity, and participation by all members of a workgroup, including management and workers alike, create a healthy and open workplace.

Conclusion and Recommendations

Maintaining a healthy and safe workplace is a major management responsibility. Effective leadership, in conjunction with meaningful program implementation by the safety director, the safety committee, and every employee will yield the best results. Safety milestones, such as one million safe work hours without a lost-time accident, are major goals in a facility's history. Cultural issues, such as respect for others, clear vision of organizational mission, trust, elimination of fear, and a commitment to continuous quality improvement, should work in partnership with traditional elements of a safety program.

Celebration and recognition should also be part of a facility's health and safety culture. However, celebration should be promptly followed by a renewed effort to implement the requirements of the health and safety programs, including the plans, procedures, and policies that were so carefully developed in the beginning. The workplace culture must include a continuous improvement process that allows employees to adjust safety program requirements to meet changing work activities, to improve in areas of weakness, and to demonstrate and maintain regulatory compliance and organizational effectiveness. In this way, valuable human and institutional resources will be respected, conserved, and protected.

Discussion Questions

1. How would you go about implementing a workplace safety program? Identify the issues involved.
2. Describe how workers and workplace safety measures are implemented in your organization. Are those measures effective? Explain your answer.
3. Describe some strategies to eliminate toxins.

References

American Society for Healthcare Services. 1997. *Health Care Safety Management: A Regulatory Update for 1997.* Professional Development Series. Washington, DC: American Society for Healthcare Services.

Chaff, L. F. (ed.). 1994. *Safety Guide for Health Care Institutions, Fifth Edition.* Chicago: American Hospital Association and the National Safety Council.

Government Institutes, Inc. 1997. *OSHA CFRs Made Easy.* Title 29, 1900–1910. END, (CD-ROM 1997 version), Product Code #4084. Rockville, MD: Government Institutes, Inc.

Kilpatrick, A. O. 2000. "A New Social Contract for the Next Millennium." *Journal of Public Administration and Management: An Interactive Journal 4 (2).* http://www.pamij.com.99_4_2.html.

Moeller, D. W. 1997. *Environmental Health, Revised Edition.* Cambridge, MA: Harvard University Press.

Wilson, T. H. 1998. *OSHA Guide for Health Care Facilities.* Washington, DC: Thompson Publishing Group.

Appendix B: Selected Resources for Workplace Safety and Health Issues

Publications

Basic Industrial Hygiene—A Training Manual. 1975. Richard S. Brief. Exxon Corporation. This is a practical guide for assessing safety hazards such as those associated with inhalation, noise, mechanical injury, ergonomics, and so on.

Environmental Health, Revised Edition. 1997. Dade W. Moeller. Harvard University Press. The revised edition of *Environmental Health* contains discussion on topics such as toxicology, epidemiology, injury control, and disaster response.

Health Care Safety Management: A Regulatory Update for 1997. Professional Development Series, American Society for Healthcare Services. This guide gives information on developing checklists for evaluating work practices, workplace hazards, waste management, and other environmental hazard management requirements.

OSHA CFRs MADE EASY. Title 29, 1900–1910.END (CD-ROM 1997 version). Government Institutes, Inc. This CD-ROM version gives complete information on Title 29 Code of Federal Regulations.

Safety Guide for Health Care Institutions, Fifth Edition. 1994. Linda F. Chaff. American Hospital Association and the National Safety Council. This reference provides a description of basic safety issues and practices for a number of functional categories, including safety for patients, employees and volunteers, visitors, clinical services, support services, and physical plant operations.

Web Sites

Occupational Health and Safety Administration, http://www.osha.gov. The Occupational Health and Safety Administration's web site includes general information about OSHA, a news room, regulations and compliance information, and an outreach area.

South Carolina Department of Health and Environmental Control, http://www.scdhec.net. This web site has links to major topical areas that fall within the mission of the agency, including environment, health, contact information, calendar of events, commissioner/board information, and news releases.

U.S. Department of Energy, http://www.doe.gov. The Department of Energy web site is linked to many important technical resources, including Oak Ridge National Lab, Argonne National Labs, Lawrence Livermore Lab, and so on.

U.S. Environmental Protection Agency, http://epa.gov. The Environmental Protection Agency's web site provides links to areas, including EPA projects and programs, laws and regulations, publications, and other resources.

USGS, Guide to Federal Environmental Law and Regulation, http://water. usgs.gov/public/eap/env_guide/index.html. This guide is a tool to aid government agencies at the federal, state, and local levels; private industry; academia; the general public; and public interest groups. Areas covered by the guide include air quality, endangered species, fish and wildlife conservation, public land resources, and water resources.

Agencies and Professional Associations

American College of Occupational and Environmental Medicine, http://www.acoem.org. The American College of Occupational and Environmental Medicine's web site includes general information, membership information, education/conferences, position statements/guidelines, *Journal of Occupational and Environmental Medicine*, and links to other OEM resources.

American Health Information Management Association, http://www.ahima. org. The American Health Information Management Association's web site includes the following areas: professional support, consumer advice, online publications, and library services.

American Hospital Association, http://www.aha.org. This web site provides up-to-date information and resources for members and nonmembers of the American Hospital Association. The web site provides links to current issues, member services publications, current events, and so on.

American Industrial Hygiene Association, http://www.aiha.org. The web site contains information about membership and the foundation, publications catalog, education public relations, safety links, and an online journal.

American Public Health Association, http://www.apha.org. The American Public Health Association's web site includes information of interest to its members and links regarding legislative affairs and advocacy, news and publications, science, practice and policy, and public health resources.

Conference of Radiation Control Program Directors, Inc., http://www. crcpd.org. The Conference of Radiation Control Program Directors, Inc.'s web site has more than a dozen links to radiation protection information.

The Health Physics Society, http://www.hps.org. The Health Physics Society's web site includes radiation fact sheets, Health Physics Society Newsletter, and links to affiliate sites.

National Center for Environmental Health, http://www.cdc.gov/nceh/. The National Center for Environmental Health's web site provides information on the Center's programs, publications, news, and so on.

National Clearinghouse for Worker Safety and Health Training, http://www. atsdr.cdc.gov. The National Clearinghouse for Worker Safety and Health Training's web site contains an online database of its collection of documents pertaining to hazardous materials and occupational safety and health.

National Safety Council, http://www.nsc.org. The National Safety Council's web site provides information on occupational health and safety services, public policy update, air quality, hazardous chemical profiles, radioactive wastes, and environmental publications.

National Institute of Environmental Health Sciences, http://www.niehs.nih. gov. The National Institute of Environmental Health Sciences's web site provides multiple links to resources important to environmental health. It contains information about environment-related disease and health risks, news and events, and scientific research.

National Safety Council, http://www.nsc.org. The National Safety Council's web site provides information on occupational health and safety services, public policy update, air quality, hazardous chemical profiles, radioactive wastes, and environmental publications.

National Toxicology Program, http://ntp-server.niehs.nih.gov/main_pages/ about_NTP.html. The National Toxicology Program was established by the secretary of Health and Human Services. The web site covers topics such as testing information and study results, how regulatory agencies use NTP data, and chemical health and safety information.

U.S. Department of Energy, Office of Environmental Management, http:// www.em.doe.gov. The Environmental Management program is a division of the U.S. Department of Energy. The web site contains areas on public information, regulatory and budget information, waste management, environmental restoration, and so on.

EMPLOYEE AND EMPLOYER RIGHTS

Beverly Lynn Rubin, J.D.

Learning Objectives

After completing this chapter, the reader should be able to:

- Discuss employee rights and responsibilities, and distinguish among statutory, regulatory, and common law rights
- Define employment-at-will concept, and discuss the concept of public policy exceptions
- Describe the contractual implications of employee handbooks, employment agreements, personnel manuals, separation agreements, and disciplinary documents
- Define the concepts of dismissal for cause and due process
- Describe the types and roles of alternative dispute resolution methods in the workplace
- Discuss the legal backdrop for a variety of healthcare-specific employee rights and responsibilities issues
- Define the idea of progressive discipline and know the steps required for employee termination
- Discuss employee privacy issues and know when to consult legal counsel when privacy issues arise

Introduction

Most people who work outside the home spend a majority of their waking hours in the workplace. In fact, Americans work an average of 43.2 hours per week (Kundu 1999). To some people, the office or job site is a microcosm of home and family and may be the source of self-esteem, social interaction, anxiety, and insecurity. The workplace, however, cannot function like a family. Employees must perform their jobs, and employers must adhere to the rules and requirements applicable to the workplace. The laws that govern the relationship between employer and employee reflect the attempt to achieve the complex balance necessary to make one's job free from personal injury, prejudice, duress, and unwanted sexual advances while allowing the employer to pursue its business goals. Because labor and employment laws involve the protection of societal values, individual rights, and the pursuit of capitalism, it is a very confusing and often conflicting area of law.

In this chapter, we define the legal basis of employer and employee rights and identify the major federal and state sources of these rights; discuss the special situation of public employees with respect to their right to due process in termination; discuss healthcare-specific issues such as job-related stress, workplace substance abuse, and impaired professionals; and discuss strategies to prevent the need for discipline.

Statutory, Regulatory, and Common Law Rights

The respective rights and responsibilities that govern the workplace appear in federal and state statutes, administrative agency regulations, case law interpretations of various federal legislation and regulations, written and verbal employment agreements, and employee handbooks. The following are some key federal employment law statutes:

- Age Discrimination in Employment Act (age 40 and over)
- Americans with Disabilities Act (disability)
- Civil Rights Act of 1964, Title VII (age, race, gender, etc. See Figure 12.1)
- COBRA—Consolidated Omnibus Budget Reconciliation Act (health insurance)
- Consumer Credit Protection Act (credit privacy)
- Drug-Free Workplace Act of 1988 (drug testing)
- Employee Polygraph Protection Act of 1988 (polygraphs)
- Employee Retirement Income Security Act of 1974 (defined benefit plans)
- Equal Pay Act of 1963 (salary equality)
- Executive Order 11246 (government contractors)
- Fair Labor Standards Act (overtime)
- Family and Medical Leave Act of 1993 (childbirth or serious health condition)
- Immigration Reform and Control Act of 1986 (transfer of foreign national employees to the United States)

FIGURE 12.1
Civil Rights
Act of 1964,
Title VII

Title VII governs, among other things, gender discrimination and entitles an employee to be free from sexual harassment in the workplace. The two forms of sexual harassment are quid pro quo and hostile work environment. Employers should adopt a policy consistent with law, train employees on the policy, and be serious about investigating claims and enforcing the policy.

- Occupational Safety and Health Act (OSHA) (workplace safety)
- Worker Adjustment and Retraining Notification Act (mass layoffs)

State law provides additional rights and responsibilities. In North Carolina and many other states, contrary to instinct, an employer may not withhold money from a paycheck if an employee owes money to the employer (NC Gen. Stat. § 95-25.7). Other states, such as California, have enacted statutes supplemental to federal statutes—in the area of pregnancy leave (CA Govt. § 12945), for example. An employer familiar with well-publicized federal law inadvertently may ignore supplemental state law and deprive an employee of protected rights.

At-Will Employment and Public Policy Exceptions

Generally in the United States, employment is at will, which means that either party to the employment relationship may terminate the relationship for any reason, without cause and without notice. A substantial caveat to this rule, however, is that an employer cannot terminate an employee for a reason the law has deemed illegal; illegal grounds for dismissal include the employer's violation of federal and state restrictions. Examples of illegal grounds for termination include pregnancy, race, age, and disability status.

An at-will employee may challenge termination based on violation of public policy. An employee, for instance, can claim wrongful discharge when terminated solely for refusing to commit perjury or for reporting the employer's violation of OSHA. These situations are difficult if the employee's performance is also poor, as the employer may have difficulty showing the termination was based *solely* on performance and not on the employee's whistle-blowing activities.

Many wrongful discharge cases arise from an employer requiring an employee to violate federal or state law on the employer's behalf. Courts have allowed employees to pursue such claims because there is a public interest in protecting individuals who complain about an employer's illegal acts that could be harmful to the public in general (e.g., nuclear reactor safety issues) or to employees of the company (e.g., locked fire and emergency exits). This public policy exception creates a cause of action for wrongful discharge when an employer fires a worker for reasons that violate or offend public policy (Yamada 1998); see Figure 12.2 for example.

Whistleblowing

Employee whistleblowing is a common cause of a wrongful discharge. A **whistleblower** is an employee who discloses or otherwise exposes illegal activity in the workplace to law enforcement or a government agency. Such illegal acts could involve discrimination, fraud, or embezzlement. Employees who blow the whistle on their employers are protected by the law, and an employer cannot legally retaliate against or mistreat an employee for whistleblowing. The False Claims Act (U.S.C. §§ 3730–33 1991), only one of the myriad

FIGURE 12.2
Illustration of
Wrongful
Discharge

Consider the scenario of a company that hires individuals who are not authorized to work in the United States. An at-will employee reports this illegal practice to the Immigration and Naturalization Service (INS) and, subsequently, gets terminated. In this situation, the complaining employee may be successful in pursuing a claim for wrongful or bad-faith discharge based on the public policy exception.

*A **whistleblower** is an employee who discloses or exposes illegal activity in the workplace, such as discrimination, fraud, or embezzlement*

of laws in this area, governs actions in cases in which a company or individual has financially defrauded the federal government (Allen 2001). In 1997, 54 percent of whistleblower cases were based on healthcare fraud (*Modern Healthcare* 1999).

Various state whistleblower laws only provide protection to the whistleblower if the individual has reported the problem to his or her supervisor, allowing for a reasonable amount of time to correct the problem, or if the individual has reason to believe the problem will not be corrected if reported (Title 26 MRSA, Section 839). Whistleblowers often face an ethical and moral dilemma when trying to decide whether to disclose information. They must consider the consequences of being deemed "disloyal" to their company and whether disclosure benefits the public, and the potential detriment to career and the personal stakes are high. The laws described above seek to alleviate such concerns.

Employee Handbooks, Personnel Manuals, and Disciplinary Documents

If an employer's personnel policies, contained in handbooks or other policy documents, contain promises to employees, these policies may restrict the employer's ability to discharge employees at will. Additionally, disciplinary documents prepared by inexperienced managers or human resources personnel may contain language that implies a promise to continue employment. Consider, for example, an employee who has been absent from work without excuse for several consecutive days. His or her manager prepares a disciplinary document stating that the employee must maintain a better attendance record over the subsequent 12-month period to keep his or her job. Through this documentation process, the employee may have an implied promise of employment for 12 months, provided he or she maintains a good attendance record.

One way to avoid such an implied promise is for a manager, with good human resources knowledge or with legal advice, to include in a disciplinary document language such as the following: "Nothing contained herein alters the at-will nature of your employment or constitutes a promise of future employment." Employee handbooks and personnel policies must contain similar language in an acknowledgment page signed by the employee and placed in the employee's personnel file.

An employment agreement contains a specified term of employment; the term of the agreement can be stated in oral or written form or a combination of the two. An employer may verbally tell an employee upon hire, transfer, or promotion that the employee has a guaranteed position for one year. However, a verbal agreement is not recommended for either party. Some standard items in employment agreements appear in Figure 12.3.

Employment Agreements

Early termination of a fixed-term employment agreement usually entitles the employee either to collect severance payments or liquidated damages specified under the agreement or to pursue a breach-of-contract claim in court. An employer has few rights when an employee terminates an employment agreement prior to the end of the term because the courts will not force an employee to continue working against the employee's will. Damages caused by the employee's departure also may be difficult to calculate.

For an employee who poses a competitive risk to the employer, including **non-competition** and **non-solicitation clauses** in the agreement may be the only way to protect the employer. An employee presented with an agreement that contains these clauses should consult an attorney prior to signing the documents because these clauses often significantly limit an employee's ability to work after termination of employment. Likewise, employers should seek legal counsel in preparing contracts with such clauses because they may be unenforceable[1] under state law or because they are unreasonable (see Figure 12.4).

*A **non-competition** **clause** prohibits an employee from providing service that competes with the employer after termination of work relationship, while a **non-solicitation** **clause** usually prevents employee from soliciting customers or employees from the employer.*

Furthermore, in the healthcare context, non-compete clauses may go against public policy for physicians in specialty practice areas in which services are subject to limited availability in the restricted geographic region (see Figure 12.5).

---

1. Start date
2. Title
3. Salary
4. Reporting relationship
5. Job duties or description
6. Term
7. Notice and renewal periods
8. Termination for cause provisions
9. Severance payments
10. Bonus
11. Fringe benefits
12. Confidentiality and work product provisions
13. Non-competition and non-solicitation provisions
14. Assignment clauses
15. Choice of law

FIGURE 12.3
Standard Items in Employment Agreements

FIGURE 12.4
Non-
Competition
Clause

To be enforceable, most courts require that non-competition clauses protect a legitimate business interest of the employer and are reasonable in terms of geography, time, and scope. For example, a hospital that prohibits a payroll clerk from working for any hospital in the United States for three years following termination probably would not be protecting its legitimate business interest, and the court would find the clause unreasonable in terms of geography, time, and scope.

FIGURE 12.5
Covenants not
to Compete
and Public
Policy

In *Medical Specialist, Inc. v. Sleweon,* 652 N.E.2d 517 (Ind. App. June 1995), the plaintiff was an infectious disease specialist employed by a physician group practice; the plaintiff's employment agreement with the practice included a covenant not to compete. After resigning from his position, the defendant group practice sought to enforce the covenant not to compete. The plaintiff brought suit against his former employer, alleging the covenant was unenforceable based on public policy grounds. The court ruled against the plaintiff because there was no showing of a shortage of such specialists in the restricted area.

***Separation
Agreements***

At the termination of employment, the employee and employer occasionally will enter into a separation agreement. Such agreements often are required as a condition of receiving certain post-termination benefits such as severance, health benefit payments, or outplacement services. The separation or severance agreement will be enforceable in court only if supported by valid consideration; that is, each party to the agreement must receive some benefit for which she or he otherwise was not entitled to under a law, regulation, personnel policy, or employment agreement.

The benefits to an employer in obtaining a severance agreement are a release of legal claims and a covenant not to sue by the terminated employee. (Because of the highly technical requirements of a release, the employer should consult experienced human resources personnel or legal counsel.) For example, in certain states, the severance agreement must specify state statutes to serve as a valid release of particular claims. Furthermore, to obtain a valid release for an age discrimination claim, an employer must follow the requirements of the Age Discrimination Employment Act (ADEA) (29 U.S.C. §§ 621-34), which include the following: (1) written agreement, (2) consideration, (3) advise employee in writing to seek advice of counsel prior to signing, (4) allow employee 21 days to consider before signing, and (5) allow employee seven days to revoke after signing. Severance agreements also can require the employee to reaffirm or the employer to waive employment obligations, such as non-competition and non-solicitation provisions.

For-Cause Dismissal

As stated above, in the absence of an agreement or representation to the contrary, employers are not required to show cause to dismiss an employee. In many employment agreements, circumstances that constitute a basis for for-cause termination are defined. The following are situations that could lead to for-cause termination:

- Misconduct, including fraud, embezzlement, and commission of a criminal act
- Violation of corporate policy or practice
- Material failure to perform employment obligations
- For professionals, loss of license

Public Employees' Right to Due Process

Despite the exceptions described above, at-will employment prevails for private employees. The same is not true, however, for public sector employees, even in at-will states. Public employees enjoy certain due process rights and cannot be fired without a good reason or without notice and a hearing.

When considering the discharge of a public employee, remember that all public employees are protected by specific federal and state statutes and the federal and state constitutions. All federal and most state government employees must be provided with written notice of the basis for any proposed disciplinary action. These employees also may be entitled to a hearing to defend against termination for cause. Because of these additional rights, management *must* seek professional assistance when terminating a public employee.

Alternative Dispute Resolution

Given the volume of employment litigation, some employers are attempting to control the escalating costs and media attention associated with litigation by including mandatory arbitration or *alternative dispute resolution (ADR) clauses* in employment contracts. Any disagreement or claim that arises from the terms of employment will be subject to ADR. ADR agreements, however, do not preempt any rights that the Equal Employment Opportunity Commission (EEOC) or various state employment rights commissions may have to investigate claims of discrimination (Moore 2000). Additionally, ADR agreements do not apply to unemployment or workers compensation claims or relieve an employer of its obligation to conduct investigations of claims such as racial discrimination or sexual harassment.

The two main types of ADR are mediation and arbitration. **Mediation** is generally a nonbinding process in which opposing parties conduct semiformal settlement negotiations assisted by a neutral third-party mediator. **Arbitration**, much like a trial, is a more formal process in which both sides can

Mediation is generally a nonbinding process in which opposing parties conduct semiformal settlement negotiations assisted by a neutral third-party mediator

Arbitration is a formal process, much like a trial, in which both sides can present evidence and call witnesses

present evidence and call witnesses, and it is typically binding and enforceable by the courts. Employers usually exclude from ADR clauses their right to seek injunctive relief for violation of non-competition and non-solicitation provisions.

Healthcare-Specific Issues

Employers, especially in the healthcare industry, cannot allow their employees to perform job duties while impaired or suffering from extreme stress. Public health as well as liability problems are associated with employers not taking proactive measures. Employers should have confidential employee assistance programs available free of charge to all employees. Managers, with advice from human resources or the legal department, also should discipline or terminate impaired employees.

Job-Related Stress

Healthcare professionals and staff experience greater levels of stress because of the nature of their work (Rowe 1998; Weinberg and Creed 2000). These stressful conditions can be exacerbated if they suffer from depression or anxiety. People who suffer from these disorders have greater incidence of prior psychiatric disorders and are less likely to have someone in whom to confide, which add to the stress of the job. Other work-related stress inducers include job insecurity, managers who are not supportive, and limited potential for job promotion.

Workplace Substance Abuse

According to the American Association of Occupational Health Nurses (American Association of Occupational Health Nurses 2001), substance abuse is characterized as unlawful, unauthorized, or improper use of alcohol, over-the-counter drugs, or products that have mind-altering properties. Changes in the impaired professional's performance, appearance, and behavior are likely to be obvious. The impact these changes have on professional's ability to carry out work-related duties without endangering the safety of themselves, patients, or coworkers is a substantial concern because:

- Professionals tend to not self-report because they fear loss of licensure.
- Professionals "are often in positions of accountability and high visibility, and the consequences of their addiction problems can be both painfully isolated and personal, but also can eventually affect their work and the care of their patients."
- "Healthcare professionals (HCPs), especially physicians and nurses, have access to prescription medications that are highly addictive. Even when healthcare professionals enter treatment highly motivated, their ongoing

exposure and access to these medications puts them at considerable risk for relapse."

- "HCPs are notoriously 'poor' patients. They have a tendency to self-treat and self-prescribe. They view illness as weakness and failure, and they have difficulty accepting and complying with medical advice from other professionals when it pertains to themselves" (Rush University 2001).

Discipline

Progressive Discipline

Although not required by law, some employers will provide at-will employees an opportunity to correct a performance problem. Under the concept of progressive discipline, an employee is made aware of the problems and what he or she must do to correct them. The employee sometimes has a reasonable amount of time to correct the problem and is made aware of the consequences of inaction.

Termination

Once termination of an employee is determined to be the proper course of action, several steps must be followed to ensure the termination is facilitated properly, including:

- *Analyze risk.* Prior to termination, review carefully the personnel file and examine all facts and circumstances surrounding the termination. Ensure that human resources or management has investigated all valid complaints raised by the employee. Also examine the employee's personal situation or status—for example, pregnancy, disability, or age.
- *Avoid procrastination.* Do not delay an employee's termination after satisfying the risk analysis process.
- *Strategically choose the termination date.* Employees that are fired on Fridays have the weekend to think about the termination and about possible recourse against the employer; therefore, termination of an employee on Fridays should be avoided. In addition, termination on significant dates to the employee, such as a birthday, anniversary, or holiday, should be avoided.
- *Consult human resources.* The human resources department requires notification to enable them to consider the possibility of a severance agreement or the necessity of communicating the termination to affected internal employees to avoid disruption of work or service. Human resources also can process final paychecks and answer benefits questions.
- *Take action.* The individual who informs the employee of the termination should be direct (University of Vermont 2001).

Preventing Discipline

Effective Recruitment and Selection

Effective screening of potential employees is a necessary step in minimizing employer liability and preventing employee discipline. The amount of screening to be performed must be balanced against the level of risk associated with the open position. Employers are expected to perform more thorough screening of candidates for positions that carry greater risk; these positions include those that give the employee access to master keys, narcotics, or finances and the chance to work with children, elderly, or disabled individuals. However, many pre-employment screening tests have risks or may be objectionable to applicants, such as a drug test or a criminal background check (see Figure 12.6 for a more comprehensive list of the tools used in screening). The employer must consider the risks and discomfort factors and must consider applying screening tests on a consistent and nondiscriminatory basis. At a minimum, employers should check references, education, and professional license status.

Training, Performance Appraisal, and Compensation

Training and development programs operate to increase an employee's level of competence through alterations in knowledge base, attitude, and skills. Training can reduce or prevent the need for discipline by enhancing employees' job skills and improving managers' ability to supervise employees. Training also enhances the value of the working relationship because training shows an employer's commitment to and investment in its employees.

Appraising an employee's performance and providing feedback is one of the primary techniques used to enhance employee performance or to inform an employee of potential problems. Managers should prepare appraisals with human resources assistance and review. Employees should receive appraisals at regular intervals and have the opportunity to comment.

When deciding to accept a job, an employee should examine *compensation* surveys available through consultants or on the Internet (see www.salary.com). Employees must further consider the total compensation package,

---

FIGURE 12.6
Possible Tools for Screening Candidates

- Detailed application form
- Interview
- Honesty test
- Handwriting analysis
- Drug screening
- Criminal background check
- Credit report
- Reference check
- Motor vehicle record check
- Educational records
- Personality tests

---

rather than the base salary in isolation. A satisfactory employment relationship is more likely to occur when total compensation is within a reasonable range.

Employee Privacy Rights and Workplace Searches

Approximately 27 percent of employers review employee e-mail messages, and 37 percent track the telephone numbers their employees have called (American Management Association 2001). The number of employers who use electronic monitoring in some form has increased from 35 percent in 1997 to 74 percent in 2000 (*USA Today* 2000). A private employee has limited privacy rights against the search of a desk, office, or work area. In *Schowengerst v. General Dynamics Corp.* (823 F.2d 1328 (9th Cir.), cert. denied 117 L.Ed.2d 650, 1987), the court ruled that a private employee who has no property interest in an area searched continues to have privacy rights. In *O'Connor v. Ortega* (480 U.S. 709, 720, 94 L.Ed.2d 714, 725, 107 S.Ct 1492, 1987)—a case in which a state-employed (public) physician's desk and file cabinet were searched—one of the arguments was that workplace searches conducted without consent or a valid search warrant may still be valid if the search meets a "standard of reasonableness under all of the circumstances." However, a majority of the U.S. Supreme Court justices agreed that the physician had a reasonable expectation of privacy in his office and unanimously agreed there was a reasonable expectation of privacy in the physician's desk and file cabinet. See Figure 12.7 for possible methods that employers can employ to avoid legal conflict over privacy violations.

Privacy and Electronic Monitoring

Employers use monitoring in the workplace to investigate organizational problems, particularly loss of productivity as a result of wasted time e-mailing coworkers and friends and family outside the workplace. Use of company systems to send discriminatory or harassing materials also can lead to litigation if the employer fails to take proper precautionary or corrective measures. Listed below are additional reasons why employees monitor their employees (Ramsey 1999):

- Develop a policy statement instructing employees that privacy in the workplace should not be assumed
- Use private information for justifiable reasons only
- Restrict the distribution of employee's personal information to company officials on a need-to-know basis
- Maintain employee medical records separately from the employee file
- Obtain a signed consent or waiver when using the employee's name or picture in an advertisement, promotional material, or training film

FIGURE 12.7

Measures an Employer Can Adopt to Minimize the Possibility of Litigation Over Privacy Violations

- Ensure and promote safety;
- Protect trade secrets;
- Enhance productivity;
- Prevent theft or other unlawful activity;
- Assess the quality and regularity of customer service;
- Search for drug use; and
- Limit employer liability by detecting and recording discriminatory behavior.

The techniques that employers use can be as simple and obvious as a desk search or can involve sophisticated hidden cameras and microphones. Some employers will install such devices when they suspect a specific employee to be conducting improper transactions or generally because of unexplained missing inventory. Listed below are common techniques most often used by employers (Ramsey 1999):

- Installing hidden cameras and microphones;
- Monitoring e-mail, voice-mail, and facsimile;
- Recording telephone conversations;
- Monitoring mail;
- Searching desk or drawers;
- Examining computer use; and
- Searching company property such as lockers or briefcases.

The Employee Polygraph Protection Act (EPPA), with many exemptions, prohibits employers from:

- requiring employees to take lie detector tests;
- using the results of lie detector tests;
- taking action against an employee for refusing to take a lie detector test; or
- retaliating against an employee for complaining about any of the above.

Significant exemptions to EPPA (29 USC §§ 2001–2009) apply to the healthcare industry and to the handling of controlled substances.

Employers' surveillance of employees is widespread and increasing as indicated by research conducted by the American Management Association (AMA). In a survey by the AMA, almost three-fourths of major American businesses examined report having employee surveillance practices (Greenberg 2000). A breakdown of the percentage of firms following specific practices in 1997 and 2000 is demonstrated in Figure 12.8.

Drug Testing

In the healthcare industry, employees have access to controlled substances, and statistics reveal problems with substance abuse among employees in healthcare. Employers may choose to initiate a pre-employment, for-cause, and random drug testing program. A number of states have laws that regulate

FIGURE 12.8
Electronic
Monitoring and
Surveillance

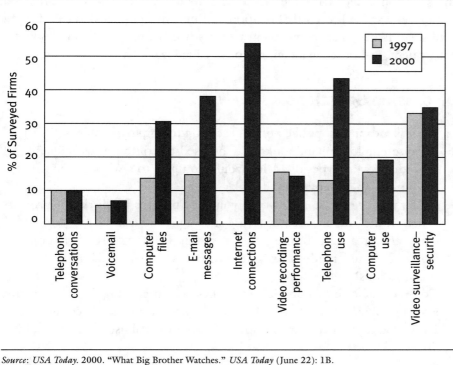

Source: USA Today. 2000. "What Big Brother Watches." USA Today (June 22): 1B.

the circumstances under which an employer may test for drugs; therefore, if an employer has multistate employees, it must check for the specific requirements of each state. Testing must be done on a confidential basis, and employers must determine what will occur if the employee's results reveal drug use. Examples of an employer's options include (1) taking disciplinary actions, (2) referring the employee to the Employee Assistance Program (EAP), or (3) referring the employee to a treatment/rehabilitation program.

Employers should consult experienced human resources personnel or legal counsel prior to initiating an employee drug testing program. Employers also should use a certified laboratory to conduct the testing. A laboratory experienced in such testing will reduce the likelihood of claims by employees for invasion of privacy.

Conclusion

Attorneys and human resources professionals have written volumes regarding each topic in this chapter. Many of the laws and regulations mentioned herein are complex, interdependent, and often conflicting. Managers should not rely on instinct alone in these areas, especially in handling whistleblowing, discrimination, or other types of highly sensitive employment situations. Mishandling any situation could harm the employer's ability to attract and retain good employees and lead to costly litigation and negative publicity. When dealing with these issues, management must seek advice from the human resources department, in-house legal counsel, or outside legal advisors.

Discussion Questions

1. What is meant by a public policy exception to employment at will?
2. Because employee handbooks may be used to contest a disciplinary procedure, what types of advice would you give to a work group that is assembling an employee handbook?
3. Under what circumstances would you use a progressive discipline process? When would you choose not to use such a procedure?
4. Given the great risks to the public resulting from impaired healthcare workers, should random drug testing be used in all healthcare organizations?
5. Consider the case of a physician who has been practicing for 15 years and is well established as one of only a few physicians in a small community. How would you deal with information about his abuse of alcohol and drugs?

Note

1. Except as provided in this chapter, every contract by which anyone is restrained from engaging in a lawful profession, trade, or business of any kind is to that extent void (California Business & Professional Code § 16600).

References

Allen, M. 2001. "Whistle Blowing." [Online article on Kennesaw State University web site; retrieved 8/7/01]. http://science.kennesaw.edu/csis/msis/stuwork/whistleblowing.html.

American Association of Occupational Health Nurses. 2001. [Online information; retrieved 8/7/01]. http://www.aaohn.org/cemodules/jan00art.htm.

American Management Association. 2001. [Online information; retrieved 8/7/01]. http://www.amanet.org/press/research/check-email.htm.

Greenberg, E. R. 2000. "Workplace Testing: Monitoring and Surveillance." [Online article on American Management Association web site; retrieved 8/7/01]. http://www.amanet.org/research/pdfs/monitr_surv.pdf.

Kundu, K. 1999. "Hours of Work: A Matter of Choice for Most Working Americans." [Online article on Employment Policy Foundation web site; retrieved 10/99]. www.epf.org/ff/ff991014/htm.

Modern Healthcare. 1999. "Healthcare Tattletales." *Modern Healthcare* 299 (November): 47.

Moore, E. C. 2000. "Arbitration Clauses in Employment Disputes: Staying Out of Court." [Online article on Health Services Benefit Administrators, Inc., web site; retrieved 10/00]. www.hsba.hosteme.com/labor_employment/arbitration.htm.

Ramsey, R. 1999. "The 'Snoopervision' Debate: Employer Interest vs. Employee Privacy." *Supervision* 60 (8).

Rowe, M. M. 1998. "Hardiness as a Stress Mediating Factor of Burnout Among Healthcare Providers." *American Journal of Healthcare Studies* 14 (1): 16.

Rush University. 2001. [Online information; retrieved 8/7/01]. http://www.rush.edu/patients/mental/pubs/professional.html.

University of Vermont. 2001. [Online information; retrieved 8/7/01]. http://www.bsad.emba.uvm.edu/hrm/Discipline/article1.htm.

Weinberg, A., and F. Creed. 2000. "Stress and Psychiatric Disorders in Healthcare Professionals and Hospital Staff." *The Lancet* 355 (9203): 533.

Yamada, D. C. 1998. "Voices from the Cubicle: Protecting and Encouraging Private Employee Speech in the Post Industrial Workplace." *Berkeley Journal of Employment and Labor Law* 19: 22.

THE DYNAMICS OF ORGANIZATIONAL CHANGE

Sharon Topping, Ph.D.

Learning Objectives

After completing this chapter, the reader should be able to:

- Distinguish between incremental and revolutionary change
- Discuss change as a continuous process
- Describe the steps in the change process
- Describe the relationship between the forces of change and the forces of inertia
- Discuss the roadblocks to organizational change
- Describe human resources strategies that can be used in the implementation of organizational change

Introduction

In previous chapters, we described the many changes that have occurred in the external environment of healthcare organizations, including numerous advances in biotechnology, increased pressure to lower costs, the rise of managed care and a more restrictive reimbursement environment, demographic changes including the aging population, and development of integrated networks. As a result, change has become a way of life in most healthcare organizations. However, with these external changes came major internal transformations that have shaped healthcare organizations. Many believe that to withstand profound change, especially those predicted to happen during the next decades, organizations must be flexible with loose boundaries and the ability to adapt and respond to the environment and its many stakeholders (Kanter, Stein, and Jick 1992; Nadler and Tushman 1997; Sherman and Schultz 1998). Consequently, change is one of the greatest problems that healthcare executives have to face in their roles as managers and decision makers.

This chapter explores change and its many consequences for healthcare organizations and the human resources function, including the forces of organizational change, the process of change and its ongoing nature, the forces that resist and promote organizational change, and implementation of a change agenda.

Certain words carry specific connotations depending on a person's experience. Change is one of those words. When most healthcare managers are asked the question, "What is **organizational change**?" they generally think of deliberate or intentional change; that is, they imagine organizations going through a transition from one state to another. Kurt Lewin (1947), one of the founding fathers of social psychology, graphically depicted change as a transition that occurs in stages of unfreezing, changing, and refreezing. This perspective may be too simplistic, however, leaving one with the notion that change is a planned, linear process with a discrete beginning and end. In reality, change is best characterized as an ongoing dynamic journey in which a sequence of events unfolds over time. This view allows managers to understand the continuous nature of change and thereby to learn how to better aid their organizations in times of turmoil and crises. Furthermore, it allows them to consider the myriad human resources issues that accompany change.

Organizational change is a continuous process that involves multiple and often incomplete transactions and uncertain future states that lead organizations to transition from one state to another

Furthermore, a person's view of change often depends on whether he or she is creating the change or is affected by it. To better understand and manage change, healthcare managers need to look at it from both perspectives. Often, change is forced on organizations, such as the 1997 Balanced Budget Act that significantly reduced reimbursement to hospitals that transfer certain patients to step-down units. Because of this federal-level decision, many hospitals were forced to close their skilled nursing units and downsize their operations. On the other hand, healthcare managers are just as likely to act as change agents themselves, so they must understand the effects of the implementation as well as the perspective of the clinical and administrative staffs who are affected. Many in the organization will view change as an opportunity, but at the same time, others will see it as a disruption and even a threat. Both viewpoints are valid and should be understood as part of the change process.

The Forces of Organizational Change

For change to occur, the need for it must be triggered; therefore, the healthcare manager has to scan the environment and interpret signals for change correctly. The scanning function acts much like the organization's window or lens to the external environment. The lens is continuously moved across an array of external organizations (e.g., regulatory, political, economic) in search of current and emerging trends (Ginter, Swayne, and Duncan 1998).

Much of the information when first encountered is diverse and unorganized, so an organization must continuously categorize and organize while monitoring and evaluating. During much of this process, the information is subject to human judgment and subjectivity. In her book, Herzlinger (1997) discusses the **forces of change** that have reshaped massive parts of the American economy (e.g., retailing, information, automotive, and manufacturing) and are now at work on healthcare; she believes that this force comes in the form of well-educated consumers who are empowered by information and are assertive in their demands to take part in their treatment. Given this view, healthcare managers must understand how to recognize this type of change in the environment and interpret it correctly.

Forces of change are forces both inside and outside the organization that combine to trigger change

One of the most difficult situations in which to make valid interpretations is when events are highly uncertain and extremely unfamiliar, such as the passage of Medicare prospective payment legislation for hospitals in 1983 (Barr 1998). In such a situation, the manager will make vague interpretations initially, looking for patterns that can be connected to something familiar. Unfortunately, managers have not historically been very good at interpreting the environment and recognizing the need for change (Nutt 1991); they tend to make erroneous assumptions about the magnitude and effect of change. For instance, Mechanic and Rosenthal (1999) discuss how medical directors in MCOs do not view trust-building programs as strategic tools even in the face of a public increasingly distrustful and hostile to managed care. Topping and Ginter (1998) describe how HCA (formerly Columbia/HCA) based its overall marketing strategy on the false assumption that the hospital sector of the healthcare industry was a national market.

One factor that has considerable impact on the healthcare manager's perception of change is the organizational context itself. Organizations that have high levels of information-processing capacity—that is, high levels of employee interaction and participation—generally process more information about the environment, which, in turn, can be used in decision making. Thomas and McDaniel (1990) studied how hospital CEOs interpreted opportunities and threats in the environment. CEOs in hospitals oriented toward high levels of information processing were more likely to interpret an environmental change as positive, viewing it as an opportunity for hospital gain. From their findings, they recommended that if managers want to alter their interpretation, they may wish to examine their organization's information-processing capacity, determining how information is collected, processed, and conveyed.

Employees, like most people, frequently have a vested interest in maintaining the status quo, so they may be blinded to reality. Sometimes, they are even able to block out the change, perceiving no threat from the environment. One of the most interesting cases of this phenomenon occurred after deregulation of the savings and loan industry when CEOs were asked what strategic change had taken place in response to the new environment (Javidan 1984). Most CEOs answered none, explaining that deregulation was only temporary and the industry would be back to its old regulated self in a couple of years. This example can be easily extrapolated to the healthcare industry and the initial reaction to managed care. Some managers interpreted managed care as a threat and lobbied legislators to limit MCO activity in their states. Others believed that managed care would go away if they ignored it, while some viewed it as an opportunity and aligned their hospitals with primary care physicians.

As shown in Figure 13.1, external forces in the environment act to trigger change, while inertial forces, often inside the organizations, act to retard change. If the inertial forces influence the interpretation, those in the organization will see no need to change and thus will resist. This type of resistance to change and how it operates will be discussed in more detail in the following sections.

The Process of Change

According to Kanter, Stein, and Jick (1992), change is messy, it is difficult, and it does not happen in isolation. Nadler and Tushman (1997) describe change as involving multiple and often incomplete transactions and uncertain future states. Therefore, the process is more like a continual journey toward some elusive, flickering goal with some right turns and some wrong turns, and where sometimes you will have a sense of just "muddling through"— taking small incremental steps—while at other times, giant transformations are seemingly happening all around. This section describes these different types of organizational change and how they fit into the process.

Incremental Versus Revolutionary Change

In conceptualizing change as a process, understanding how organizational change actually occurs is important. Change is typically described in terms of "waves" or "spurts and pauses." In this context, it may result in a complete

FIGURE 13.1

Forces of Change

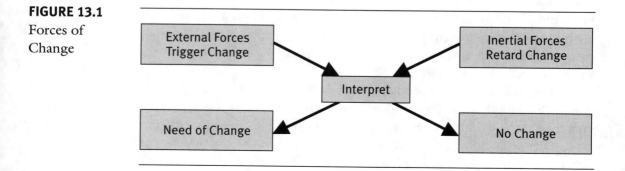

reversal—a revolution—of an organization's direction, which is similar to "drastic leaps forward." A public sector hospital or clinic that enters into a partnership with a for-profit MCO may experience revolutionary change when efficiency standards and cost reductions become an important priority. To truly be revolutionary, organizational change must involve transformation of structure, culture, and strategy—"frame breaking." This type of change can pose major complications for healthcare organizations and their employees. As a result, the change process must be thought through very carefully.

Although **revolutionary change** is important, change also occurs incrementally or in a series of small steps. Findings from change research indicate that this type of change predominates in most organizations. **Incremental change** is less disruptive, giving the organization and the employees time to adjust to the change process. It also allows for fine tuning that is very useful when implementing change, especially in a new environment. Furthermore, incremental change can be tied in with the strategic planning process and used to evaluate progress. Incremental change is still not very useful in times of crisis. When survival is the goal, revolutionary change is needed. However, healthcare managers have to be careful about waiting until a crisis to implement change. Although times of adversity and crisis may generate innovation, it is usually the time when successful implementation is less likely because that is when resources are scarce and time is a luxury.

Change as a Continuous Process

Revolutionary change represents a dramatic and sharp shift of organizational direction, while incremental change involves small steps that represent adjustments to environmental changes or fine tuning of the direction of the healthcare organization. The former can be disruptive; the latter generally is not, so long periods of calm and relatively smooth adjustments result. However, strategic shifts in organizations can take years if not decades to accomplish, and the change is typically a combination of both revolutionary and incremental change. Consider Duke Children's Hospital (DCH) and the turnaround it initiated (Meliones 2000). A decision to implement a balanced scorecard approach came about when DCH faced a $7 million increase in annual losses in four years.

Figure 13.2 depicts the continual nature of the organizational change process. This model of change is based on Tushman and Romanelli's (1985) **punctuated equilibrium model of change** that posits that organizations proceed through long periods of incremental change interrupted by revolutions. To summarize this model, given a trigger of change, DCH's $7 million increase in annual losses, responses are generally crude and experimental because stability and certainty are diminished by the impact of this jolt. This leads to a **period of ferment** in which healthcare organizations attempt to make sense out of the change, which is a kind of testing the waters approach. During

Revolutionary change is a complete reversal of an organization's direction that involves a transformation of the structure, culture, and strategy

Incremental change is a series of small steps that represent adjustments to environmental changes or fine tuning of the direction of an organization

Punctuated equilibrium model of change is a model of change that is based on the assumption that organizations proceed through long periods of incremental change (adjustments) that are interrupted on a very infrequent basis by revolutionary or drastic change

Period of ferment is a time period in which organizations test new responses to the environment by making incremental changes

FIGURE 13.2
The Dynamics
of Change

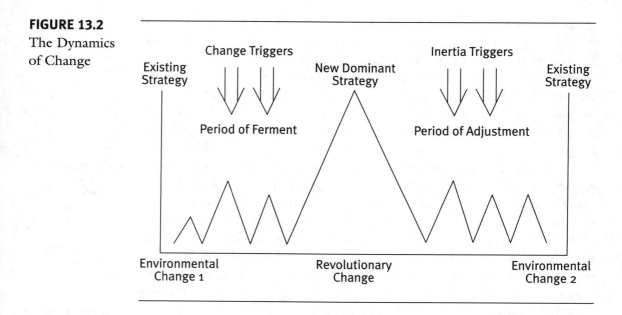

the period of ferment, incremental change predominates, such as trying a few cost-cutting measures while beginning discussions with employees about the seriousness of the problems. Thus, the forces of change begin to build, and the momentum eventually triggers revolutionary change within the organization. At this time, a dominant new strategy is recognized (e.g., the implementation of the balanced scorecard). This new strategy or recipe may be pioneered by the healthcare organization itself (being the first mover) or copied from some other first-mover organizations. In the case of DCH, the balanced scorecard method had been used successfully in many Fortune 500 corporations, and DCH was to become the healthcare leader in this approach. After the dominant strategy (revolutionary change) is accepted and implementation begins, it is followed by a period of adjustment or incremental change in which the managerial innovation has to be refined and readjusted to fit the particular organization.

In all phases, resistance to change will be experienced, but the triggers of inertia begin in earnest during the period of adjustment or implementation. These are powerful forces that obscure threats and create resistance in organizations and can lead to failure if not managed correctly. One study (Hambrick and D'Aveni 1988) investigated 57 large bankruptcies occurring between 1972 and 1982 and found that few were sudden. Most followed a ten-year decline in accounting performance, but forces of inertia had built up a powerful momentum to block change. One of the best safeguards is to know where the roadblocks are in your organization; you need to ask:

Forces of inertia are powerful forces that obscure threats and create resistance to change in organizations and can lead to failure of a change agenda if not managed correctly

• Are the **forces of inertia** in my healthcare organization powerful enough to block change?

- What human resources tools and strategies can be implemented to prevent this from happening?

The roadblocks to change are discussed in more detail in the next section.

Roadblocks to Change

Chris Argyris (1985) has stated that "almost any action that disturbs the status quo or represents a threat to the usual way of doing things will invoke resistance or a defensive reaction." Thus, the implementation of organizational change is a difficult and complex phenomenon, probably more than most healthcare managers realize. The failure of organizations to implement change is legendary. Any situation that involves change can generate a great deal of tension between those initiating change and those implementing change and between those implementing it and those on the receiving end. Why does this conflict occur? Primarily, because people fear uncertainty and change brings with it surprise and confusion, staff members in a healthcare organization may view change as a loss of control and a threat to current jobs. They may see it as an infringement on their turf or a way of requiring more effort and work from them. Peter Senge (1999) in *The Dance of Change* believes that this resistance is a natural response of the system fighting to maintain its internal balance. However, many times, healthcare managers fight against this balancing process, rather than try to understand the cause of the imbalance. They push harder, and the system pushes back just as hard; therefore, regardless of the reason, resistance is inherent in the change process and it cannot be eradicated, so managers must know from where the resistance will come and why.

Some of the roadblocks that serve as barriers to organizational change include:

- bureaucratic hierarchies and administrative systems;
- organization's culture;
- organization's history, including past performance and current strong leader;
- organization's size and age;
- lack of resources; and
- employees and organizational politics.

One strong barrier to change is the *bureaucracy* in an organization. Generally, organizations develop competencies or areas in which they excel. The Kaleidoscope Program in Chicago is known for its work with troubled youth and families; consequently, it has built its competencies around the provision of unconditional, individual care in providing in-home family support services and therapeutic foster care to this population (VanDenBerg 1999). To capitalize on these competencies, Kaleidoscope has put into place certain rules and routines, such as a team structure, decision-making rules, and treatment procedures, that act as a complement to the competencies. Once these administrative systems and bureaucratic hierarchies are in place, they reinforce the status quo and act as a barrier to change. In addition to controls, the organizational culture plays a major role in resistance. *Culture* is a set of beliefs, norms, and values that are shared by the organization's members and serve as a basis for behavior. In this role, the culture of the healthcare organization can be a very effective barrier to change.

Another roadblock to change is the *history of the organization*. If the past performance of a healthcare organization has been successful, the tendency of that organization is to continue the status quo. When a particular strategy is successful over a long period of time, the inclination is to continue down that road regardless of environmental jolts to the contrary. After all, who wants to change something that has been so effective for so long? Related to this roadblock is the influence of a successful, long-time healthcare leader, which is termed the "founding effect." In this phenomenon, a strong leader in a healthcare organization will put his or her imprint on the organization, making change difficult to implement. *Size and age* are also roadblocks because resistance increases as healthcare organizations become larger and older. With age and size come rules and routines, which make implementing change even more difficult.

Many organizations put off change until a crisis occurs, and too frequently, the crisis is financial. They find themselves without the necessary resources to implement change, presenting another, often large, barrier to change. Finally, a source of resistance is the misunderstanding that others in the organization may have about the need for change. Change is a disruption that people may resist because they do not want to alter what they have been doing for years. Consider academic health centers and the resistance to policy recommendations to increase medical training in primary care (Topping et al. 1999). Of course, where there are people, there are politics, and when change becomes part of the agenda, politics intensify. The motivation to preserve the healthcare organization can serve to entrench current leaders who are already anti-change.

Another element of this is the cynicism that develops about change in an organization (Reichers, Wanous, and Austin 1997). This cynicism usually is a response to a history of change attempts that have not been successful, leading to a real lack of faith in the leaders of change. Resistance to change should be seen as a management challenge. When faced with resistance from staff, many healthcare managers react forcefully. The best advice is not to fight the resistance because you cannot control it, stop it, or make it go away. Healthcare managers must accept the fact that every change creates resistance and, consequently, the forces of resistance must be explored willingly for causes. Others in the organization have different points of view, so their understanding of the need to change will be different. The next section describes the implementation process and various human resources strategies that can be used to facilitate change.

Strategies for Implementing Change

Management and implementation are probably two of the most troublesome and challenging tasks related to change. How do you keep regular operations going while also trying to implement the change agenda? Many things can be done to help improve the implementation process, but often healthcare managers believe that they do not have time. Senge (1999) considers the "not enough time" excuse as one of the greatest challenges to change—one that signals a lack of flexibility and ability to prioritize. Yet, by automatically anticipating resistance to change, a healthcare manager can develop strategies ahead of time that will lead to successful implementation. What are some of the other forces that can be used to promote change? Strategies that facilitate change in organizations by focusing on the human resources element of the organization are listed below:

- develop open channels of communication;
- set up change teams;
- identify champions within the organization;
- develop internal systems such as shared culture and incentive systems;
- form stakeholder coalitions;
- have a change plan;
- use outside consultants; and
- build networks and alliances.

Encouraging Open Communication with Employees

One of the most important strategies in implementing change is to encourage open communication so administrative and clinical staffs feel they can express different opinions without repercussions. Developing open communication should happen early in the change process. In this way, everyone participates in the discussion of the issues, thereby allowing a common definition of the problem to develop. Using this strategy, healthcare managers utilize resistance as an opportunity—a chance to get everyone thinking the same way. Unfortunately, viewing resistance in this manner is seldom the case. In one example of a hospital merger, most employees surveyed felt uninformed and more than 50 percent did not feel they had been well prepared by management (Petchers, Swanker, and Singer 1992).

One method of enhancing communication is by holding forums where questions are asked, ideas are contributed, and confrontation of each other's underlying assumptions can occur. Listening and responding to concerns will aid understanding of what is happening in all parts of the organization. This takes time and effort. Jack Welch, former CEO of General Electric, is probably one of the most successful change agents in the world. He described the process as labor intensive yet worth the effort. Healthcare managers need to try walking the halls and sharing lunch with staff as Welch used to do. In addition, they should always remember to keep surprises at a minimum by keeping people informed. To do this, they must take into consideration the timing of announcements because people need information, especially when they are likely to be surprised or caught off guard by an event.

Winning Over Stakeholders

Most healthcare managers must realize that they are limited in terms of how much they can accomplish alone. This is particularly true in the healthcare delivery environment today, in which multiple stakeholders exist and conflicts of interest are becoming more and more apparent (Blair and Fottler 1998). Therefore, a critical mass of support for change is needed; this is accomplished by winning over key power groups such as state legislators, consumer groups, and federal agencies.

When considering various stakeholder groups, one of the significant forces of change is the use of champions. Studies on diffusion of practice protocols to physicians in the field have found that adoption requires a champion—usually someone visible and of prominent status in the medical community. Topping and Hartwig (1997) found that the development of a HIV/ AIDS clinic in a very conservative rural community was expedited by the involvement of respected, high-status champions. Along with the champions, Rogers (1983) suggests that managers identify opinion leaders in the organization and elicit their help in supporting the change agenda; that is, a change agent, such as a public health department manager, should identify persons in the organization (e.g., physicians, nurses, social workers) who are able to influence the attitudes and behaviors of other individuals in the organization. The change agent then seeks the support of these opinion leaders and works to initiate change through them. Another strategy that can be used is bringing in outsiders to help set the stage for change and guide the implementation; many healthcare organizations use outside consultants for this very purpose. Not only do outside consultants bring new ideas and excitement to a change agenda, but also they bring a sense of independence, which validates the need for change.

Multiple stakeholders at all levels of the healthcare organization are involved in making change happen, and their assumptions, perspectives, and even agendas do not always converge. Although managers cannot control some of the environmental forces discussed earlier in other chapters, they can manage the way staff members interact. If all of those affected by the change share an understanding of what change is needed, why it is needed, and how they will be affected, the change is far more likely to succeed. Yet, because each person will view the change differently, everyone should be treated with consideration as individuals. Kanter, Stein, and Jick (1992) believe that three groups should be considered in the change process. The first group consists of the "strategists," who lay the foundation and craft the vision. This group needs allies in the change process who should be brought in before the plan is made public. The second group includes the "implementers," who manage the day-to-day operational process of change. Because they confront resistance daily, the implementers need strategies to counter these forces, such as allowing each unit to develop its own implementation plan within the change guidelines or developing reward systems commensurate with the change. The third group comprises the "recipients," who either adopt or fail to adopt the change plan. Understanding how the individuals in this group perceive the change and experience it is extremely important. Each of the three groups has a specific role in the process of change, and strategies must be devised that enhance the participation of each.

Using Teams for Innovation

One of the most crucial times for any healthcare manager is during a crisis, such as the downsizing of a healthcare organization. The challenge becomes one of solving the problem while simultaneously stopping it from interfering with the operation of the organization. The tendency during a crisis is to centralize control or to manage with tighter reigns. Although the need for fast decision making may necessitate this, centralizing control is risky. Leaders need help facing crises; they need teams that are small enough to work with easily and to communicate with rapidly (Fried, Topping, and Rundall 2000). They need teams composed of stakeholders in the organization who can contribute to the solution of the problem while also influencing others positively in the change process. At the same time, by using teams, employees are involved in the change process, allowing them time to prepare psychologically for the change. Nadler and Tushman (1997) describe how Kaiser Permanente's Northern California Region Hospitals and Health Plan responded to the changing healthcare environment in the early 1990s by adopting a customer focus in all operations. To implement this major change in orientation, a new organizational design was required that removed walls between departments and functions while opening up the flow of information and coordination. This structural change was accomplished using a strategic design team to fully assess the need and to recommend a full-scale plan for reorganization.

Mullaney (1992) describes how one hospital used a highly visible steering committee to develop and implement a comprehensive downsizing plan. One important aspect of this downsizing plan was the inclusion of the human resources manager on this team who was significant in the development of a lay-off process. In the case of downsizing, human resources problems intensify because morale decreases substantially and a sense of guilt arises among the survivors. At the same time, those employees laid off experience considerable psychological distress that may result in depression, feelings of betrayal, and sometimes violence. The degree to which clinical and administrative staffs are affected is a function of how the downsizing is handled (Whetten, Keiser, and Urban 1995); the downsizing of Middletown Psychiatric Center located in New York provides an excellent example (Citrome 1997). An orderly process was implemented that involved the dissemination of information ahead of rumors, notification of staff whose positions were targeted for elimination, and provision of employee assistance in resume writing and contacting potential employers.

Motivating Constructive Behavior Internally

A shared culture is an additional force that can be used to support and motivate change. Members of the organization must share the same explicit set of values about the direction of the organization and the reasoning behind the shift. Shared values promote a shared vision of the future and thus inspire commitment and cooperation. In addition, if change occurs, the staff must be reoriented and redirected, which requires education and training. Another important element is the development of structure and process that can be used to implement change. A surprising number of healthcare organizations start full-scale change programs with no idea of how coordination is to be accomplished and who is accountable for various tasks. Many public health programs, for instance, have been implemented with little thought on how community-based services would be coordinated among the various agencies involved in the care. Another aspect of the internal operations is the provision of signals that the change is important. A reward system that recognizes the extra work that change requires is crucial.

Building Networks and Alliances

Often, in the process of change, having financial, managerial, and technological resources is a major factor. A good way to increase availability of resources is to build relationships with other organizations. However, successful collaboration requires hard work and care. For alliances and partnerships to be successful, healthcare managers must view the relationships as strategically important. Management must exhibit attention and commitment; serve as sponsor of the alliance; and promote compatible cultures, clear objectives, and an understanding of mutual benefits between partners. Managers must also work to integrate the organizations to maintain communication and control. Furthermore, for these relationships to endure, trust must exist between organizations. Partnerships have to be built on ethical values that are clearly articulated, communicated, and enforced (Sifonis and Goldberg 1996).

Successful partnerships involve providers from agencies who believe in the same philosophy of care and basic values. An example of such an alliance is the Health Care for the Homeless (HCH) program set up to take care of the homeless in Jacksonville, Florida (Bogue and Hall 1997). This alliance involves not only an onsite medical clinic, but also, because of the high incidence of mental illness, an onsite program with the Mental Health

Resources Center. Three full-time mental health counselors work with the clinic staff to provide case management. Because many of the homeless have comorbid disorders, mental health care includes on-site drug and alcohol rehabilitation programs, support groups, and referrals to permanent housing and group facilities.

Conclusion

This chapter provides an understanding of organizational change and the change process and discusses some of the skills needed to implement a change agenda in healthcare organizations. The future challenge for healthcare managers is to be able to interpret the environment to be able to respond effectively to the inevitable changes that will transpire. For instance, the move of managed care into the public domain brings with it many threats and opportunities. Yet, to take advantage of the latter, the healthcare manager must think in terms of fresh and innovative approaches to the new environment, such as forging partnerships and alliances with organizations that differ in culture and goals. At the same time, stakeholder diversity and empowerment have created and will continue to cause upheavals in healthcare organizations. The treatment role has changed, the potential for stakeholder influence has intensified, and the role of stakeholder management has taken on added significance. The healthcare manager who does not realize this and act accordingly will not survive. The roles of other organizations that are interdependent with a particular healthcare organization are also changing. Consider the position of community hospitals and the role of MCOs and HMOs and the impact they are having on the healthcare sector. New relationships and structures, such as joint ventures and partnerships, are inevitable. Often, these kinds of changes lead to human resources problems in gaining the acceptance of such a change agenda.

Healthcare managers need to think in terms of how to accomplish the process of change. Proper planning of a change agenda is important, especially the inclusion of influential stakeholders and the integration of formulation and implementation. Resistance is inevitable, so accommodating it should be part of the plan as well. As this chapter has demonstrated, strategies can be developed that decrease resistance while enhancing acceptance. The effective healthcare manager always has the time to develop a proper change agenda if he or she wants to see change accomplished. As Peter Senge (1999) implies from his book title, change agents must learn the "dance of change," and not only how to do it but also when and where.

Discussion Questions

1. Why should healthcare managers be concerned with organizational change?

2. Describe the steps involved in the change process.
3. Access information on the web site for the Center for Studying Health System Change (www.hschange.com). Give examples of organizational change.
4. Why do forces of inertia develop when organizations are attempting change?
5. Describe how the external environment acts as a force of change.
6. What is the difference between incremental and revolutionary change?
7. What are some of the roadblocks to change?
8. Why is open communication an important strategy to use in implementing change within an organization? How does the use of teams fit into this strategy?
9. Should all stakeholders be treated the same when implementing change? If not, how should they be treated?
10. What are the advantages and disadvantages of using collaboration (networks and alliances) as a strategy for implementing change?

References

Argyris, C. 1985. *Strategy, Change, and Defensive Routines*. Cambridge, MA: Ballinger.

Barr, P. S. 1998. "Adapting to Unfamiliar Environmental Events: A Look at the Evolution of Interpretation and Its Role in Strategic Change." *Organization Science* 9 (6): 644–69.

Blair, J. D., and M. D. Fottler. 1998. *Strategic Leadership for Medical Groups: Navigating Your Strategic Web*. San Francisco: Jossey-Bass.

Bogue, R., and C. H. Hall. 1997. *Health Network Innovations: How 20 Communities Are Improving Their Systems Through Collaboration*. Chicago: American Hospital Publishing, Inc.

Citrome, L. 1997. "Layoffs, Reductions-in-force, Downsizing, Rightsizing: The Case of a State Psychiatric Hospital." *Administration and Policy in Mental Health* 24 (6): 523–33.

Fried, B., S. Topping, and T. G. Rundall. 2000. "Groups and Teams in Health Services Organizations." In *Health Care Management: Organization, Design, and Behavior, Fourth Edition*, edited by S. Shortell and A. Kaluzny. Albany, NY: Delmar.

Ginter, P. M., L. E. Swayne, and W. J. Duncan. 1998. *Strategic Management of Health Care Organizations*. Malden, MA: Blackwell.

Hambrick, D. C., and R. A. D'Aveni. 1988. "Large Corporate Failures as Downward Spirals." *Administrative Science Quarterly* 33: 1–23.

Herzlinger, R. E. 1997. *Market-Driven Health Care: Who Wins, Who Loses in the Transformation of America's Largest Service Industry*. Reading, MA: Addison-Wesley.

Javidan, M. 1984. "The Impact of Environmental Uncertainty on Long-Range Planning Practices of the U.S. Savings and Loan Industry." *Strategic Management Journal* 5: 381–92.

Kanter, R. M., B. A. Stein, and T. D. Jick. 1992. *The Challenge of Organizational Change*. New York: Free Press.

Lewin, K. 1947. "Frontiers in Group Dynamics." *Human Relations* 1: 5–41.

Mechanic, D., and M. Rosenthal. 1999. "Responses of HMO Medical Directors to Trust Building in Managed Care." *The Milbank Quarterly* 77 (3): 283–303.

Meliones, J. 2000. "Saving Money, Saving Lives." *Harvard Business Review* (November–December): 5–11.

Mullaney, A. D. 1992. "Downsizing: How One Hospital Responded to Decreasing Demand." In *Human Resource Management in Health Care*, edited by M. Brown, pp. 197–204. Gaithersburg, MD: Aspen.

Nadler, D. A., and M. L. Tushman. 1997. *Competing by Design: The Power of Organizational Architecture*. New York: Oxford University Press.

Nutt, P. C. 1991. "How Top Managers in Health Organizations Set Directions that Guide Decision Making." *Hospital & Health Services Administration* 36 (1): 57–75.

Petchers, M. K., S. Swanker, and M. I. Singer. 1992. "The Hospital Merger: Its Effect on Employees." In *Human Resource Management in Health Care*, edited by M. Brown, pp. 181–6. Gaithersburg, MD: Aspen.

Reichers, A. E., J. P. Wanous, and J. T. Austin. 1997. "Understanding and Managing Cynicism About Organizational Change." *Academy of Management Executives* 11 (1): 48–59.

Rogers, E. M. 1983. *Diffusion of Innovations, Third Edition*. New York: Free Press.

Senge, P. 1999. *The Dance of Change: The Challenges of Sustaining Momentum in Learning Organizations*. New York: Doubleday.

Sherman, H., and R. Schultz. 1998. *Open Boundaries: Creating Business Innovation Through Complexity*. Reading, MA: Perseus Books.

Sifonis, J. G., and B. Goldberg. 1996. *Corporation on a Tightrope: Balancing Leadership, Governance, and Technology in an Age of Complexity*. New York: Oxford University Press.

Thomas, J. B., and R. R. McDaniel. 1990. "Interpreting Strategic Issues: Effects of Strategy and the Information-Processing Structure of Top Management Teams." *Academy of Management Journal* 33 (2): 286–306.

Topping, S., and L. Hartwig. 1997. "Delivering Care to Rural HIV/AIDS Patients." *Journal of Rural Health* 13 (3): 226–36.

Topping, S., and P. Ginter. 1998. "Columbia/HCA Healthcare Corporation: A Growth and Acquisition Strategy." In *Strategic Management of Health Care Organizations, Third Edition*, edited by P. M. Ginter, L. E. Swayne, and W. J. Duncan, pp. 811–24. Cambridge, MA: Blackwell.

Topping, S., J. Hyde, J. Barker, and F. Woodrell. 1999. "Academic Health Centers in Turbulent Times: An Examination for Survival." *Health Care Management Review* 24 (2): 7–18.

Tushman, M. L., and E. Romanelli. 1985. "Organizational Evolution: A Metamorphosis Model of Convergence and Reorientation." In *Research in Organizational Behavior*, edited by B. M. Staw and L. L. Cummings, pp. 171–222. Greenwich, CT: JAI Press.

VanDenBerg, J. 1999. "History of the Wraparound Process." In *Promising Practices in Wraparound for Children with Serious Emotional Disturbance and Their*

Families, edited by B. J. Burns and S. K. Goldman, pp. 1–8. Washington, DC: Georgetown University National Technical Assistance Center for Children's Mental Health.

Whetten, D. A., J. D. Keiser, and T. Urban. 1995. "Implications of Organizational Downsizing for the Human Resource Management Function." In *Handbook of Human Resource Management*, edited by F. R. Ferris, S. D. Rosen, and D. T. Barnum, pp. 282–96. Cambridge, MA: Blackwell.

CHAPTER 14

MANAGING WITH ORGANIZED LABOR

Donna Malvey, Ph.D.

Learning Objectives

After completing this chapter, the reader should be able to:

- Examine the relationship of organized labor and management in healthcare
- Distinguish the different phases of the labor relations process
- Describe the evolving role of unions in the healthcare workforce
- Examine legislative and judicial rulings that affect management of organized labor in healthcare settings
- Review emerging healthcare labor trends

Introduction

The **labor relations process** occurs when management (as the representative for the employer) and the union (as the exclusive bargaining representative for the employees) jointly determine and administer the rules of the workplace. A *union* is an organization formed by employees for the purpose of acting as a single unit when dealing with management about workplace issues, hence the term *organized* labor. Unions are not present in every organization because employees must authorize a union to represent them. Unions typically are viewed as threats by management because they interfere with management's ability to make and implement decisions. Once a union is present, management may no longer unilaterally make decisions about the terms and conditions of work. Instead, management must negotiate these decisions with the union. Similarly, employees may no longer communicate directly with management about work issues but instead must go through the union. Thus, the union functions as a middleman, which is relatively expensive to maintain for both parties. Employees pay union dues, and management incurs additional costs for such things as contract negotiations and any increases in salaries and benefits negotiated by the union (Freeman and Medoff 1984). Subsequently, management has a vested interest in keeping unions out of the organization.

Labor relations process is the process in which management and the union jointly decide on and administer terms and conditions of employment

However, given recent trends of unionization in healthcare, managers are increasingly forced to work with unions.

This chapter examines the phenomenon of healthcare unionization and provides direction for managing with organized labor. In addition, we discuss the possible behaviors and strategies that comprise the labor management relationship; develop an understanding of the generic labor relations process of organizing, negotiating, and administering contracts; explore developments in organizing a relatively unorganized healthcare workforce; consider the impact of labor laws, amendments, and rulings on human resources strategies and goals; and discuss the trend toward physician unions and how changes in employment status will affect the growth of these unions.

Managing with organized labor involves the application and maintenance of a positive labor relations program within the organization. A productive and positive labor management relationship can only be accomplished through integration with other human resources functions. For example, employees expect management to provide environments that are clean and safe from workplace hazards and related concerns such as AIDS and hepatitis B. If management allows the environment to deteriorate, union organizers will focus on these issues (Becker and Rowe 1989; Fennell 1987). In addition, the labor relations process occurs across all levels of the organization and involves all levels of management. Upper-level management will develop objectives and strategies regarding wage rates, while mid-level managers and first-line supervisors will implement these objectives.

Developing strategies and goals to implement a positive labor relations program in healthcare requires an understanding of the generic labor relations process of organizing, negotiating, and administering contracts with a union as well as specific knowledge of emerging healthcare labor trends such as physician unions. A productive and positive labor management relationship involves compromise by both parties because of the adversarial nature of the relationship. Just because a union has won the right to represent employees does not mean that management has to accept all of its terms. All parties, management, unions, and employees have a vested interest in the success and survival of the organization; yet they also have opposing or conflicting interests. For example, unions will look toward improving the benefits package for employees while management, faced with budget cutbacks and declining reimbursements, will have concerns about containing costs. Thus, the challenge for management is working with the union to reconcile differences in a fair and consistent manner.

As Figure 14.1 suggests, the labor management relationship reflects a continuum of possible behaviors and strategies. These range from the most positive, or collaborative, (in which management and the union share common goals oriented in the organization's success) to the most negative, or oppositional, and self-serving. Even if the relationship is neutral and both parties cooperate to maintain the status quo, a variety of factors can cause the

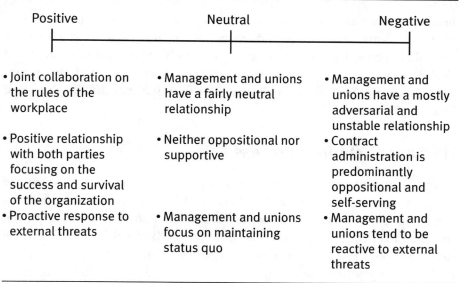

Positive	Neutral	Negative
• Joint collaboration on the rules of the workplace	• Management and unions have a fairly neutral relationship	• Management and unions have a mostly adversarial and unstable relationship
• Positive relationship with both parties focusing on the success and survival of the organization	• Neither oppositional nor supportive	• Contract administration is predominantly oppositional and self-serving
• Proactive response to external threats	• Management and unions focus on maintaining status quo	• Management and unions tend to be reactive to external threats

FIGURE 14.1
The Labor Management Relationship in Healthcare

relationship to shift in either direction. For instance, a merger may create uncertainty for both the union and management and, as a result, may reposition their relationship along the continuum. However, the direction in which the relationship moves will depend largely on the knowledge and understanding of the labor relations process on both sides of the issue.

Overview of Unionization

Union membership has been declining steadily for decades. In the 1950s to 1970s, union membership represented 25 to 30 percent of the U.S. workforce. In 2000, unions represented only 16.3 million or 13.5 percent of workers in the United States. Meanwhile, the healthcare workforce of 9.8 million is relatively unorganized; of the 4.3 million workers currently employed in hospitals, only 471,000 belong to a union. In addition, 246,000 of the 5.4 million workers employed in other health services industries such as nursing homes and clinics are unionized (Bureau of Labor Statistics 2000a). Thus, the healthcare workforce represents one of the largest pools of unorganized workers in the United States and a prime target for union organizers.

Union election activity has been declining nationally. The AFL-CIO (American Federation of Labor-Congress of Industrial Organizations), the largest labor organization in the United States, reported having slightly more than 13 million members in 1999, not much more than when it was founded in 1955. In addition, the union must recruit about 400,000 new members annually just to keep pace with attrition (Swoboda 1999). Overall, during the 1980s and 1990s, organized labor's influence and bargaining power continued to decline as the nature of U.S. industries shifted from factories and traditional union strongholds to service and technologies (Fottler et al. 1999). Recently, unions have been more successful in organizing workers in the public sector than in the private sector, with the exception of state and local government whose membership has edged downward, and in healthcare rather than in other industries (Bureau of Labor Statistics 2000b; Scott and Lowery 1994).

The Labor Relations Process

In an attempt to protect workers' rights to unionize, Congress passed the *National Labor Relations Act (NLRA)* in 1935, which serves as the legal framework for the labor relations process. Although the NLRA has been amended over the years, it remains the only legislation that governs federal labor relations. The law contains significant provisions intended to protect workers' rights to form and join unions and to engage in collective bargaining. The law also defines unfair labor practices, which restrict both unions and employers from interfering with the labor relations process. The NLRA delegates to the *National Labor Relations Board (NLRB)* responsibility for overseeing implementation of the NLRA and investigating and remedying unfair labor practices. NLRB rulemaking occurs on a case-by-case basis.

Key participants in the labor relations process include management officials, who serve as surrogates for the owners or employers of the organization; union officials, who are usually elected by members; the government, which participates through executive, legislative, and judicial branches occurring at federal, state, and local levels; and third-party neutrals such as arbitrators. The process also involves three phases that are equally essential: the recognition phase, the negotiation phase, and the administration phase.

Recognition Phase

During this phase unions attempt to organize employees and gain representation through either voluntary recognition of the union or a representation election, which certifies that the union has the authority to act on behalf of employees in negotiating a collective bargaining agreement. In rare cases, the NLRB may direct an employer to recognize and bargain with the union if evidence exists that a fair and impartial election would be impossible. During the past two decades, management strategies and tactics have become more aggressive during the recognition phase as management has endeavored to keep unions from becoming the employees' representative. For example, management may institute unfair labor practices such as filing for bankruptcy, illegally firing union supporters, and relocation. Although unions may file grievances with the NLRB over these practices and the use of any illegal or union-busting tactics, legal resolution usually occurs years after the fact and long after union elections have been held. Thus, both unions and management understand that the battle lines are drawn in the recognition phase, and both sides will be fervently engaged in shoring up support.

The desire to unionize is believed to result from three issues: wages, benefits, and employee perceptions about the workplace. Because ascertaining the desires of employees is difficult, management must rely on *signals* or indicators in the workplace. Table 14.1 summarizes some of the behaviors that might indicate organizing activities or the potential for organizing employees. For example, high turnover of approximately 40 percent characterizes healthcare institutions such as hospitals (Swoboda 1999). However, when employees are leaving their jobs for a local competitor, management must investigate the underlying reasons for turnover. Even simple issues such as an increase in requests for information on policies and procedures can indicate problems and should not be discounted.

During the recognition phase, the union solicits signed authorization cards that designate the union to act as the employees' collective bargaining representative. When at least 30 percent of employees in the bargaining unit have signed cards, the union requests the employer to *voluntarily* recognize the union. Voluntary recognition is rarely granted by employers, however, and occurs less than 2 percent of the time in healthcare organizations. When employers refuse voluntary recognition of the union, the union is then eligible to petition the NLRB for a representation election. In response to the petition, the NLRB verifies the authenticity of the signatures collected by the union, determines the appropriate bargaining unit, and sets a date for a secret ballot election.

Bargaining Units in Healthcare

The NLRB determines which employees are eligible to be in a bargaining unit. Currently, the NLRB permits a total of eight bargaining units in healthcare settings. The implications of this number and some historical perspective are provided later in this chapter; that section summarizes legislative and judicial rulings. Although the NLRB has modified its criteria over the years, it has not changed its outlook on managerial or supervisory employees, who are ineligible for membership in a bargaining unit. Under a provision of the NLRA, 29USCS 152(11), an employee is a "supervisor" if the employee has the authority, in the interest of the employer, to engage in specific activities, including responsible direction of other employees, where exercise of such authority requires the use of independent judgment. The U.S. Supreme court in the case of the *NLRB v. Kentucky River Community Care, Inc.* reached a decision about the legal question of which nurses qualify as supervisors. In its ruling on May 29, 2001, the court determined that registered nurses who use independent judgment in directing employees are supervisors and thus exempt from being organized into collective bargaining units. This ruling is expected to have a significant impact on the ability of nurses to form unions

TABLE 14.1
Warning
Indicators for
Healthcare
Organizations

Item	Increase/ Decrease	Comment
Turnover— especially to competitors	Increase	Turnover in healthcare organizations typically is much higher than in organizations in other industries because of enhanced mobility from licensing and standardization. However, if employees are moving to competing organizations in the local area, such movement may indicate dissatisfaction rather than career opportunities
Employee-generated incidents	Increase	Staff members are fighting among themselves, theft or damage to organization's property, and insubordination related to routine requests by supervisors
Grievances	Increase	More grievances are being filed with the HR office compared with informal settlements of supervisors and employees
Communication	Decrease	Staff members are reluctant to provide feedback and generally become quiet when management enters the room. Suggestion boxes are empty and employees are less willing to avail themselves of the "open door" system or other mechanisms to air dissatisfaction/problems
HR office informational requests	Increase	Employees are interested in policies, procedures, and other matters related to the terms and conditions of employment, and they want this information in writing. Verbal responses no longer satisfy them
Off-site meetings	Increase	Employees appear to be congregating more at off-site premises
Grapevine activity	Increase	Rumors increase in number and intensity
Absenteeism and/or tardiness	Increase	Employees are engaging in union-organizing activities prior to and during working hours

because employers will try to claim more registered nurses are supervisors when they direct the work of others such as practical nurses and aides.

Generally, the union election is scheduled to occur on workplace premises during working hours. The union is permitted to conduct a pre-election campaign in accordance with solicitation rules that are proscribed for both unions and management. For example, patient care areas such as treatment rooms, waiting areas used by patients, and elevators and stairs used in transporting patients are off limits; but kitchens, supply rooms, business areas, and employee lounges are permissible locations. During the campaign, management may not make threats or announce reprisals regarding the outcome of the election such as telling nurses that layoffs will result if the union is elected or pay raises will be given if the union loses. Management also may not directly ask employees about their attitudes or voting intentions or those other employees. Management is allowed, however, to conduct *captive audience* speeches, which are meetings during work time to inform employees about the changes that certifying a union will mean for the organization and persuade employees to give management another chance.

To win the election and be certified by the NLRB as representing the bargaining unit, the union must achieve a simple majority or 50 percent *plus one* of those voting. When the union wins the election, it assumes the duties of the exclusive bargaining agent for all employees in the unit even if those employees choose not to join the union and pay membership dues. Similarly, any negotiated agreements will cover all employees in the bargaining unit. If the union loses, however, it can continue to maintain contact with employees and provide certain representational services such as informing them of their rights. The union may lose the right to represent employees through a **decertification** election.

Negotiation Phase

After winning the election, the union will begin to negotiate a contract on behalf of the employees in the bargaining unit. Federal labor laws encourage collective bargaining on the theory that employees and their employers are best able to reach agreement on issues such as wages, hours, and conditions of employment through negotiating their differences. The process of negotiating this contract is referred to as **collective bargaining**. The NLRA defines collective bargaining as:

> . . . the performance of the mutual obligation of the employer and the representative of the employees to meet at reasonable times and confer in good faith with respect to wages, hours and terms and conditions of employment or the negotiation of an agreement, or any question arising thereunder, and the execution of a written contract incorporating any agreement reached requested by either party to agree to a proposal or require the making of a concession (NLRA, Section 8 [d], 1935).

Decertification is a NLRB procedure available for employees when they believe, usually as a result of an election, that the union no longer represents the interests of the majority of the bargaining unit

Collective bargaining is an activity whereby union and management officials attempt to resolve conflicting interests in a manner that will sustain and possibly enrich their continuing relationships

The NLRA requires an employer to recognize and bargain in good faith with a certified union, but it does not force the employer to agree with the union or make any concessions. The key to satisfying the duty to bargain in good faith is approaching the bargaining table with an open mind and negotiating with the intention of reaching final agreement (LLR 3115: 7888).

Issues for bargaining have evolved over a period of years as the result of NLRB and court decisions. Those issues are categorized as either illegal, mandatory, or voluntary (permissive). Illegal subjects, such as age discrimination employment clauses, may not be considered for bargaining. **Mandatory bargaining issues** are related to wages, hours, and other conditions of employment; Table 14.2 provides a partial list of these issues. Mandatory subjects must be bargained if they are introduced for negotiation. **Voluntary, or permissive bargaining, issues** carry no similar restriction. Examples of voluntary issues include strike insurance and benefits for retired employees.

Mandatory bargaining issues are topics related to wages, hours, and other conditions of employment that must be bargained

Prior to bargaining, management will formulate ranges for each issue, which is similar to an opening offer, followed by a series of benchmarks that represent expected levels of settlement. Of course, management must calculate a resistance point beyond which it will cease negotiations. Fisher and Ury (1981) have developed a principled method of negotiation based on the merits or principles of the issues. The following four basic points are involved:

Voluntary (permissive or nonmandatory) issues are topics, such as benefits for retired employees, that can be bargained only if both parties so desire

1. People: Separate the people from the problem.
2. Interests: Focus on interests, not the positions that people hold.
3. Options: Generate a variety of alternative possibilities.
4. Criteria: Insist that solutions be evaluated using objective standards.

According to this method, management will formulate a best alternative to a negotiated agreement for each issue. In this manner, negotiators evaluate whether the type of agreement that can be reached is better than no agreement at all. By considering mutual options for gain, the negotiator offers a more flexible approach toward bargaining and increases the likelihood of achieving creative solutions.

Collective bargaining is both a laborious and a time-consuming endeavor. Bargaining requires not only listening to others but attempting to understand the motivational force behind the dialog. Successful negotiators make every effort to understand fully what truly underlies bargaining positions and why they are so fiercely held, and they are receptive to any signals that are being communicated, including nonverbal communication such as body language (Fisher and Ury 1981).

Bargaining, as depicted in Figure 14.2, can be conceptualized as a continuum of bargaining behaviors and strategies. At one end of the continuum is *concessionary bargaining*, in which the employer asks the union to eliminate, limit, or reduce wages and other commitments in response to financial constraints. This type of bargaining is likely to occur when the organization is

- Wages
- Arbitration
- Duration of agreement
- Reinstatement of economic strikers
- Work rules
- Lunch periods
- Bonus payments
- Promotions
- Transfers
- Plant reopening
- Bargaining over "bar list"
- Arrangement for negotiation
- Plant closedown and relocation
- Overtime pay
- Company houses
- Union-imposed production ceiling
- No-strike clause
- Workloads
- Cancellation of security upon relocation of plant
- Employer's insistence on clause, giving arbitrator right to enforce award
- Severance pay
- Safety
- Checkoff
- Hours
- Holidays (paid)
- Grievance procedure
- Change of payment (hourly to salary)
- Merit wage increase
- Pension plan
- Price of company meals
- Seniority
- Plant closing
- Employee physical examination
- Truck rentals
- Change in insurance carrier/benefits
- Profit-sharing plan
- Agency shop
- Subcontracting
- Most-favored-nation clause
- Piece rates
- Change of employee status to independent contractor
- Discounts on company's products
- Clause providing for supervisors' keeping seniority in unit
- Nondiscriminatory hiring hall
- Prohibition against supervisors doing unit work
- Partial plant closing
- Discharge
- Vacations (paid)
- Layoff plan
- Union security and checkoff
- Work schedule
- Retirement age
- Group insurance (health, life, and accident)
- Layoffs
- Job-posting procedures
- Union security
- Musician price list
- Change in operations resulting in reclassifying workers from incentive to straight time, cut workforce, or installation of cost-saving machine
- Motor carrier union agreement
- Sick leave
- Discriminatory racial policies
- Work assignments and transfers
- Stock-purchase plan
- Management Rights clause
- Shift differentials
- Procedures for income tax withholding
- Plant rules
- Superseniority for union stewards
- Hunting on employer forest preserve where previously granted

TABLE 14.2
Mandatory Bargaining Issues

Note: This is a list of major items for bargaining; the list does not include subcategories.

FIGURE 14.2
Collective
Bargaining
Continuum

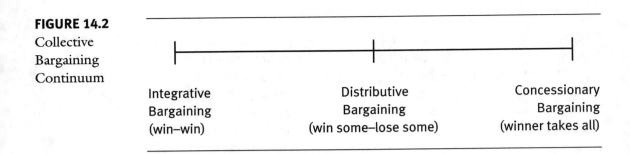

Even when both parties negotiate in good faith and fulfill the covenants
of the NLRA, an agreement still may not be reached at times. When this

in financial jeopardy and struggling to survive. At the opposite end is *integrative bargaining*, which seeks win-win situations and solutions that creatively respond to both parties' needs. This type of bargaining requires the trust and cooperation of both parties. In the center is *distributive bargaining*, which is a win-lose type in which each party gives up something to gain something else. This type of bargaining is likely when negotiations are contentious and full of conflict.

Even when both parties negotiate in good faith and fulfill the covenants of the NLRA, an agreement still may not be reached at times. When this happens, parties are said to have reached an **impasse**. To resolve an impasse, a variety of techniques may be implemented. These techniques involve third parties and include **mediation**, in which a mediator evaluates the dispute and issues nonbinding recommendations. If either party rejects the mediator's recommendations, arbitration is an alternative. Arbitrators, similar to mediators, are neutral third parties, but their decisions are legally binding. For example, arbitrators may recommend that either party's position be accepted as a final offer or they can attempt to split the differences between the two parties' positions.

If these techniques fail to resolve the impasse, employers or the union can initiate work stoppages that may take the form of lockouts or strikes. A lockout occurs when the employer shuts down operations either during or prior to a dispute. A strike, on the other hand, is employee initiated. **Lockouts** or **strikes** can occur during negotiations and also during the life of the contract. Special provisions for these work stoppages in healthcare settings are discussed in the section below on the history of judicial and legislative rulings.

In addition, no-strike and no-lockout clauses can be negotiated in the agreement. No-strike clauses essentially prohibit strikes, either unconditionally or with conditions. An unconditional no-strike clause means that the union and its members will not engage in either a strike or work slow-down while the contract is in effect. A conditional no-strike clause bans strikes and slow-downs except in certain situations and under specific conditions, which are delineated in detail in the agreement. Comparable clauses for lockouts exist for employers.

Impasse is a deadlock in negotiating between management and officials over terms and conditions of employment

Mediation is a process whereby a third-party neutral attempts to help union and management officials resolve a grievance

Lockout is an act by an employer when it shuts down its operation during or before a labor dispute

Strike is a temporary stoppage of work by a group of employees for the purposes of expressing a grievance or enforcing a demand

Administration Phase

When an agreement between the union and the employer is reached, it must be recorded in writing and executed in good faith, which means that the terms and conditions of the agreement must be applied and enforced. This agreement will include disciplinary, grievance, and arbitration procedures, many of which have been discussed in earlier chapters. The collective bargaining agreement imposes limitations on the disciplinary actions that management may take. The right to discharge, suspend, or discipline is clearly enunciated in contractual clauses and in the adoption of rules and procedures that may or may not be incorporated in the agreement.

Management may discipline up through discharge only for sufficient and appropriate reasons and must base all procedures on **due process**. The union's role in the process is to defend employees and to determine the propriety of management action. The burden of proof rests with management to prove that whatever action was taken was proper and consistent with progressive discipline. If the grievance proceeds to arbitration, arbitrators will usually support management if they find evidence of progressive discipline and evidence that employees were fully aware of the standards against which their behavior was to be measured. These standards include very basic rules and regulations outlining offenses that will subject employees to disciplinary action and the extent of such action.

Due process is the procedural aspect of disciplinary cases, such as following time limits prescribed in the labor agreement, providing union representation, and notifying an employee of a specific offense in writing

The heart of administering the collective bargaining agreement is the grievance procedure. This procedure is a useful and productive management tool that allows implementation and interpretation of the contract. A **grievance** must be well defined and restricted to violations of the terms and conditions of the agreement. However, other conditions may give rise to a grievance, including violations of the law or company rules, a change in working conditions or past company practices, or violations of health and safety standards.

Grievance is any employee's concern over a perceived violation of the labor agreement that is submitted to the grievance procedure for eventual resolution

The grievance process usually contains a series of steps. The first step always involves the presentation of the grievance by the employee (or representative) to the immediate, first-line supervisor. If the grievance is not resolved at this step, broader action is taken. Because most grievances involve an action by the immediate supervisor, the second step necessarily must occur outside the department and at a higher level; thus, the second step will involve the employee (or representative) and a department head or other administrator. Prior to this meeting the grievance will be written out, dated, and signed by the employee and the union representative. The written grievance will document the events as the employee perceived them, cite the appropriate contract provisions that allegedly had been violated, and indicate the desired resolution or settlement prospects. If the grievance is unresolved at this point, a third step becomes necessary, involving an in-house review by top management. A grievance that remains unresolved at the conclusion of the third step may go to arbitration if provided for in the contract and if the union is in agreement.

Most collective bargaining agreements restrict the arbitrator's decision to application and interpretation of the agreement and make the decision final and binding upon both parties. Most agreements also specify methods for selecting arbitrators. If the union agrees to arbitration, it must notify management, and an arbitrator is jointly selected. In evaluating the grievance, arbitrators focus on a variety of criteria, including the actual nature of the offense, the past record of the grieving employee, warnings, knowledge of rules, past practices, and discriminatory treatment. Thus, a large number of factors interact, making arbitration a complex process.

An arbitration hearing permits each side an opportunity to present its case. Similar to a court hearing, witnesses, cross-examinations, transcripts, and legal counsel may be used. As with a court hearing, the nature of arbitration is adversarial. Thus, cases may be lost because of poor preparation and presentation. Generally, the courts will enforce an arbitrator's decision unless it is shown to be unreasonable, unsound, or capricious relative to the issues under consideration. Also, if an arbitrator has exceeded his or her authority or issued an order that violates existing state or federal law, the decision may be vacated. Consistent and fair adjudication of grievances is the hallmark of a sound labor management relationship.

In healthcare settings, the strike is the most severe form of a labor management dispute. A critical part of planning for negotiations is an honest assessment of strike potential. This involves identifying strike issues that are likely to be critical for all parties. Although estimating the impact of possible strikes, including economic pressures from lost wages and revenues, is essential, the key to a successful strike from the perspective of the union is to impose enough pressure on management to expedite movement toward a compromise. Pressure may be psychological as well as economic. In healthcare settings, the real losers in a strike are the patients and their families. Patients may be denied services or forced to postpone treatment, be relocated to another institution, or even be discharged prematurely.

Management must be aware of critical factors that affect its ability and willingness to withstand a strike. When attempting to estimate the impact of these factors, managers will evaluate several key indicators, including revenue losses, timing of the strike, and availability of replacements for striking workers. However, management must also contemplate factors that affect the union, such as the question of whether striking employees will be entitled to strike benefits, especially health benefits. If so, for how long? Both parties must also consider the impact of outside assistance to avoid or settle a strike.

A Review of Legislative and Judicial Rulings

Table 14.3 summarizes important legislative and judicial rulings and their impact on healthcare settings. The Taft Hartley Act (Taft Hartley) amended the NLRA in 1947. The primary intent of these amendments was to strike

Year	Legislation/Judicial Ruling	Impact on Healthcare Organizations
1947	Taft Hartley amendments to NLRA	Exempted not-for-profit hospitals from NLRA coverage, including collective bargaining
1962	Executive order #10988	Permitted federally supported hospitals to bargain collectively
1974	Healthcare amendments to NLRA	Extended NLRA coverage to private, not-for-profit hospitals and healthcare institutions; special provisions for strikes, pickets, and impasses
1976	NLRB ruling: Cedars-Sinai Medical Center, Los Angeles, CA	Ruled that medical residents, interns, and fellows (house staff) are students and excluded from collective bargaining
1989/ 1991	NLRB ruling/Supreme Court affirmation on multiple bargaining units: PL. 93-360	Expanded the number of bargaining units in acute care hospitals from three to eight
1999	NLRB Ruling: Boston Medical Center	Reversed Cedars-Sinai Medical Center decision and ruled that house staff are employees, not students, and can therefore be included in collective bargaining
2001	Supreme Court decision regarding nurse supervisors: *NLRB v. Kentucky River Community Care, Inc.*	Court ruled that registered nurses who use independent judgment in directing employees are supervisors. Expected impact: limiting unions' ability to organize nurses
Beyond 2001	Congressional legislation to exempt physicians who practice as independent contractors from anti-trust provisions	Outcome would open the floodgates for physicians in independent practice to join unions. Currently only employed physicians may unionize

TABLE 14.3
Summary of Important Legislative and Judicial Rulings

a balance in the NLRA because most of its protections and rights applied to workers, and employers needed a means for redress. Taft Hartley also gave states federal permission to enact **right-to-work laws**, which essentially prohibit employees from being forced to join unions as a condition of employment. Currently, 21 states, mostly in the South and West, have enacted such laws. Unions oppose right-to-work laws in part because under the NLRA,

Right-to-work laws are laws in 21 states that have implemented point 14(b) of the National Labor Relations Act, which prohibits union membership (and related union security clauses) as a condition of employment

unions are responsible for representing all employees in the bargaining unit, even those members who choose not to join the union and consequently pay no dues to the union. (Nonunion members of the bargaining unit are often referred to as "free riders" because they acquire all of the benefits of union membership without any cost. Meanwhile, proponents of right-to-work laws maintain that no one should be forced to join a private organization, especially if that organization is using dues money to support causes that contravene an individual's moral or religious beliefs.)

Although the NLRA, as it was initially enacted in 1935, did not exempt healthcare employees explicitly, court interpretations tended to exclude healthcare workers from its regulations until later amendments asserted jurisdiction over a variety of healthcare institutions. The Taft Hartley Act had a significant impact on healthcare workers because Section 2 (2) specifically excluded from the definition of "employer" those private, not-for-profit hospitals and healthcare institutions. However, the NLRB asserted jurisdiction over proprietary hospitals and nursing homes when the 1974 Health Care Amendments, Public Law 93-360, brought the private, not-for-profit health industry within the jurisdiction of federal labor law.

Approximately two million additional healthcare workers became eligible for representation with the 1974 Health Care Amendments (Stickler 1990). These amendments afforded stringent protections regarding work stoppages to safeguard patient care. Table 14.4 summarizes the provisions for strikes and **pickets** as well as impasse requirements. In drafting the 1974 amendments, the congressional committee specifically included a ten-day strike and picket notice provision, a requirement that had not been applied to other industries. The committee did so to ensure that healthcare institutions would have sufficient advance notice of a strike. Furthermore, the committee report of the amendments held that a union would be in violation if it struck a facility more than 72 hours after the designated notice time unless the parties agreed to a new time or the union issued a new ten-day notice. In addition, if the union does not begin the strike or other job action at the time designated in the initial ten-day notice, it must provide the healthcare facility with at least 12 hours notice before the actual beginning of the action. Thus, the 12-hour "warning" must fall completely within the 72-hour notice period. Repeatedly serving ten-day notices on the employer also constitutes evidence of a refusal to bargain in good faith and is a violation of the NLRA.

Picketing is outside patrolling by union members of any employer's premises for the purpose of achieving a specific objective

The reprisals for violating the ten-day notice are substantial. For example, workers engaged in work stoppage in violation of the ten-day strike notice lose their status as employees and are subsequently unprotected by the NLRA provisions. Exceptions to the requirements for unions to provide notices are provided as well. If the employer has committed a flagrant or serious unfair labor practice, notices would not be required. In addition, the employer may not use the ten-day notice period to essentially undermine the bargaining relationship that would otherwise exist. For example, the facility would be

1974 Healthcare Amendments to the Taft Hartley Act	General NLRA Provisions
30-day "reasonable" time to picket following which a representation petition must be filed by the union with NLRB	Similar requirement
90-day notice for modifying an existing collective bargaining agreement	60-day requirement
60-day notice to FMCS of impending expiration of existing collective bargaining agreement	30-day requirement
Following FMCS notification, contract must remain in effect for 60 days without any strikes or lockouts	30-day requirement
30-day notice of a dispute must be given to FMCS and appropriate state agency during initial negotiations	No similar requirement
The director of FMCS is authorized to appoint a board of inquiry in the event of a threatened or actual work stoppage	No similar authority
10-day written notice to employer and FMCS of strikes or pickets required of healthcare unions. (Note: this notice cannot occur before either (1) the end of the 90-day notice to modify the existing contract or (2) the 30-day notice in the case of an impasse during negotiations of the new contract	No similar requirement
A new section 19 provides for an alternate, a contribution to designated 501(C)(3) charities, for the payment of union dues for persons with religious convictions against making such payments	No similar requirement

TABLE 14.4 Comparison of Provisions for Strike or Picket Notification and Impasse Requirements

able to receive supplies, but it would not be free to stockpile supplies for an unduly extended period. Similarly, the facility would not be able to bring in large numbers of personnel from other facilities for the purpose of replacing striking workers (Metzger, Ferentino, and Kruger 1984).

In 1989 a NLRB ruling established eight units for the purpose of collective bargaining in acute care hospitals; the units are (1) physicians, (2) nurses, (3) all other professionals, (4) technical employees, (5) business office clerical employees, (6) skilled maintenance employees, (7) guards, and (8) all other nonprofessionals; Table 14.5 provides more detail on the various occupations that fall within the eight designated categories. As with all bargaining unit determinations, supervisors are excluded from unit membership.

TABLE 14.5

Eight
Categories
of Workers
Specified
in NLRB
Bargaining
Rules

1. Physicians
2. Nurses:
   • registered nurses
   • graduate nurses
   • non-nursing department nurses
   • nurse anesthetists
   • nurse instructors
   • nurse practitioners
3. All professionals, except for registered nurses and physicians:
   • audiologists
   • chemists
   • counselors
   • dietitians
   • educational programmers
   • educators
   • medical artists
   • nuclear physicists
   • pharmacists
   • social workers
   • technologists
   • therapists
   • utilization review coordinators
4. Technical employees:
   • infant-care technicians
   • laboratory technicians
   • licensed practical nurses
   • operating room technicians
   • orthopedic technicians
   • physical therapy assistants
   • psychiatric technicians
   • respiratory therapy technicians
   • surgical assistants
   • x-ray technicians
5. Business office clerical employees
6. Skilled maintenance employees
7. Guards
8. All other nonprofessional employees

The AHA strongly opposed the ruling and appealed to the U.S. Supreme Court, protesting that eight units would lead to a proliferation of bargaining units in the hospital, further fragmenting healthcare collective bargaining, increasing bargaining costs, making implementation of hospital-wide policies more difficult, and ultimately inflating the cost of healthcare and rendering the bargaining process more complicated, lengthy, and subject to legal appeals and challenges (American Hospital Association 1991). The Supreme Court disagreed, affirming the NLRB's ruling in 1991. Although little empirical evidence specifically evaluates the impact of the eight-unit ruling (Hirsch and Schumacher 1998), election activity and the union win rate have increased since 1995. Table 14.6 presents election information for the period 1995–1999.

Developments in Organizing Physicians and Nurses

Physicians

At their annual meeting in June 1999, the AMA House of Delegates approved a controversial resolution creating a national "bargaining unit" for physicians. The unit is called *Physicians for Responsible Negotiations (PRN)*. PRN would permit employed physicians to bargain with health plans and insurers. The resolution was controversial because the AMA had in the past staunchly opposed unions. In endorsing PRN, the AMA has not altered its view of physicians' unions; that is, much of the AMA membership views unionism in general as antithetical to professionalism and unions as economic devices that extract benefits for their members at the expense of patient trust and confidence (Cohen 1999). However, the AMA now maintains that collective bargaining is an acceptable professional mechanism for interacting with government and other third-party payers. The action of the AMA House of Delegates is worth noting because it was taken against the recommendation of the AMA's own board of trustees and against the advice of both the AMA Section of Medical Schools and the AMA Council on Medical Education (Association of American Medical Colleges Executive Council 1999). Estimates on current physician union membership vary from 30,000 to 50,000. At least 25 physician unions exist nationwide, although some of these unions include nonphysicians such as dentists (Sobal and Hepner 1990).

The majority of physicians are independent contractors and technically ineligible for union membership because only "employed" physicians, including those employed in academic settings, are authorized to bargain collectively. Physicians who practice as independent contractors are restricted from collective bargaining by the Sherman Anti-trust Act of 1980, which prohibits all business combinations that restrain free trade. Therefore, these physicians cannot legally talk with one another about price of service. Subsequently,

Year	Total Elections	Union Wins
1995	291	156
1996	370	205
1997	407	258
1998	486	290
1999	517	333

TABLE 14.6 Summary of Election Activity in Health Services Elections, 1995–1999.

Source: Industrial Distribution of Representation Elections Held in Cases Closed, FY 1995–1999. Annual Reports of the NLRB.

independent contractors who engage in collective bargaining with entities such as health plans and insurers risk exposure to federal anti-trust suits.

Of the roughly 600,000 physicians that currently treat patients in the United States, approximately one in seven is employed and therefore eligible for collective bargaining. Although most physicians currently are ineligible to join a union, the proportion of employed physicians is growing. In a recent physician study for the period 1983–1994, the percentage of physicians practicing as employees increased from 24.2 percent to 42.3 percent while those self-employed in solo or group practices fell from 40.5 percent to 29.3 percent and from 35.3 percent to 28.4 percent, respectively (Kletke, Emmons, and Gillis 1996).

In addition, efforts are under way to redefine "employed." The existing legal definition is being challenged by several physician unions with claims that managed care contracts are the equivalent of employment agreements. Under the proposed new definition, about half of all practicing physicians, or approximately 300,000, actually may become eligible for collective bargaining; that physician membership is expected to grow by at least 15 percent annually (Anthony and Erf 2000; Greenhouse 1999; Havighurst 1999; Thompson 2000).

Federal legislation (HR 1304, the Quality Health Care Coalition Act) sponsored by Representative Tom Campbell, R-California, and endorsed by the AMA would have amended anti-trust laws to permit independent physicians to bargain collectively with health plans, MCOS, and insurers. However, the legislation failed to pass the Senate, and Representative Campbell is no longer a member of Congress; thus, similar legislation is unlikely to be reintroduced. In addition, physicians have been advocating at the state level for laws that would allow local collective bargaining. Texas and Washington have both passed laws designed to protect private practice physicians from federal anti-trust suits, enabling them to negotiate with health plans under state supervision.

House Staff (Medical Residents, Interns, and Fellows)

In 1999, the NLRB ruled that house staff members at Boston Medical Center were employees and not students. The impact of this ruling is that house staff in private hospitals now have the legal right to bargain collectively. This determination was a reversal of a 1976 ruling for Cedars-Sinai Medical Center in Los Angeles (Yacht 2000). Opponents of house staff unionization suggest union activity will create adversarial relationships between house staff and instructors. For example, unions could negotiate resident promotions and fight against disciplinary actions and dismissal of poorly performing house staff (Levenson 1999).

Nurses

In hospitals, nursing represents the largest service, providing patient care 24 hours a day, seven days a week. Historically, nurses have struggled with conflict among their obligation to their patients, their profession, and union representation. Despite uneven salary levels across the profession and widespread persistent discontent with working conditions, the majority of nurses do not belong to unions. Recent evidence suggests that for nurses to vote in favor of a union, they must believe that joining a union will help them gain greater control over patient care (Clark et al. 2000). Because only 17 percent of the nation's 2.2 million RNs belong to unions, the RN population is a promising target for union organizers. However, union organizers appear to be concentrating on nurses who already belong to unions. Subsequently, many of the battles waged over nurses' membership are not to add new members, but to lure existing members from one union to another (Greene 1998; Leung 1999). Unions may also find an uphill battle in organizing registered nurses because the U.S. Supreme Court recently determined that registered nurses who use independent judgment in directing employees, such as aides and practical nurses, are supervisors and thereby ineligible to join unions.

Management Guidelines

1. Whether a healthcare organization is union or nonunion, it should have a policy on unionism, and this policy should be communicated to current and prospective employees. A positive labor management relationship begins with the screening process. All prospective employees should be given information about the institution's position toward unions, including goals and strategies of fair and consistent dealings with unions. Employee handbooks and orientation represent other opportunities to communicate management's commitment to provide equitable treatment to all employees concerning their wages, benefits, hours, and conditions of employment. Furthermore, management must also communicate that each employee is important and deserving of respect and that adequate funds and management time have been designated to maintain effective employee relations (Rutkowski and Rutkowski 1984).

2. While management must have effective policies and procedures for selection of new employees, it must also ensure proper fit of personnel with specific jobs. Subsequently, job analyses, job descriptions, and job evaluations, as well as fair wage and salary programs, are essential for establishing a fundamental basis for **fair representation**. Management must not make promises that cannot be fulfilled; at the same time it should strive to do whatever is possible to improve employee relations. Monitoring of employee attitudes through surveys is essential; otherwise, management is dependent on the union for communicating any problems or change in attitudes.

3. Management must also ensure that it is fulfilling its roles and responsibilities by providing necessary training for employees, especially

Fair representation is a union's legal obligation to evenhandedly represent all bargaining-unit employees, both union members and nonmembers alike

first-line supervisors who are instrumental in determining how policies are implemented and in serving as liaisons between management and employees. If these supervisors are not properly trained, grievances are less likely to be settled quickly and are more likely to escalate into substantive formal disputes. Training is especially critical in healthcare settings because of constant and rapid changes in technology and safety issues. Management commitment to training is consistent with fair and honest treatment of employees. Similarly, if management fails to establish objective performance policies and does not ensure that they are done routinely, the labor-management relationship will be affected. Employees may perceive inequities and unfairness and experience problems of declining morale and productivity because rewards are not matched with performance.

4. Inconsistent and unfair application of disciplinary policies and procedures can create unnecessary grievance problems. At a minimum, the principle of just cause should guide the disciplinary process. When employees file grievances, they expect prompt attention to their requests. If management delays the process or turns a deaf ear to complaints, such actions signal to employees that management does not care about their problems and essentially cannot be trusted. Furthermore, management's credibility with employees will deteriorate, creating an imbalance in the labor-management relationship such that employees perceive the union's position as the most honest.

5. Each phase of the labor relations process is interrelated and can affect the outcome of other phases. For example, if the union is able to obtain representation through voluntary recognition, negotiating the collective bargaining agreement will very likely be less adversarial than if a representation election had occurred. Similarly, if the negotiations for a collective bargaining agreement are contentious, difficulties may occur in administering the contract. Thus, having a full understanding of each phase and its potential to enhance or impede the overall process of labor relations is essential.

Conclusion

As this chapter describes, managing with organized labor is challenging. Unionism has been declining nationally for decades, but the relatively unorganized healthcare workforce has become a target for unions. Because union membership and election activity have increased in healthcare settings, managers must devote high-level attention to the application and maintenance of a positive labor relations program that integrates human resources functions. Strategies and goals to implement a positive labor relations program must be based on a solid understanding of the labor relations process and of emerging trends and legislation. The growth of physician unions, in particular, signals major changes for human resources practices and for the labor relations process.

Discussion Questions

1. Why should management have a policy on unionism? What purpose does it serve?
2. Describe the three phases of the labor relations process. Why are all phases equally important?
3. What are some of the behaviors that might indicate to managers that organizing activities are occurring?
4. Is the growing trend toward physician unionization a good thing for physicians, patients, and the healthcare system?

References

Association of American Medical Colleges Executive Council. 1999. "AAMC Statement on Negotiating Units for Physicians." *AAMC Reporter* 9 (2): 7.

American Hospital Association. 1991. *Legal Memorandum Number 16: Collective Bargaining Units in the Health Care Industry.* Chicago: American Hospital Association.

Anthony, M. F., and S. Erf. 2000. "Can Physician Unionization Succeed?" *Healthcare Executive* (March/April): 50.

Becker, W. L., and A. M. Rowe. 1989. "Update on Union Organization in Health Care." *Review of Federation of American Health Systems* 22 (5): 11–2, 14–6.

Bureau of Labor Statistics. 2000a. Unpublished Tabulations from Current Population Surveys, Union Membership Tables, 1999 Annual Averages. Washington, DC: U.S. Government Printing Office.

———. 2000b. "Union Membership Edges Up but Share Continues to Fall." [Online news release; retrieved 12/5/01]. http://stats.bls.gov/opub/ted.

Clark, D. A., P. F. Clark, D. Day, and D. Shea. 2000. "The Relationship Between Health Care Reform and Nurses' Interest in Union Representation: The Role of Workplace Climate." *Journal of Professional Nursing* 16 (2): 92–6.

Cohen, J. J. 1999. "Unions Are Bad Medicine for Doctors." *Academic Medicine* 74 (8): 905.

Fennell, K. S. 1987. "The Unionization of the Healthcare Industry: General Trends and Emerging Issues." *Journal of Health in Human Resources Administration* 10 (1): 66–81.

Fisher, R., and W. Ury. 1981. "Getting to Yes—Negotiating an Agreement Without Giving In." In *Harvard Negotiation Project,* edited by B. Patton, pp. 21–53. Boston: Houghton Mifflin.

Fottler, M. D., R. A. Johnson, K. J. McGlown, and E. W. Ford. 1999. "Attitudes of Organized Labor Officials Toward Health Care Issues: An Exploratory Survey of Alabama Labor Officials." *Health Care Management Review* 24 (2): 71–82.

Freeman, R. B., and J. L. Medoff. 1984. *What Do Unions Do?* New York: Basic Books.

Greene, J. 1998. "Nurses' Aid." *Hospitals and Health Networks* 72 (12): 38–40.

Greenhouse, S. 1999. "Angered by H.M.O.'s Treatment, More Doctors Are Joining Unions." *New York Times* (February 4).

Havighurst, C. A. 1999. "Union Answer." [Online article on *American Medical News*; retrieved 1/11/01]. http://www.ama-assn.org/sai-pubs.amnews.

Hirsch, B. T., and E. J. Schumacher. 1998. "Union Wages, Rents and Skills in Health Care Labor Markets." *Journal of Labor Research* 19 (Winter): 125–47.

Kletke, P. R., D. W. Emmons, and K. D. Gillis. 1996. "Current Trends in Physicians Practices Arrangements: From Owners to Employees." *Journal of the American Medical Association* 276 (7): 555–60.

Leung, S. 1999. "More Nurses Join Unions Across State." *Wall Street Journal* (September 15).

Levenson, D. 1999. "Private Hospitals Worry NLRB Ruling Will Spark Intern, Resident Disputes." *AHA News* 35 (47): 1–2.

Metzger, N., J. Ferentino, and K. Kruger. 1984. *When Health Care Employees Strike.* Rockville, MD: Aspen.

Rutkowski, A. D., and B. L. Rutkowski. 1984. *Labor Relations in Hospitals.* Rockville, MD: Aspen.

Scott, C., and C. M. Lowery. 1994. "Union Election Activity in the Health Care Industry." *Health Care Management Review* 19 (1): 18–27.

Sobal, L. V., and J. O. Hepner. 1990. "Physician Unions: Any Doctor Can Join, but Who Can Bargain Collectively?" *Hospital & Health Services Administration* 35 (3): 327–40.

Stickler, K. B. 1990. "Union Organizing Will Be Divisive and Costly." *Hospitals* (July 5): 68–70.

Swoboda, F. 1999. "A Healthy Sign for Organized Labor; Vote by L. A. Caregivers Called Historic." *The Washington Post* (February 27).

Thompson, E. 2000. "Organized Doctors." *Modern Healthcare* (February 28): 35–6, 38, 40.

Yacht, A. C. 2000. "Unionization of House Officers: The Experience at One Medical Center." *The New England Journal of Medicine* 342 (6): 429–31.

CREATING CUSTOMER FOCUS

Myron D. Fottler, Ph.D., and *Robert C. Ford, Ph.D.*

Learning Objectives

After completing this chapter, the reader should be able to:

- Describe the significance of customer service in the highly competitive healthcare market
- Distinguish healthcare organizations that exhibit high levels of customer service from those that do not
- Describe the role of human resources management practices in enhancing customer service
- Describe six specific human resources strategies that can enhance customer service

Introduction

Healthcare organizations have not traditionally been focused on the needs, wants, or desires of their patient customers. As a result of their history and reimbursement sources, these organizations have concentrated on meeting the expectations of their medical staff and the third-party payers. The medical staffs, historically, have had the power to decide where their patients would go for healthcare services, and healthcare providers have gone to great lengths to make them happy. Because third-party payers pay the bills, healthcare organizations have also spent considerable effort in satisfying these customers.

This definition of the customer has resulted in healthcare organizations focusing on increasing market share, decreasing costs, and expanding revenues to retain the support of its third-party payers while providing sophisticated technology and in-house amenities for the doctors. At the same time, the patient has been overlooked and underappreciated as the ultimate healthcare customer. Indeed, even the term "patient" implies a passive person who patiently waits for service from experts who know what that patient needs and often provide it without consultation or explanation.

This paradigm has led to an increasingly unhappy and vocal patient. A survey commissioned by Voluntary Hospitals of America (VHA) and another survey published in *Fortune* magazine reported the following consumer attitudinal trends toward healthcare organizations (*Alliance* 1998):

- Over the past five years, public trust in healthcare organizations has markedly declined, with health plans losing more ground than physicians or hospitals. The decline in trust is especially pronounced among consumers age 40 to 59; those with higher income and education levels; and those who have recently changed, added, or selected a physician or hospital.
- Consumers gave hospitals only a 67 percent satisfaction rating; compared with 31 other industries, hospitals rank 27th. This ranking placed hospitals just above the Internal Revenue Service and 10 percentage points below the tobacco industry.

Moreover, other data from the National Coalition on Health Care indicate that 80 percent of Americans agree that hospitals have cut corners to save money and 77 percent agree that these cuts endanger patients (Health Care Advisory Board 1999; National Coalition on Health Care 2000).

None of these findings is surprising, given that services paid for by private insurers and government are not likely to reflect consumer preferences for convenience and personal control (Herzlinger 1997, 95). The increasingly involved consumer-patient and the newly evolved competitive market are forcing healthcare organizations to consider who their customers really are. They are starting to rethink the old paradigm of "take care of the doctors and third-party payers and all good things will follow" to a new paradigm of "don't forget the patient as customer" (Ford and Fottler 2000). Today's medical consumers have much more knowledge and access to information about the value and quality of their healthcare alternatives. They are now more savvy about what they are getting for their healthcare dollar and are increasingly involved in the decisions about how those dollars are spent. Because they have many alternative choices for their insurance coverage and healthcare providers, their voice is being heard. In addition, increasingly vocal consumer groups have changed patients' attitudes from being a patient into an active participant in their own healthcare decisions (Herzlinger 1997). Regina Herzlinger (1997, 3–4) describes this new healthcare consumer:

> They want what they want, they want it fast, and they want it when they want it. Well-informed, overworked, and overburdened with child and elder-care responsibilities, they are a new breed of consumer, and their demands for convenience and control have caused many American businesses to greatly enhance their quality and control their costs. . . . The consumer revolutionaries want their health-care system to provide them with the same kinds of convenience and mastery they

have found with Home Depot, *Consumer Reports,* and Nordic Track, so that their health status and costs will improve even further.

This chapter identifies six key human resources management strategies that benchmark guest-focused organizations have discovered as critical for their success in meeting and exceeding their guest's expectations from the guest-service experience. These lessons learned by the hospitality industry can be readily adopted as guiding principles by the healthcare industry as it moves from the old paradigm to the new paradigm. If the competitive market demands that healthcare providers treat patients as important primary customers, instead of patient bystanders to their own healthcare experience, these principles of hospitality can make the difference.

Exemplars of customer-driven organizations, such as Disney, Marriott, or Southwest Airlines, know that their success is based on meeting and exceeding their guests' expectations. This means that they spend considerable time and energy trying to identify and measure the key drivers in their guest's judgments about the quality and value of the service experience. The benchmark organizations manage the entire experience to the degree possible so that their guests' expectations are met and, they hope, exceeded. They have learned that the best predictors of intention to return and satisfaction with the guest-service experience can be identified and managed. They make sure that the key drivers in their guests' decision processes (i.e., what is most important to the guests) become the key drivers in the organizations' decision processes.

Knowing the guests' key drivers is especially important because the service product is largely intangible. Just as benchmark hospitality organizations know that the quality and value of their service experience is in the minds of the guests, so too must healthcare organizations recognize this simple truth. Healthcare customers have expectations that not only will the surgeon successfully remove the diseased organ, but he or she will also show empathy and concern before and after the surgery. They also have expectations that the operating room and the in-patient room will not only be sterile, but that the physical surroundings are cheerful, the nursing staff responsive, and the patient services prompt.

An Emerging Customer Focus

Although no one would argue that physicians and third-party payers are unimportant, the patient is becoming increasingly critical in determining the success or failure of the healthcare organization. Consequently, today the patient and patient's family are increasingly being recognized by the more successful competitors in the healthcare market as the real customer. These providers are spending increasing amounts of time and energy convincing their customers that the healthcare product they provide has both quality and value.

The results of this change in customer focus can be seen in a number of ways. Third-party payers are increasingly willing to pay for homeopathic treatments, acupuncture, and even chiropractic treatments, in spite of established medical practice resistance. Pharmaceutical companies now spend enormous sums of money on television and print advertisements to market directly to patients to influence their utilization of branded drugs. The direct marketing has proven to be a very effective strategy to influence doctors to prescribe certain drugs and circumvent HMO drug guidelines. Hospitals, too, have begun to offer such patient amenities as chef-prepared foods for patients and their families, valet parking, and comprehensive single-nurse care to influence the patient to request admission to the hospital that offers these benefits.

While consumers now have access to more information through such resources as provider report cards and the Internet, the question remains why providers should be more responsive to consumers than they have been in the past. Arnold (1991) suggests that the major environmental forces that lead to the increase in competition and greater provider responsiveness to consumers include excess capacity, the consumer movement, deregulation of the healthcare industry, changes to reimbursement systems, declines in occupancy rates, and corporate restructuring and diversification. Such increased competition among healthcare providers has resulted in greater interest in redesigning healthcare organizations to make them more customer focused.

An even more potent factor is the changing views of corporate America toward its role in healthcare cost management. After long relying on managed care companies as their defense against rising employee healthcare benefit costs, some U.S. employers are undergoing a fundamental change in their healthcare cost management strategy by turning healthcare decisions over to their employees. This idea is driven by a confluence of interacting forces, including the backlash against managed care, the popularity of 401(k) plans, the use of Web-based information to help consumers make more informed healthcare decisions, the recent increase in healthcare costs (despite the efforts of managed care organizations), and a growing feeling among many that the nation's healthcare market will not work well until patients themselves hold the purse strings (Weber 1997). The new trend to let employees handle their own healthcare benefits, just as they do their retirement money, adds momentum to the growing customer involvement in healthcare decisions (Winslow and Gentry 2000). Other employers have created web sites to help employees make health benefit decisions and sign up for plans. Entrepreneurs are responding to this trend by developing Web-based services that would greatly reduce the need for employers to manage this information. In addition, these entrepreneurs are more creative in providing customers with new tools to navigate the healthcare system and take decisions into their own hands (Winslow and Gentry 2000).

Corporations are also self-insuring in increasing numbers. This means that healthcare services are increasingly paid for by the corporations' own administrators instead of insurance companies. One of the significant advantages of self-insurance is that it allows greater flexibility in the health plans offered. When the employer manages its healthcare plans, the employee has a significantly greater voice in what these plans provide and how they provide it. Employees or their union representatives need only to persuade their employer of the need to change their choices of healthcare provider or health plan. Thus, the increasing use of self-insurance leads to an increasing voice for customers in decisions about their healthcare choices. All of these trends lead to a need for organizations to understand and utilize the successful best practices of the guest-service industry to gain a potential competitive advantage in this new patient-as-customer environment.

The result of the growing trend to rank and publicize the scores of healthcare organizations is also having a significant impact on the attitudes of healthcare providers toward the importance of the patient as customer. Data generated by the Healthcare Advisory Board (1999) suggest that healthcare executives are beginning to respond to the forces discussed above. Interviews with 321 health industry executives in 1998 found they agree (i.e., a response average greater than 4.0 on a five-point scale) with each of the following statements:

1. Individual consumers' new predominance in the healthcare marketplace is increasingly influencing policy, strategy, operations, and investment decisions of healthcare organizations within all segments of the industry.
2. Healthcare organizations will provide education and readily available data to encourage and empower consumers to be direct purchasers of care.
3. Healthcare organizations will develop new products, offer more choices, and provide service enhancements to respond directly to consumer preferences.
4. Healthcare organizations will increasingly invest in feedback mechanisms to ensure they are in touch with consumer needs and are meeting customer expectations.

Moreover, national magazines like *U.S. News and World Report* publish lists of "best hospitals," while local television and newspaper outlets rate the best physicians. Local magazines in cities like Boston and Philadelphia provide an annual list of the best regional physicians and hospitals (Clark 1999), and the Department of Public Health offers ratings of skilled nursing facilities in Massachusetts on its web site and updates it every six months. Major clinical users track seven satisfaction measures, and the results are publicized in newspapers and on television (Frye 1998).

Only recently have healthcare executives begun to expand their focus to meeting the needs, wants, and desires of their customer-patients, not only for a positive clinical experience but for a positive healthcare experience (Ford, Bach, and Fottler 1997; Fottler et al. 2000; Pines and Gilmore 1998). When the customer-patient has choices, just being the best medical provider at the lowest price is not enough. Now, the need is also to persuade the customer-patient that the service is most responsive to his or her needs and meets his or her healthcare expectations for a total healthcare experience. The business of healthcare must change to understand how to relate to its patients as customers and not merely as clinical material. The healthcare industry is facing a whole new paradigm.

The New Paradigm

The patient's determination of the value and quality of the total healthcare experience comprises more than the success or failure of the medical procedure or clinical service itself. Such a determination is a holistic perception that begins before admission and ends after discharge and bill payment. Indeed, in a sense, it may never end, as the ongoing nature of a healthcare provider's relationship with the customer-patient requires continued reminders through advertisements and other communications that the healthcare organization is a high-quality provider and one that the patient should seek to return to if a healthcare need arises again. As it has for the famous retailer Nordstrom and all hospitality organizations, the idea of worrying about repeat customer usage has begun to emerge as an important consideration for healthcare organizations.

Who the organization defines as its customer determines how it makes a variety of important decisions. Table 15.1 summarizes the human resources differences between the two paradigms, with the traditional healthcare organizations being the "old paradigm" and the new evolving customer-focused organization being the "new paradigm."

Customer-Focused Strategies Under the New Paradigm

Below, we discuss how the six strategies of the new paradigm might be implemented in a healthcare environment, citing examples from both the guest-services and the healthcare industry (Ford and Fottler 2000). Increasingly, customer-oriented healthcare organizations will need to incorporate these six strategies into their human resources strategy to ensure they recruit, select, train, appraise, and reward the people in charge of providing an outstanding patient experience.

Strategy 1: Identify customer key drivers.   Start identifying customers' needs, wants, and expectations (key drivers) by asking the customers themselves; successful customer-focused organizations extensively survey their customers to find out how they define a quality service experience. Knowing what is important to the customer-patient can then serve as the starting point for all organizational decisions. The customer-patients, not the strategic planners sitting in their isolated offices, define what determines the value and quality of the service product. From customer input, the organization can then develop

Human Resources Strategy	Old Paradigm	New Paradigm
1. Customer's Key Drivers	Clinical effectiveness and cost efficiency	Patient/customer perceptions of quality and value
2. Patient/Customer Coproduction Involvement	Limited involvement in coproduction	Maximum patient/customer coproduction of service experience
3. Culture	Provider driven	Patient/customer driven
4. Staff Selection and Training	Focused only on clinical skills	Focused on both clinical and patient/customer service skills
5. Motivational Strategies	Rewards for technical proficiency	Rewards for both technical proficiency and customer service
6. Measures of Effectiveness	Costs, clinical processes, and medical outcomes	The total service experience

TABLE 15.1

Human Resources Management Strategies of Old Paradigm Organizations Versus New Paradigm Organizations

its organizational plans and operational strategies for meeting and exceeding guests' expectations.

A theme park, for example, may find that its guest research identifies several key drivers: One may be cleanliness, another may be friendliness and helpfulness of employees, and a third may be length of wait in lines. Thus, the strategically appropriate response for the theme park is to put its effort and financial resources into keeping the park clean, training employees to be friendly, and building enough capacity to keep the waiting lines minimal. This attention to key drivers is especially important when the relationship between these key drivers and guests' intention to return and their overall satisfaction with the park experience is very high.

Similarly, a healthcare organization could survey its patients to identify their key drivers. For example, it may determine that its customer-patients' key drivers are perceived quality of food; their physician's communication skills; and courtesy, warmth, and friendliness of hospital staff. Once these are identified and shown to be significantly related to overall patient satisfaction with the healthcare experience and intention to use this service again, the organization would know exactly how to improve its customers' satisfaction by directing its time and resources to enhancing each of their key drivers. This could translate into more training for physicians and staff or an increased emphasis on the culinary aspects of patient menus.

In the past, joint replacement patients at the University of Alabama at Birmingham Hospital were required to arrive early in the morning and received only the service of surgery. As a result of patient input, patients are now able to purchase an entire three-night package, which includes staying three nights in redesigned rooms similar to high-quality hotels, arriving the day prior to surgery, having gourmet meals in a communal setting with other joint replacement patients, and having special nursing staff assigned to the patient. The hospital is so pleased with its patients' reactions that it is considering expanding this type of service package to other procedures.

All of the key drivers will have human resources management implications. In addition, satisfying the customers' key drivers will often have particular implications for employee selection, training, and performance appraisal. Meeting the customer-patient expectations should be an important evaluation criterion for all human resource functions. Clinical skill alone is not enough in an increasingly competitive healthcare market.

Strategy 2: Encourage customer participation.   Think of the patient as a partial employee responsible for coproducing the healthcare experience. Most customer-focused organizations know the importance and value of letting their customers participate in the service experience. The obvious benefit to encouraging customer participation is that anything customers do for themselves represents one less thing that the organization has to pay someone to do for them. In other words, the patient or patient's family may be a partial substitute for employees in delivering a service. For this to occur, employee job descriptions need to clearly define the respective roles of employee and customer, and training must prepare employees to delegate certain functions to customers.

Other advantages are evident as well. Patients who coproduce the service experience also are more satisfied with the service product because criticizing what they produce for themselves to suit their own tastes and needs is more difficult than criticizing someone else. A person making his or her own salad at a salad bar has little basis for complaint if the salad was not prepared exactly as desired. In a similar way, including the customer as a coproducing partial employee has other advantages for the organization; the customer can help supervise the guest-service employees. Because the service is being produced with the customer watching, the unsmiling server at the cafeteria can be sent a strong verbal or nonverbal message that this is an inappropriate, unfriendly behavior even without a supervisor watching. Indeed, a loyal repeat customer can even train the server in lieu of managers and even train other customers about how to enjoy or best benefit from the service experience.

For healthcare organizations to consider the patient as a partial employee responsible for coproducing the healthcare experience is a novel concept. Most physicians, employees, and healthcare organizations tend to see their patients as passive and submissive objects that the experts do something to instead of with. However, the reality is that the patient is increasingly involved in participating in his or her own health and is increasingly making demands and suggestions about how that healthcare should be provided and delivered. People are less willing to lie passively in bed while the experts do things to them.

While most healthcare employees know that the patient has to get up and walk after surgery, the psychiatric patient has to participate in the therapy, and the sick person has to tell the doctor where it hurts, most organizations have not considered the full ramifications of including the patient in the treatment process as a full coproducer of the healthcare experience. Although the healthcare literature and the lawyers discuss repeatedly the value of the medical staff communicating and consulting with the patient as the most effective way to enhance patient satisfaction, still far too little attention is paid to the need to bring the patient into the production of wellness. Until the patient fully comprehends and agrees to the regimen of care, the best doctors and best treatment facilities in the world will not help him or her prevent illness or get well.

Perhaps the most advanced example of how coproducing can be effective is the current practice of hospices, in which the patient is actively engaged in the care along with the patient's family and loved ones. Another example is the installation of painkiller pumps, which allows the patient to control pain medication and which often results in quicker healing with less discomfort. In addition, costs are lower because the patient typically uses less painkiller than would have been previously prescribed.

The Shouldice Hospital in Toronto focuses on the repair of abdominal hernias (Herzlinger 1997, 159). Its operating procedures are the products of intense deliberation about patient comfort, convenience, and health status. Shouldice has an integrated operating system carefully designed so that each of its activities reinforces the others. The operating system purposefully places considerable demands on the patients: meals are served only in the dining room, and the patients' rooms lack a telephone or television. Patients even prepare themselves for surgery by shaving the area to be operated on, and they are expected to walk from the operating room. They are also discouraged by all staff members from lingering in bed and are encouraged to engage in aerobic exercise. The Shouldice system creates higher levels of patient satisfaction because of their empowerment and also results in lower costs and higher quality than general hospitals.

Strategy 3: Develop a customer-focused culture. Redefine the organizational culture. The culture of any organization drives how its employees behave in that organization. Culture is generally defined as the beliefs, values, and ways of doing things that are unique to that organization and that differentiates it from others. Culture communicates to all employees what is important and what is not, what is appropriate behavior and what is not, and how people should deal with others both inside and outside the organization. In other words, culture is both "the way we do things around here" and "why we are what we are." Leaders teach and communicate the culture by what they reward, recognize, punish, or praise. They can do this not only through formal reward and recognition systems but also through informal stories they tell about organizational values, the heroes they create to illustrate points of importance, and the legends they perpetuate to communicate what the organization stands for.

A classic illustration of perpetuating legends in the guest-service industry is the story about the Olive Garden chain of restaurants. In its early years, when it was trying to establish a strong customer-service culture and teach it to all employees, a situation occurred that became a legend. A portly customer named Larry had written to the president of Olive Garden telling him of the delightful meal, the great service, and wonderful dining experience that he had at an Olive Garden. Unfortunately, however, the one complaint he had was that, being somewhat stout, he had found the armchairs used in the restaurant to be uncomfortably narrow for him and suggested they might want to do something to better accommodate people like himself. The president immediately responded by ordering two chairs for each restaurant that did not have arms to accommodate their heavier guests. These chairs, known throughout the chain as "Larry chairs," not only came to symbolize an opportunity to better serve the customers but also generated an inspiring story told to all new employees to illustrate how dedicated the company was to providing exceptional customer service.

Healthcare organizations also can use stories, legends, and heroes as an effective way of conveying the new service culture that the modern customer-patient expects. In the past, the healthcare staff told only stories about how the hospital had responded to physicians' needs and demands or how it had sought to accommodate the expectations of a HMO. In other words, the stories, legends, and heroes were all about accommodating the needs and wants of third-party payers or physicians. The change to the new customer paradigm must be accompanied by the creation of new stories, heroes, and legends that extol the healthcare employee who provided unusually effective patient care or service that somehow enhanced that patient's overall satisfaction with the healthcare experience. One nursing home, for example, told the story of a nurse's aide. The aide discovered that an elderly patient who was having a hard time sustaining interest in eating had a passion for peanut butter milkshakes. This aide went out of her way, on her own time, to make such a concoction so the patient would eat something. A top manager told this story in an employee gathering and recognized this person with a customer satisfaction award. This had an enormous impact on defining the culture of doing whatever it takes to create patient satisfaction.

Today's healthcare organizational cultures can be classified by where they fall on a spectrum of service from "bureaucratic" to "polite" to "empathetic." The differences between these three levels are primarily a matter of staff attitude. Staff members are the healthcare organization's first marketing tool; when staff cares about guests, that care shows in their attitudes and the way they provide care. Opportunities to display a caring, empathetic attitude occur during thousands of interactions between staff and customers that take place out of the sight of direct supervision. These can be managed only by influencing the values and attitudes of staff members who create the organization's reputation for service throughout the day as they make numerous contacts with patient-guests, family members, and other visitors. Bureaucratic cultures tend to be nonresponsive to individual patient needs. Polite staff members respect patient privacy, inform the patient, provide a caring environment, and give quick and punctual service. Empathetic staff members anticipate patient needs and attempt to exceed their expectations.

Culture begins at the top: the commitment to customer service should start at the executive level. The lessons of behavior taught by top managers on a continuing basis are more important than slogans and communications. The CEO and senior management must "walk the talk" of customer service if the message is to be believed throughout the organization. Executive-level reinforcement of the customer-focused culture in turn requires appropriate employee selection and training, as discussed below.

Strategy 4: Select and train customer-focused employees.   Hire people who are customer-service oriented. The guest-service literature suggests that only a certain percentage of people really care about giving high-quality guest service. In his book, *Positively Outrageous Service*, Scott Gross (1991) calls employees who love to provide great service "lovers"; these employees can provide their customers with a "feel good" level of service. It feels good because the employee somehow connects with the customer in a way that builds a relationship. Although the service encounter may be very brief, this relationship makes the customer feel that the service experience is special and memorable.

The challenge for healthcare executives is to recruit such employees, continuously train all staff members in guest service, and provide positive incentives to maintain and improve that service. Indeed, Scott Gross estimates that people who love to serve represent only one in ten of the available workforce. He states that the "ten percent" cannot get enough of their customers. This group is in contrast with five percent of those interviewed, who want to be left alone by customers, and the majority in the center whose attitude toward customers is that they can "take 'em or leave 'em" (Gross 1991, 159). If Gross's percentages are accurate, he raises two major challenges for healthcare executives. First, they need to develop a process that will systematically recruit and select those ten percent who are truly committed to providing excellent service. Second, they must work even harder to teach their other employees how to provide the same quality of service the "lovers" do naturally. In other words, the successful service organizations know how to "select the best and train the rest."

Guest-service organizations, such as Disney, Marriott, and Southwest Airlines, have learned this lesson well. They spend countless dollars recruiting, selecting, and training their guest contact employees to provide excellent customer service. They know that the impact of their service is created at the moment when the customer initiates a relationship or encounter with the employee. The challenge for them is especially great because so often the customer-contact employee is a minimum wage, low-skilled, entry-level employee. Ensuring that this employee is effective in providing an excellent guest-service experience is vital for both meeting their guests' expectations and influencing their intent to return. The important point is that the outstanding service organizations recognize and commit time and money to ensure that the people they put in front to their guests are not only well trained in the necessary job skills but also have the personality, disposition, and individual willingness to provide a high-quality guest-service experience.

Healthcare organizations in the traditional paradigm tend to select employees based on experience and clinical credentials only; seldom is an expectation of customer service skills considered. Although an obvious need exists to ensure that all new employees have the requisite clinical skills, those organizations that seek to move to the patient-as-customer paradigm must also develop ways to identify those potential employees who treat their customer-patients as guests. Both Irving Medical Center in California and Lutheran General Hospital in Illinois use testing and structured interviews to analyze a job applicant's fit with institutional values such as service orientation and servanthood (*Hospitals* 1991). Some hospitals and healthcare providers have begun to offer courses in guest relations, but these represent only a beginning. The willingness of management to provide such training is, however, a strong statement of how it values this critical customer orientation part of the total employee responsibility in healthcare.

The Emergency Department of Inova Fairfax Hospital in Falls Church, Virginia, initiated customer service training in 1994 (Mayer et al. 1998). All emergency department (ED) staff involved in patient contact (i.e., physicians, nurses, ED technicians, registration personnel, core secretaries, social workers, ED radiology, and ED respiratory therapy) are required to attend an eight-hour customer service training program. The program covers basic customer service principles, recognition of patients and customers, service industry benchmarking leaders, stress recognition and management, communication skills, negotiation skills, empowerment, customer service proactivity, service transitions, service fail-safes, change management, and specific customer service core competencies. Additional mandatory customer service updates were offered three times a year and included modules on conflict resolution, customer service skill updates, advanced communication skills, and assertiveness training.

Results showed that all 14 key quality characteristics identified in the survey increased during the one-year study period—May 1, 1994 to April 30, 1995 (Mayer et al. 1998). The most dramatic improvement came in the areas of likelihood of returning, overall satisfaction, and ratings of physician and nurse skill. In addition, patient complaints declined more than 70 percent, and patient compliments increased more than 100 percent. The clear implication of this data is that customer service training offers a competitive market advantage to healthcare organizations.

Specific topics for customer service training in healthcare might include the following:

- standard operating procedures for dealing with the customer-patient;
- team orientation;
- training and use of multiskilled health practitioners;
- flexibility in responding to customer concerns;
- training for communications with customers;
- responsibility for customers;
- incorporation of results of focus groups with customers;
- sharing patient information across organizational units;
- scripting greetings of customers and making eye contact;
- addressing customers by name; and
- response to customers' needs and requests.

Strategy 5: Motivate employees to be customer focused.   Redesign and redirect reward and motivational strategies to refocus everyone's attention on providing excellent customer and guest service. In the guest-services industry, many efforts are in place to recognize and reward not only technical excellence in the job but also guest satisfaction. Serving a gourmet meal is not enough if the server was so unpleasant that the guest was insulted or ignored, or providing a safe plane ride is not satisfactory if the flight attendant was rude. Because the customer service aspect of the total job performance is so important, managers of guest-service organizations are evaluated on the extent to which their customers are satisfied with the way the service was provided in addition to the quality of the service itself. Countless hours are spent finding ways to motivate their employees to be both technically proficient *and* guest focused.

In the guest-service industry, a demonstrated statistical relationship exists between happy employees and happy guests (Ford and Heaton 2000). If the employees are having a fun, enjoyable experience serving the guests, they will influence the experience of the guests they are serving in a positive way. This is a fundamental philosophy of CEO Herb Kelleher of Southwest Airlines. Managers in guest-service organizations know the importance of keeping their employees upbeat, happy, and positive so that they not only deliver the service product in the way they were trained but do it in a way that promotes an exceptional guest experience.

Traditionally, healthcare management systems have measured and reinforced only excellent healthcare as defined by the providers or accreditation agencies. Managers and entire healthcare organizations were evaluated only on aggregate statistical measures or accreditation standards of the Joint Commission, which typically measured the organization's structure, processes, or clinical outcomes. For example, if a hospital had a below-average mortality rate, a surgeon had a high survival rate for heart transplants, or a HMO had a large percentage of its female patients receiving mammograms, these individuals or institutions were considered of higher quality than their counterparts. Thus, the reward and reinforcement mechanism were focused on these provider-dominated measures of its success.

Strategy 6: Measure all aspects of the service experience.   Measure anything that is important to the guest's satisfaction with the guest-service experience. In the new patient care paradigm, managers, healthcare staff, and healthcare organizations overall must also be measured and rewarded on the extent to which they provide guest-patient satisfaction. Because *that which gets measured gets managed,* the motivation and reward systems must include measures of patient satisfaction as well as employee attitudes to ensure that the managers spend the necessary time and effort managing these vital aspects of customer service.

Excellent service organizations, such as Marriott Hotels, Walt Disney World, Nordstrom, and Southwest Airlines, spend countless dollars and expend extraordinary effort to capture from their guests their level of satisfaction with the guest-service experience through a variety of survey techniques. They send questionnaires, interview departing guests, and pay people to sample the guest-service experience in highly systematic investigations to gather the necessary data to understand and assess the quality and value of their guests' perception of their service experience. These organizations have learned that the only way to know whether the guest is satisfied is to ask.

This is especially important for service organizations for three reasons. First, the service experience is an intangible product that is produced at the moment it is consumed. Second, each guest is not only different from other customers, but each guest may exhibit different behaviors from one guest-service experience to the next. Because the quality and value of the service experience is defined by the customer, the only way to assess quality and value is to measure them through the eyes of the customer. Third, only by knowing and then developing measures of what is important to the guest can management effectively manage the critical aspects of customer service. Again, that which gets measured gets managed, but most dimensions of customer satisfaction in healthcare organizations today are neither measured nor managed. Patients' perceptions of convenience, comfort, and service quality are ignored. The healthcare equivalent of comparative surveys of consumer perceptions, such as the Zagats' survey of restaurants and the J. D. Power surveys of automobile quality, has yet to appear (Herzlinger 1997, 94).

Moreover, accreditation of hospitals and industry-developed ratings of HMOs do not appear to be highly correlated with independent surveys of user satisfaction (*Consumer Reports* 1996). Some healthcare organizations, however, are beginning to use measurement techniques to understand their patients' perceptions of their healthcare experience. Increasingly, hospitals, healthcare centers, and even individual physicians send out surveys after care to identify the extent to which their patients are satisfied with the service and to identify the flaws in the service delivery system that may impede the ability of the organization to provide the desired level of guest service. The service industry has increasingly recognized the consequences of failing the guest twice by not correcting errors in the service experience. Therefore, discovering how and when the healthcare provider is failing the patient is becoming an equally important part of the new paradigm. Measurement tactics currently being used in healthcare include mystery shoppers, comment cards, focus groups, and elaborate surveys of the patient service experience (Ford, Bach, and Fottler 1997). The Campbell Health System in Weathford, Texas, for example, reinforces its patient satisfaction data by using mystery shoppers who report the intimate details of their service encounters in a way that is meaningful and motivating for its staff (Millstead 1999).

Healthcare organizations can measure and reward superior service by establishing a baseline of patient satisfaction in every unit and continually sampling patient attitudes. This approach can help to identify both problems and opportunities. Salnik Health Care, which operates outpatient cancer centers, has meticulously maintained patient records from which it has worked up detailed practice guidelines to standardize and refine the treatment of numerous types of cancer (Bianco 1998). As a result, this company has been able to achieve better clinical outcomes, higher levels of guest satisfaction, and lower costs of care.

The key human resource issue is to link customer expectations and satisfaction back to the factors that are measured in the organization's performance appraisal system. This will undoubtedly mean some significant differences in the criteria for different positions. Success in meeting customer expectations should also be reinforced through economic and noneconomic rewards.

Conclusion

We have presented the six human resource strategies developed and proven by successful service organizations to show how they can be successfully applied to healthcare organizations that desire to remain competitive in this new paradigm in which the customer is the patient. These six strategies are all important and indivisible, and none is more important than the others in providing superior service. They must be linked together as a complete strategy to provide the level of service excellence increasingly demanded by more sophisticated and knowledgeable healthcare consumers. The six strategies learned by the successful guest-service organizations can help a healthcare organization make the transition to the new paradigm. The healthcare industry has become too competitive to ignore its customer-patients.

Patients today are increasingly assertive in demanding health services that are convenient, cost effective, high quality, and customer focused. Furthermore, as mentioned earlier, the healthcare system is becoming increasingly responsive to these demands. The growth of medical savings accounts should enhance that trend (Goodman and Musgrave 1992).

Achieving competitive advantage in this hypercompetitive market requires developing organizational capabilities that are difficult for competitors to duplicate quickly. Capabilities represent integrating and coordinating mechanisms that bring together resources and competencies that are superior to those of competitors (Henderson and Cockburn 1994). Our six human resources strategies, implemented as a total system, represent one such integrative and coordinating mechanism for achieving competitive advantage through increased customer satisfaction.

These strategies have been derived from the best practices of the guest-service industry as developed and modified over many years. Some healthcare leaders may argue that because healthcare deals with more serious issues of life, death, and health status, their customers are not as interested in the amenities of service delivery as are customers of guest-services organizations. However, no data support this claim, and the success of healthcare organizations that provide both excellent clinical care and excellent customer satisfaction with the total service experience would argue otherwise.

Implementation of these six strategies from identification of the customer's key drivers to measurement of customer-oriented employee performance will require a champion (i.e., CEO or vice president) who will identify benchmark service organizations, cross organizational boundaries, and make total customer service the highest value in the organization. This process may take considerable time (several years), and success is not guaranteed. Most healthcare organizations today have made some progress in implementing some of the principles. However, we do not know of any to have successfully implemented all of them as a total system.

If these strategies can be successfully implemented, they will provide capabilities that can become a core competency of the organization (Prahalad and Hamel 1990). In such a case, the core competency is the collective learning about how to coordinate diverse operational skills and integrate multiple activities toward enhancing customer satisfaction. The long-term nature of the process of implementing our principles would create difficulty for a competitor that is trying to emulate them over a short period of time.

Discussion Questions

1. Why is customer service becoming more important to healthcare organizations? What are the negative implications of failing to address this issue?
2. Think about your own experience or that of a family member in receiving health services. To what degree was the healthcare provider customer oriented? Why? What lessons can you derive from that experience that will help you to enhance customer service in the future?
3. Describe one human resources practice that can enhance customer service in healthcare. How would you go about implementing it, and what problems do you anticipate? If successfully implemented, what positive outcomes would you expect and why?
4. If you found yourself in the position of CEO of a healthcare organization that was *not* customer oriented, how would you change the culture to be customer oriented? What are the potential obstacles, and how would you overcome them? Provide a step-by-step plan for reforming your culture.

References

Arnold, A. 1991. "The Big Bang Theory of Competition in Healthcare." *Forum* 15 (4): 6–9.

Alliance. 1998. "Consumer Attitudes." *Alliance* (May/June): 11.

Bianco, A. 1998. "Bernie Salnik's Business in Cancer." *Business Week* (June 22): 76–84.

Clark, R. H. 1999. "Marketing Health Services." In *Health Care Administration*, edited by L. P. Wolper, pp. 161–82. Gaithersburg, MD: Aspen.

Consumer Reports. 1996. "How Good Is Your Health Plan?" *Consumer Reports* 61 (8): 34–5.

Ford, R. C., S. A. Bach, and M. D. Fottler. 1997. "Methods of Measuring Patient Satisfaction in Healthcare Organizations." *Health Care Management Review* 22 (2): 74–89.

Ford, R. C., and M. D. Fottler. 2000. "Creating Customer-Focused Health Care Organizations." *Health Care Management Review* 25 (4): 18–33.

Ford, R. C., and C. P. Heaton. 2000. *Managing the Guest Experience in Hospitality*. Albany, NY: Delmar.

Fottler, M. D., R. C. Ford, V. Roberts, and E. Ford. 2000. "Creating a Healthy Environment: The Importance of the Service Setting in the New Customer Oriented Health Care System." *Journal of Healthcare Management* 45 (2): 91–106.

Frye, L. 1998. "Patient Services Shows How Mass. Hospitals Stack Up." *Boston Globe* (November 13): A1.

Goodman, J., and G. Musgrave. 1992. *Patient Power*. Washington, DC: Cato Institute.

Gross, T. S. 1991. *Positively Outrageous Service*. New York: Warner Books.

Health Care Advisory Board. 1999. *Hardworking for Service Excellence: Breakthrough Improvements in Patient Satisfaction*. Washington, DC: Health Care Advisory Board.

Henderson, R., and I. Cockburn. 1994. "Measuring Competence." *Strategic Management Journal* 15 (1): 63–84.

Herzlinger, R. 1997. *Market Driven Health Care: Who Wins in the Transformation of America's Largest Service Industry*. Reading, MA: Addison-Wesley.

Hospitals. 1991. "Hospitals Probe Applicants' Values for Organizational Fit." *Hospitals* 65 (20): 34.

Mayer, T. J., R. J. Cates, M. J. Mastorovich, and D. L. Royalty. 1998. "Emergency Department Patient Satisfaction and Ratings of Patient and Nurse Skill." *Journal of Healthcare Management* 43 (4): 427–40.

Millstead, J. B. 1999. "Satisfying Your Customers: Mystery Shopping in Your Organization." *Healthcare Executive* 14 (3): 66–7.

National Coalition on Health Care. 2000. "How Americans Perceive the Health Care System." [Online article]. http://www.nchc.org/perceive.html.

Pines, B. J., and J. H. Gilmore. 1998. "Welcome to the Experience Economy." *Harvard Business Review* 78 (4): 97–105.

Prahalad, C. K., and G. Hamel. 1990. "The Core Competence of the Corporation." *Harvard Business Review* 68 (1): 78–90.

Weber, D. 1997. "The Empowered Consumer." *Healthcare Forum Journal* (September/October): 28.

Winslow, R., and C. Gentry. 2000. "Medical Vouchers: Health Care Trend—Give Workers Money, Let Them Buy a Plan." *Wall Street Journal* (February 8): A1, A12.

INDEX

ABOUT THE AUTHORS

Dolores Gurnick Clement, Dr.P.H., serves as associate dean of the School of Allied Health Professions of Virginia Commonwealth University (VCU) and is a professor in the Department of Health Administration on the Medical College of Virginia Campus of VCU. Dr. Clement earned a Dr.P.H. in health policy and administration from the University of California, Berkeley, and a M.S. in health systems management from Rush University, Chicago. Previously, Dr. Clement served as director of Professional Graduate Programs from 1995 through 1997, as director of Health Information Management Program from 1989 through 1992, and as associate director of the Williamson Institute for Health Studies from 1989 through 1994. Dr. Clement continues to do research in community health and well-being and Medicare risk contracting with HMOs for the elderly.

John Crisafulli, M.H.A., M.B.A., is a healthcare management consultant. Mr. Crisafulli's prior healthcare experience is in finance and operations with Rex Healthcare in Raleigh, North Carolina; in strategic planning and facility planning with Children's National Medical Center in Washington, DC; and in clinical support services with Fair Oaks Hospital in Fairfax, Virginia. He received a M.B.A. from the Kenan-Flagler Business School at the University of North Carolina at Chapel Hill and a M.H.A. from the School of Public Health at the University of North Carolina at Chapel Hill.

Robert C. Ford, Ph.D., is associate dean for Graduate and External Programs and professor of management at the University of Central Florida's (UCF) College of Business Administration. He joined UCF in 1993 as chair of the Department of Hospitality Management after serving on the faculty of the University of North Florida and the University of Alabama at Birmingham. He has authored or co-authored over 100 articles, books, and presentations on organizational issues, human resources management, guest services management, and healthcare and related service-management topics. His recent book, *Managing the Guest Experience in Hospitality*, is a compendium of hospitality-based concepts important in managing any service organization. Previously,

Dr. Ford served the Academy of Management as director of Placement and as division chair for both the Management History and the Management Education and Management Development divisions. In addition, he chaired the Accreditation Commission for Programs in Hospitality Administration, and he was president of the Southern Management Association. He currently is the editor of *Academy of Management Executive*.

Myron D. Fottler, Ph.D., is professor and director of Health Services Administration Programs at the University of Central Florida. Previously, he was the director of the Ph.D. program in Health Services Administration at the University of Alabama at Birmingham. His publications include more than 100 journal articles, 30 book chapters, and 12 books that deal with a wide variety of health services management topics including strategic management, customer service, stakeholder management, and human resources management. In addition, he serves on a number of editorial review boards and is a coeditor of an annual book series titled *Advances in Health Care Management* (published by JAI/Elsevier Science).

Bruce J. Fried, Ph.D., is an associate professor in the Department of Health Policy and Administration in the School of Public Health at the University of North Carolina at Chapel Hill. He is the director of the Master's Degree Program in the department and a research fellow at the Cecil G. Sheps Center for Health Services Research. Dr. Fried teaches in the areas of organizational theory and human resources management and workforce issues in healthcare. His research interests include mental health services, workforce issues, and interorganizational relationships. He has worked with a variety of organizations nationally and internationally in the areas of strategic planning and human resources management. He received his undergraduate degree from the State University of New York at Buffalo, his master's degree from the University of Chicago, and his doctorate degree from the University of North Carolina at Chapel Hill.

James A. Johnson, Ph.D., is a professor of health administration and leadership at the Medical University of South Carolina (MUSC) and the Dow College of Health Professions at Central Michigan University. He is also an adjunct professor of public health at University of South Carolina in Columbia. Dr. Johnson is the former chair of the Department of Health Administration and Policy at MUSC and founding director of the nation's first executive Doctor of Health Administration (DHA) program. He currently serves on the board of directors for the Association of University Programs in Health Administration. He is the immediate past editor of the *Journal of Healthcare Management* and was the editor of the *Journal of Management Practice*. Dr. Johnson has published seven books and over 60 articles on a wide range of healthcare and organizational issues. He is active in the international community and has lectured at the World Health Organization in Geneva,

Switzerland, and Oxford University in England. He received a Ph.D. from the Askew School of Policy and Administration at Florida State University where he specialized in organizational behavior and development.

Anne Osborne Kilpatrick, D.P.A., is professor of health administration and policy at the Medical University of South Carolina, where she was the second recipient of the University's Earl B. Higgins Award for Achievements in Diversity. Dr. Kilpatrick is one of two university faculty selected to be in the Class of 2000–2001 Creating Healthy Communities Fellowship with the Health Forum/AHA. Since 1995, she has served as an internal consultant to the University's Division of Finance and Administration, facilitating a major quality initiative to change the culture and climate. She received a D.P.A. in public administration from the University of Georgia where she specialized in national health policy and organization development. Dr. Kilpatrick has published numerous articles on leadership, organizational effectiveness, burnout, healthy workplaces, and cutback management, and she is a principal researcher in a national longitudinal study of the VA leadership. Currently, she is editor of the section on health administration and policy for the *Encyclopedia of Public Administration*.

Donna M. Malvey, Ph.D., is an assistant professor in the Department of Health Policy and Management, College of Public Health, University of South Florida in Tampa, Florida. Her areas of expertise include labor-management relations and the strategic management of health services organizations. Dr. Malvey received her Ph.D. in Health Services Administration from the University of Alabama at Birmingham and her M.H.S.A. from George Washington University. Prior to assuming an academic career, she served as executive director of a national trade association that represents health professionals and as a congressional aide.

Andrew Osucha, M.B.A., is a 2001 graduate of the Manderson Graduate School of Business at the University of Alabama. During the summer of 2000, Mr. Osucha participated in an internship program with the Kelsey-Seybold Clinic in Houston, Texas. As an intern, Mr. Osucha was responsible for carrying out various tasks related to the company's managed care products. After graduation, Mr. Osucha was recruited by the Kelsey-Seybold management team and offered a position in clinical operations. The Kelsey-Seybold Clinic is a nationally recognized multispecialty care clinic that serves customers at 23 clinics throughout the Houston market.

Michael T. Ryan, Ph. D., C.H.P., is an independent consultant in radiological sciences and health physics. He is an adjunct associate professor in the College of Health Professions at the Medical University of South Carolina, and he holds adjunct appointments at Georgia Institute of Technology, the University of South Carolina, and the College of Charleston. He earned a Ph.D. from the Georgia Institute of Technology, where he was recently inducted into the Academy of Distinguished Alumni; he earned a M.S. in radiological sciences and protection from the University of Lowell under a U.S. Energy Research and Development Administration (ERDA) scholarship. Dr. Ryan is a recipient of the Francis Cabot Lowell Distinguished Alumni for Arts and Sciences Award from the University of Massachusetts Lowell. Dr. Ryan is editor-in-chief of *Health Physics Journal*. In addition, Dr. Ryan has authored many refereed articles and publications in the areas of environmental radiation assessment, radiation dosimetry, and regulatory compliance for radioactive materials. Dr. Ryan's research, grants, and contracts are in the areas of regulatory compliance, compliance data management, occupational radiation dosimetry, environmental management, and radiation protection policy.

Beverly L. Rubin, J.D., is the vice president of Global Human Resources Operations and associate general counsel for Quintiles Transnational Corp. From 1992 to 1998, Ms. Rubin was an associate at the law firm of Moore & Van Allen in Raleigh, North Carolina, where she practiced in the areas of healthcare, employment, and commercial litigation. From 1991 to 1992, she was a law clerk to the Honorable James A. Wynn, Jr., Judge for the North Carolina Court of Appeals. Ms. Rubin received her law degree from the University of North Carolina at Chapel Hill in 1991. She also served as notes editor for the *North Carolina Law Review* and was a member of the Order of the Coif.

Sharon Topping, Ph.D., is an associate professor of management at the University of Southern Mississippi. She recently was a NIMH Post-Doctoral Fellow at the Cecil G. Sheps Center for Health Services Research at the University of North Carolina-Chapel Hill and at Duke University Medical School. She has published numerous articles, cases, and chapters in management and healthcare journals and books. In addition, Dr. Topping has been awarded grants from the National Institutes of Health and other federal agencies. She is currently the principal investigator on Coordination of Services Using Multidisciplinary Teams, funded by the National Institute of Mental Health, and the senior evaluator on the Mississippi System of Care grant, funded by the Center for Mental Health Services. She received her Ph.D. in health services administration from the University of Alabama at Birmingham.

Kenneth R. White, Ph.D., FACHE, associate professor and director, Graduate Program in Health Administration, Medical College of Virginia Campus of Virginia Commonwealth University (VCU). Dr. White received a Ph.D. in health services organization and research from VCU, a M.P.H. in health administration from the University of Oklahoma, and a M.S. in Nursing from VCU. Dr. White has extensive experience in hospital administration and consulting, particularly in the areas of leadership development, marketing, medical staff development, and operations management. Dr. White is a registered nurse, a Fellow of the American College of Healthcare Executives, and co-author of *The Well-Managed Healthcare Organization*, 5th Edition.

Eric S. Williams, Ph.D., is assistant professor of healthcare management, Department of Management and Marketing, Culverhouse College of Commerce and Business Administration, University of Alabama. Dr. Williams earned a Ph.D. in management from the State University of New York at Buffalo. He was also a NRSA Post-Doctoral Fellow at the Cecil G. Sheps Center for Health Services Research at the University of North Carolina. His research interests include the evolving role of physicians; the impact of physician worklife on physician job attitudes, behaviors, and outcomes; and quality management. He has been an active member of both the Health Care Management Division of the Academy of Management and Association for Health Services Research. His articles have appeared in journals such as *Health Services Research, Medical Care, Health Care Management Review, Medical Care Research and Review, Journal of General Internal Medicine,* and *Journal of Management.* In 2000, he and his colleagues were awarded the Best Paper in the Health Care Management Division of the Academy of Management.

Derek van Amerongen, M.D., M.S., is vice president and chief medical officer for Humana/ChoiceCare in Cincinnati, Ohio. Before joining Humana, Dr. van Amerongen was national medical director for Anthem Blue Cross and Blue Shield; he was chief of Obstetrics and Gynecology for the Johns Hopkins Medical Services Corporation in Baltimore, Maryland; and he was as a faculty member in the Department of Gynecology and Obstetrics of the Johns Hopkins School of Medicine. Dr. van Amerongen received a M.D. from Rush Medical College in Chicago and performed his residency in Obstetrics and Gynecology at the University of Chicago; he earned a M.S. in medical administration from the University of Wisconsin. Dr. van Amerongen has written and presented extensively on managed care and women's health topics. His articles and letters have appeared in such publications as *The New England Journal of Medicine, Physician Executive, Health Affairs, The Journal of Reproductive Medicine, Oncology,* and others. His first book, *Networks and the Future of Medical Practice,* won the 1998 Robert A. Henry Literary Award of the American College of Physician Executives.

ALSO FROM HEALTH ADMINISTRATION PRESS

Human Resources and Organizational Behavior:
Cases in Health Services Administration
Anne Osborne Kilpatrick, D.P.A.; and James A. Johnson, Ph.D.

Softbound, 133 pp, 1999, ISBN 1-56793-104-9, Order code: BKCO-1070, $45
An AUPHA/HAP Book

The perfect complement to *Human Resources in Healthcare: Managing for Success,* this book will help current and future leaders prepare to tackle challenges arising from the changing delivery system. More than 60 concise case studies provide practice in handling a large variety of real-world problems. Ideal for group discussion, the cases facilitate rich discussions and varied interpretations.

Leadership for the Future: Core Competencies in Healthcare
Austin Ross, LFACHE; Frederick J. Wenzel; and Joseph W. Mitlyng

Hardbound, approx. 400 pp, publishing in November 2001,
ISBN 1-56793-160-X, Order code: BKCO-1130, $60

Develop the strong leadership skills that are so crucial in today's volatile healthcare environment. This book breaks down the skills a manager needs into two categories—system competencies, such as governance and strategy development, and personal leadership competencies, such as decision making and team building. Each competency is brought to life with a case or real-life example to enhance understanding.